BASIC STRUCTURES of the HEAD and NECK

a programed instruction in clinical anatomy for dental professionals

GRETCHEN MAYO REED, B.S., M.A. (Ed.), M.A. (Biology)

Department of Anatomy, Physiology and Biophysics,
College of Basic Medical Sciences, University of
Tennessee Center for the Health Sciences, Memphis

VINCENT F. SHEPPARD, A.B., M.A., M.Ed., Ph.D.

Learning Resources Center, LeMoyne-Owen College, Memphis

W. B. SAUNDERS COMPANY / PHILADELPHIA / LONDON / TORONTO

W. B. Saunders Company: West Washington Square
Philadelphia, Pa. 19105

1 St. Anne's Road
Eastbourne, East Sussex BN21 3UN, England

833 Oxford Street
Toronto, M8Z 5T9, Canada

Library of Congress Cataloging in Publication Data
Reed, Gretchen Mayo.
    Basic structures of the head and neck.

    Includes index.
    1. Head—Programmed instruction. 2. Neck—Programmed
instruction. I. Sheppard, Vincent F., 1919–   joint author. II. Title.
QM535.R4   611'.91'077   75-298
ISBN 0-7216-7516-6

Basic Structures of the Head and Neck   ISBN   0-7216-7516-6

Last digit is the print number: 9   8   7   6   5   4   3   2

PREFACE

This programed instruction textbook offers a unique presentation of the anatomy of the head and neck—one designed specifically for the requirements of persons engaged in the dental professions: students, practitioners, and teachers. The content is geared to both theoretical and clinical aspects.

Students find it difficult to sift out the general coverage of the anatomy of the head from extremely advanced textbooks. On the other hand, adequate treatment of minute details of specific areas of the head is hard to find in a single introductory manual. Attempted spot reading, especially of advanced texts, is laborious and time consuming. Here students of dentistry will find in one place a coverage which is both sufficient and as simple as the complexity of the subject will permit.

Practicing dental clinicians who feel a need for a quick reference, but whose time is limited, can select quickly the area of review desired without the need for going through the whole book or engaging in lengthy searches.

Professors in dental and allied health schools may wish to make use of this program as a classroom assignment, with stated goals set for regular progression from one unit to the next within a fixed time sequence. Others may wish to utilize the program more flexibly as a supplement to classroom instruction. Still other teachers may find it helpful to use parts or all of the program as the basic material for classroom lecture and discussion in the area of head and neck anatomy.

This program presupposes that the student will have completed a course in general anatomy of the human body. As a more advanced text, this book is intended to supplement approximately 25 hours of class instruction related directly to clinical orientation.

The program is organized into four parts: Anatomical Landmarks, Systems, Regions, and Clinical Applications. Part One presents an introductory examination of surface features, followed by a detailed look at the bones and foramina of the skull. These first two units establish points of reference for locating structures of the various systems. Part Two treats, in turn, the muscular, nervous, and vascular systems of the head and neck. Included in Part Two is some detail about the trigeminal, facial, glossopharyngeal, and vagus nerves because of the special importance of these four cranial nerves in dentistry. Part Three addresses itself to different regions of the head and neck in order to clarify spatial relationships among the structures of the various systems. The regions investigated in Part Three include the temporal and infratemporal fossae, the mouth, the nose and paranasal sinuses, and the pharynx and larynx. The culmination of the program is Part Four, which correlates anatomical topography with two important clinical applications, the spread of dental infection and the sites of dental injections.

The principal reference source for material in Units One through Sixteen is Russell T. Woodburne's *Essentials of Human Anatomy,* 4th Edition, New York, Oxford University Press. The two main sources consulted in the writing of Units Seventeen and Eighteen were *Oral Anatomy,* by Harry Sicher and E. Lloyd DuBrul, 5th Edition, Saint Louis, C. V. Mosby Company; and, *Manual of Local Anesthesia in General Dentistry,* published by Cook-Waite Laboratories, Inc., New York. The authors are particularly grateful for permission to copy illustrations contained in these three publications.

The behavioral objectives the student can expect to achieve upon completion of this program include the ability to describe:

(1) the superficial structures of the head and face,

(2) the principal bones of the skull, points of muscle attachment, foramina, and related vessels and nerves,

(3) the action, innervation, and blood supply of the muscles of facial expression and the muscles of mastication;

(4) the structures and actions related to the temporomandibular joint,

(5) the major superficial landmarks and blood supply of the brain,

(6) the location and function of the cranial nerves and their sensory and motor innervation,

(7) the major branches of the trigeminal, facial, glossopharyngeal, and vagus nerves, and the functional components of each,

(8) the branches of the external carotid artery and the structures of the head and neck which they supply,

(9) the structures in the oral cavity, relating surface anatomy to underlying muscles, blood vessels, nerves, and glands, and

(10) the cerebrospinal circulation and lymphatic drainage of the head and neck.

The student can also expect to be able to identify in the patient:

(1) areas of the oral cavity,

(2) nerve and blood supply to the teeth,

(3) gross structures of the tongue, palate, pharynx, and larynx,

(4) location of major nerves and blood vessels related to the mouth, and

(5) bony prominences of the face and head, boundaries of facial muscles, and superficial muscles of the neck.

The programed instruction method of learning enables the student to move by gradual steps from the familiar to the unknown, from a simple general overview to more minute details. As the program progresses, repetition of previously covered material in new meaningful relationships enhances understanding and memory. The student's active participation involves reading a small segment of material and organizing thoughts to answer questions on that segment. Confidence and satisfaction gained from repeated correct answers provide strong psychological reinforcement. Any erroneous answers are accompanied by a built-in system for immediate detection and clarification of misconceptions at each step.

Original illustrations and redrawings of illustrations copied or modified from other publications are the work of two artists, Lucy B. Watkins and Phillip R. Dotson. The authors acknowledge with deep appreciation the courtesy of the copyright holders of the following publications who granted permission to reproduce or redraw and modify illustrations: *Cunningham's Textbook of Anatomy*, edited by G. J. Romanes, 10th Edition, New York, Oxford University Press; Curtis, *Introduction to the Neurosciences*, Philadelphia, W. B. Saunders Company; Gatz, *Manter's Essentials of Clinical Neuroanatomy and Neurophysiology*, 4th Edition, Philadelphia, F. A. Davis Company; *Gray's Anatomy of the Human Body*, edited by Charles Mayo Goss, 29th Edition, Philadelphia, Lea and Febiger; Jacob and Francone, *Structure and Function in Man*, 3rd Edition, Philadelphia, W. B. Saunders Company; King and Showers, *Human Anatomy and Physiology*, 6th Edition, Philadelphia, W. B. Saunders Company; Leeson and Leeson, *Human Structure*, Philadelphia, W. B. Saunders Company; *Manual of Local Anesthesia in General Dentistry*, New York, Cook-Waite Laboratories, Inc.; *Morris' Human Anatomy*, edited by Barry J. Anson, 12th Edition, New York, McGraw-Hill Book Company; Sicher and DuBrul, *Oral Anatomy*, 5th Edition, Saint Louis, C. V. Mosby Company; Sicher and Tandler, *Anatomie für Zahnärzte,* Vienna, Austria, Springer Verlag AG; Truex and Carpenter, *Strong and Elwyn's Human Neuroanatomy,* 5th Edition, and Truex and Carpenter, *Human Neuroanatomy,* 6th Edition, Baltimore, The Williams and Wilkins Company; Truex and Kellner, *Detailed Atlas of the Head and Neck,* New York, Oxford University Press: Wolf-Heidegger, *Atlas of Systematic Human Anatomy,* Basel, Switzerland, S. Karger AG; Woodburne, *Essentials of Human Anatomy,* 4th Edition, New York, Oxford University Press.

The authors are indebted to the instructors and students in schools where the program was field tested: The University of Tennessee Center for the Health Sciences, Memphis, Tennessee; and Indiana State University, Evansville Campus. Special thanks go to Gordon E. Kelley, D.D.S, M.S.D., Director of Allied Health and Dental Auxiliary Education at the Evansville Campus of Indiana State University, for his assistance with the field testing and for his helpful criticisms of the field test manuscript. The authors express their thanks also to Thomas Armstrong, D.D.S., of the University of Tennessee Center for the Health Sciences, for giving generously of his time and expertise to review the clinical material in Units Seventeen and Eighteen. Numerous helpful suggestions for improvement of the entire manuscript were also given by professors in the Department of Anatomy, College of Basic Sciences, University of Tennessee Center for the Health Sciences. A final word of thanks is due the staff of W. B. Saunders Company, and especially to Mr. Carroll Cann, Dental Editor, whose tireless and expert guidance aided the preparation of this book immeasurably from inception to conclusion.

A NOTE ON VISUALIZATION

The study of anatomy involves forming mental images of the parts of the body and their positions relative to surrounding structures. The student must visualize in three dimensions as well as employ "X-ray vision" to picture structures which are normally hidden under the skin. Proper visualization can change a burdensome memory chore into an intriguing exploration with a high degree of retention of detail.

The most effective approach is to visualize in terms of structural boundaries, areas and their contents, and the position of an unfamiliar structure as it bounds or approaches a familiar one. Each time the text introduces a new structure, project your imagination to the area described. It aids imagination, in depth projection, to actually touch the appropriate areas of your own head, face, or neck. The text will always discuss an unknown structure in reference to an area which is already familiar.

Soon you will be able to close your eyes and remember the contents and relative position of such an area as the infratemporal fossa—presumably a mystery to you now—just as readily as you can close your eyes and picture the contents and arrangement of items in your desk drawer.

This textbook makes abundant use of illustrations to facilitate depth projection. Each time you are referred to a figure, it is extremely important that you stop and examine it closely. Careful study of the illustrations is essential to mastery of the program.

HOW TO
USE THIS BOOK

This book includes 18 Units, each of which is subdivided into a number of Items. Each Item presents a factual explanation of a single topic, followed by several questions. The correct answer to each question appears immediately below the question. Alternative correct answers to the fill-in questions appear in parentheses.

Do not look at the answers given in the book until you have written what you think are the correct answers. Use the piece of cardboard provided to mask the answer below each question while you write the appropriate words in the blanks of a fill-in question or encircle your choice of the alternative answers to a multiple-choice question. Then slide the cardboard cover down the page to reveal the correct answer and check the accuracy of your own answer.

Avoid guessing. If you are not sure of the answer, reread the explanatory part of the Item. The need for such rereading is to be expected occasionally and perhaps even frequently. Rereading the Item will reinforce learning, eliminate vagueness, and enhance your confidence.

Turn now to Item 1 of Unit One and begin the course.

CONTENTS

PART ONE

□

ANATOMICAL LANDMARKS

Unit One □ SURFACE ANATOMY OF THE HEAD AND NECK

STRUCTURES STUDIED IN SURFACE ANATOMY

ITEM 1

A clinician's first impression of a patient comes from the patient's surface anatomical features. The term *surface anatomy* refers to any structure detectable by view or palpation, such as muscle contour or skeletal prominence. The term *topographical anatomy* includes surface features, but also deals with underlying structures and their particular location in terms of level or depth, as projected onto the surface. This unit deals principally with surface anatomy of the face and the anterior neck.

You should cultivate the habit of identifying on others all the surface features treated in this unit. Also, you should locate each structure on yourself by looking into a mirror and by palpating the structure with your fingers. Illustrations of surface structures have been omitted from this first unit deliberately to enable you, from the outset, to form the habit of locating these structures on yourself. Your own face, seen in the mirror and palpated with your fingers, as well as faces of others, provides the most effective illustrations you can have.

Surface anatomy studies structures which can be
A. either seen or felt
B. both seen and felt

QUESTION 1

The correct answer is A. While structures dealt with in surface anatomy are often both visible and palpable, some of the surface features can be palpated even though they may not be visible. Certain muscles of the neck, for example, may not be seen directly but can be palpated easily.

ANSWER

Three-dimensional conceptualization of deep structures of the body is termed _____ anatomy.

QUESTION 2

---

topographical

ANSWER   3

ITEM 2

VARIATION OF SURFACE FEATURES

As you begin to observe surface anatomical structures of other people more consciously and closely, you will recognize considerable variation from one individual to another. A rather wide range of variation is entirely normal. A change in the usual appearance or configuration of some surface feature of a given person, however, may signal a condition of important clinical significance. It is the change of appearance in a particular individual more than variation from other individuals which is medically significant.

QUESTION 3

In observing surface anatomical structures, one should attach more clinical importance to _____ in these features in individuals than to their _____ from person to person.

ANSWER

changes . . . variation

ITEM 3

THE FOREHEAD

Just above each eyebrow is a *superciliary ridge*. The flattened area between the eyebrows is the *glabella*. In a lateral view, the prominence of the forehead, called the *frontal eminence,* is evident. The frontal eminence is usually more prominent in females, while the superciliary ridges are ordinarily more marked in males.

With your fingers, feel the frontal eminence, superciliary ridges, and glabella on your own forehead. Look at the surface projections of these structures in the mirror. Repeat the names of these surface features to yourself as you see them on other people. You will be surprised at how quickly and easily you can remember the technical names of various structures by observing them on yourself and others and repeating the names as you do so.

QUESTION 4

The glabella is a flattened area *above/between* (circle one) the eyebrows.

ANSWER

between

QUESTION 5

When the forehead is viewed laterally, a prominent projection called the _____ eminence can be seen.

ANSWER

frontal

The ridge above the eyebrow which is more prominent in males than in females is termed the _____ ridge.

superciliary

THE EYES   ITEM 4

Each eye consists of an *eyeball* and supporting structures contained within a bony socket called the *orbit*. On the eyeball itself, notice the white of the eye, which is a portion of the *sclera*. The pigmented *iris* gives eyes their various colors. In the center of the iris is the dark opening called the *pupil*. Observe the pupil in a brightly lit room and in rather dim light. It will be much larger in the dim room to admit more light, much smaller in bright light to prevent too much light from entering. The pupil reflexly dilates or constricts to accommodate to the intensity of light.

The bony socket which houses the eye in the skull is called the _____.

orbit

The pigmented part of the eye is the _____; the white of the eye is part of the _____.

iris . . . sclera

The opening within the iris through which light enters to fall on the retina is called the _____.

pupil

The pupil of the eye constricts or dilates reflexly to allow for variations in _____ of light.

intensity

ITEM 5   THE EYELIDS

Two movable *eyelids,* an upper and a lower, cover each eye. The outer angle where upper and lower lids meet is termed the *lateral canthus;* the inner angle, the *medial canthus.* The canthi are important radiological landmarks when extraoral radiography is indicated.

Examine the eyelids and lashes. Observe other people as they close and open their eyelids and notice how the upper lid does most of the movement. Observation of the lids is important, since they are often the first places where swelling becomes visible in conditions of *edema,* or accumulation of fluid in the tissues.

QUESTION 11

The lateral canthus is the _____ angle at which upper and lower eyelids meet; the medial canthus, the _____ angle at which the eyelids meet.

ANSWER

outer . . . inner

QUESTION 12

The eyelids are among the first tissues to accumulate fluid in the condition called _____ .

ANSWER

edema

QUESTION 13

In extraoral radiography, the dental clinician uses the lateral and medial _____ as landmarks.

ANSWER

canthi

ITEM 6   THE EAR

The external ear comprises the oval *auricle,* which collects sound waves, and the *external acoustic meatus,* the tubelike canal through which sound waves are transmitted to the middle ear. Overhanging the orifice of the external acoustic meatus anteriorly is the cartilaginous *tragus.* Palpation of the tragus will reveal the nature of its cartilage framework. The auricle, external acoustic meatus, and tragus are useful landmarks in dental radiology.

The tube through which sound waves are transmitted from the auricle to the tympanic membrane is called the external _____ _____.

QUESTION
14

acoustic meatus

ANSWER

The small cartilaginous prominence overhanging the beginning of the external acoustic meatus is the _____.

QUESTION
15

tragus

ANSWER

The auricle, tragus, and external acoustic meatus serve as landmarks in dental _____.

QUESTION
16

radiology

ANSWER

THE NOSE ITEM 7

The *root* of the nose is the area between the eyes. As you run a finger down onto the nose from the glabella, you can feel a depression, the *nasion*, which is used in dental radiology as a landmark for correct positioning of the beam. Inferior to the nasion, the bony structure of the *bridge* of the nose can be felt. The immovable bridge is formed by the underlying *nasal bones*. Continuing downward, you can feel the flexible tip, or *apex*, which is supported by cartilage rather than bone. From below the apex, the two nostrils, or *nares*, are visible, separated by a portion of the *nasal septum*. The nares are bounded laterally by the winglike *alae* of the nose.

The nose extends from the _____ between the eyes down to the _____ at the tip.

QUESTION
17

root . . . apex

ANSWER

The depressed portion of the nose felt between the eyes is termed the _____ _____.

QUESTION
18

nasion

ANSWER

QUESTION
19

The immovable bridge of the nose is supported by _____; the movable part is supported by _____.

ANSWER

bone . . . cartilage

QUESTION
20

The anatomical term for the nostrils is _____; for the middle partition between the nostrils, _____; for the flared winglike tissues which bound the nostrils laterally, _____.

ANSWER

nares . . . septum (nasal septum) . . . alae

ITEM 8   THE LIPS

The lips are muscular folds which are extremely labile, or mobile, because they do not have direct bony attachments. In the center of the upper lip, extending down the midline from the nasal septum, is a groove called the *philtrum*, which terminates in a thicker area of the upper lip, the *tubercle*. The lower lips extend to the horizontal *labiomental groove*, which separates the lower lip from the chin. The upper and lower lips meet laterally at the *angle of the mouth*, or *labial commissure*.

QUESTION
21

The lability of the lips is attributable to their lack of attachment to _____.

ANSWER

bone

QUESTION
22

The vertical depression running from the nasal septum down the midline of the upper lip is the _____.

ANSWER

philtrum

QUESTION
23

The thickened area in the center of the upper lip at which the philtrum terminates is called the _____.

ANSWER

tubercle

QUESTION
24

The labiomental groove is a horizontal line separating the _____ lip from the _____.

lower . . . chin   ANSWER

The labial commissure is another term for the _____ of the _____   QUESTION
_____, or the fold connecting the upper and lower lips.   25

---

angle . . . mouth   ANSWER

THE MODIOLUS AND THE NASOLABIAL SULCUS   ITEM 9

Slightly lateral to the angle of the mouth, an area known as the *modiolus* is formed by the meeting of facial muscles running in several different directions. In many persons the modiolus is strongly marked in the form of the familiar dimple when they smile or grin. The groove running upward between the upper lip and the cheeks is called the *nasolabial sulcus*.

The depressed area lateral to the angle of the mouth, referred to as a dimple   QUESTION
in lay terms and as the modiolus in anatomical language, is indented because of the   26
convergence of _____ in the area.

---

muscles   ANSWER

The groove running from the modiolus upward toward the root of the nose   QUESTION
is the _____ sulcus.   27

---

nasolabial   ANSWER

THE LOWER JAW   ITEM 10

The prominence of the chin is called the *mental protuberance*. It is usually more pronounced in males but can also be felt in females. The *body of the mandible* can be palpated at the edge of the lower jaw, as it extends posteriorly toward the earlobe, where the bony edge can be felt to swing sharply upward to form the *angle of the mandible*. The vertical arm extending superiorly from the angle is the *ramus of the mandible*.

The entire area of the lower jaw, or mandible, can be palpated. It cannot be emphasized too strongly that one of the tricks in learning anatomy is to learn the structures on yourself. One set of class notes you cannot lose is the set of notes in your own head which enable you to transfer pictures in a book to your own body. Palpate each structure, then think about it. Close your eyes and think, "hand." Easy—you know all about the hand because you see it a lot. Now think, "mandible." Palpate the mandible along its length and think to yourself the technical names of its various parts. Say "mental protuberance" to yourself as you feel the anterior prominence of your chin. Cultivate this easy habit of projecting onto yourself all the illustrations and descriptions of anatomical structures which you see and read about.

QUESTION
28

Palpate on yourself the prominent anteriormost part of the mandible; this area of the chin is called the _____ protuberance.

ANSWER

mental

QUESTION
29

Run your fingers backward along the lower part of the jaw; what you are feeling is the _____ of the mandible.

ANSWER

body

QUESTION
30

Palpate the lower jaw where it swings upward near the earlobe; you are feeling the _____ of the mandible; the vertical arm you feel is called the _____ of the mandible.

ANSWER

angle . . . ramus

ITEM 11

THE CHEEK

The cheek is that broad area of the face between the nose and upper lip and the ear, extending from the bone of the lower jaw upward to the lower margin of the orbit. Most of the cheek is fleshy, being formed by muscles and a characteristic mass of fat. Just below the lateral margin of the eye a prominent bone, the *zygoma*, can be palpated. Careful palpation posteriorly from the zygoma reveals a bony ridge, the *zygomatic arch*, which extends toward the upper part of the ear. Feel carefully downward from the zygomatic arch, just in front of the ear, as you open and close your mouth. This region is the *temporomandibular joint*, the point of articulation of the mandible with the skull.

Palpate on yourself the mass of soft tissues comprising the cheek; this tissue is soft because it is composed of bulging layers of ＿＿＿＿ and ＿＿＿＿＿ under the skin.

QUESTION
31

muscle . . . fat (in either order)

ANSWER

Palpate the bony prominence under the lateral margin of the eye; the bone you are feeling is called the ＿＿＿＿.

QUESTION
32

zygoma

ANSWER

The bony ridge you can palpate from the zygoma to the upper part of the ear is the ＿＿＿＿ ＿＿＿.

QUESTION
33

zygomatic arch

ANSWER

An area of particular clinical importance can be felt inferior to the posterior-most part of the zygomatic arch. Run your fingers downward to the only freely movable joint in the head; this is the area of the ＿＿＿＿＿ joint.

QUESTION
34

temporomandibular

ANSWER

The movable joint below the zygomatic arch is the point of articulation of the ＿＿＿＿ with the ＿＿＿＿.

QUESTION
35

mandible . . . skull

ANSWER

THE NECK   ITEM 12

A primary muscular landmark of the neck is the *sternocleidomastoid muscle*, named for its points of origin and insertion. This prominent muscle originates from the medial *clavicle* and the *sternum*. It inserts at the mastoid process of the temporal bone, just posterior and inferior to the ear. The sternocleidomastoid muscle can be easily felt with your left hand as you try to turn your head to the right against the resistance of the right hand.

Now raise your shoulders and bring them forward. You can feel a depression above the clavicle, the *supraclavicular fossa*. At the lateral end of this fossa, the edge of the *trapezius muscle* can be seen and palpated as it ascends from the lateral portion of the clavicle to the back of the skull.

QUESTION
36

The bony landmark posterior and inferior to the ear, to which the sterno-cleidomastoid muscle inserts, is the _____ process.

ANSWER

mastoid

QUESTION
37

The points of origin of the sternocleidomastoid muscle are the _____ and the _____.

ANSWER

sternum . . . clavicle (in either order)

QUESTION
38

The depression which can be felt above the clavicle when the shoulders are hunched and brought forward is the _____ fossa.

ANSWER

supraclavicular

QUESTION
39

The trapezius muscle can be felt extending from the region of the posterior part of the _____ fossa to the back of the _____.

ANSWER

supraclavicular . . . skull

ITEM 13

SKIN OF THE FACE

The skin of the face and neck, like skin in general, is attached to underlying structures by loose connective tissue. The loose consistency of this connective tissue permits considerable distortion by swelling. Skin of the face is unique in that the muscles of facial expression attach directly to it. These muscles come into play with both voluntary and involuntary movements of facial expression.

QUESTION
40

Skin of the face is freely movable because it is attached to underlying structures by _____ _____ tissue.

ANSWER

loose connective

The consistency of the connective tissue attaching skin of the face to underlying structures makes the face readily susceptible to distortion by _____.

swelling

The very great subtlety and complexity of facial expression is due, in part, to the fact that the muscles of facial expression insert directly into _____ rather than into bone.

skin

BLOOD SUPPLY TO THE FACE   ITEM 14

While intracranial structures receive their blood supply from the *internal carotid artery,* most of the blood supply to extracranial structures, including the face, is provided by the *external carotid artery*. The external carotid artery can be felt pulsating directly below the angle of the mandible. A branch of the external carotid, the *facial artery,* can usually be palpated at the point where it crosses the mandible about one finger's breadth anterior to the angle of the mandible.

Before reaching the mandible, the facial artery gives off palatine, tonsillar, glandular, and muscular branches. As the facial artery ascends obliquely toward the eye, it gives off branches to skin and muscles of the face.

Extracranial structures are supplied by the _____ _____ artery; intracranial structures, by the _____ _____ artery.

external carotid . . . internal carotid

Pulsations of the external carotid artery can be palpated just below the _____ of the _____; pulsations of the facial artery can be felt as this branch crosses bone anterior to the _____ of the _____.

angle . . . mandible . . . angle . . . mandible

ITEM 15

CUTANEOUS NERVE SUPPLY TO THE FACE

Sensory nerve supply to the skin of the face is provided by the fifth cranial nerve, or *trigeminal nerve,* which is considered in detail in Unit Six. At this point, just consider the areas of the face innervated by the three divisions of the trigeminal nerve: the *ophthalmic division,* the *maxillary division,* and the *mandibular division.* The ophthalmic division supplies the forehead, upper eyelids, and midline of the nose. The maxillary division supplies the more lateral portions of the nose, the upper half of the cheek, and the side of the forehead. The mandibular division supplies the lower jaw and the region anterior to the ear. Touch the anterior part of the forehead, the upper eyelids, and the midline of the nose, and repeat to yourself as you touch each, "ophthalmic nerve." Repeat this exercise with the portions of the face supplied by the maxillary and mandibular divisions of the trigeminal nerve (V).

QUESTION 45

The cranial nerve which provides sensory nerve supply to the skin of the face is the _____ nerve.

ANSWER

trigeminal (fifth cranial)

QUESTION 46

The forehead, upper eyelids, and bridge of the nose are supplied by the _____ division of the _____ nerve.

ANSWER

ophthalmic . . . trigeminal (fifth cranial)

QUESTION 47

The skin anterior to the ear extending downward to include the lower jaw, chin, and lower lip is innervated by the _____ division of the trigeminal nerve.

ANSWER

mandibular

QUESTION 48

The area roughly defined as lying between the eye and the angle of the mouth receives its sensory innervation from the _____ division of the trigeminal nerve.

ANSWER

maxillary

THE SCALP   ITEM 16

The term *scalp* refers to the surface of the head overlying the broad, flat bones. Five distinct layers comprise the scalp: (1) the outer skin, (2) underlying dense connective tissue, (3) a membraneous sheet called the aponeurosis, which connects muscles over the forehead with muscles over the back of the skull, (4) a layer of loose connective tissue which permits movement of the three more superficial layers, and (5) a fibrous connective tissue forming the periosteum for the outer surface of bones of the skull.

The second layer, the dense connective tissue binding the skin firmly to underlying structures, has particular clinical significance. Because the second layer of the scalp is dense and fibrous, blood vessels tend to remain open when the scalp is wounded. This fact causes scalp wounds to bleed more profusely than wounds in other locations.

The reason that bleeding from a scalp wound may be disturbingly profuse is that contraction of the injured blood vessels is impeded by the density of the _____ _____ underlying the outer layer of skin.

QUESTION
49

---

connective tissue

ANSWER

Underlying the layers of outer skin, connective tissue, and the muscles and aponeurosis of the scalp is the fourth layer, the layer of _____ connective tissue which permits movement of the three layers above it.

QUESTION
50

---

loose

ANSWER

SUMMARY OF UNIT ONE

PALPABLE LANDMARKS

Although a wide range of variation in surface anatomical features is entirely normal, sometimes the first signs of a clinically important condition are changes in the surface features—hence the importance of constant alertness to surface anatomy.

Viewing the face laterally, one notices the frontal eminence, or prominence of the forehead. From the anterior view, one sees a superciliary ridge above each eyebrow and a flattened area between the eyebrows, called the glabella.

The socket containing the eyeball is called the orbit. The white of the eye is called the sclera; the pigmented portion, the iris; and the dark center, the pupil. The outer angle where upper and lower eyelids meet is the lateral canthus; the inner angle, the medial canthus.

The visible oval part of the external ear is called the auricle. The tubelike opening extending from the auricle to the middle ear is the external acoustic meatus. The small cartilaginous prominence anterior to the external acoustic meatus is the tragus.

The depression at the root of the nose is the nasion; the short bony structure, the bridge. The cartilaginous tip of the nose is the apex; the external openings, the nares; the partition between the nares, the nasal septum; the wings, the alae.

The vertical groove in the upper lip extending inferiorly from the nasal septum is called the philtrum; the thickening of the upper lip below the philtrum, the tubercle. The horizontal line separating lower lip from chin is the labiomental groove; the juncture of upper and lower lips, the angle of the mouth, or labial commissure. The depression lateral to the angle of the mouth where muscles converge under the skin is the modiolus. The groove between the upper lip and cheek is termed the nasolabial sulcus.

The anterior prominence of the chin is called the mental protuberance. The parts of the mandible include the body, the angle, and the vertical arm or ramus.

The bony prominence of the cheek inferior to the lateral canthus of the eye is the zygoma. The ridge extending from the zygoma posteriorly to the ear is the zygomatic arch. Inferior to the zygomatic arch and anterior to the ear, the mandible articulates with the skull in the temporomandibular joint.

BLOOD AND NERVE SUPPLY TO THE FACE

The thin, vascular skin of the face adheres loosely to underlying structures to permit great mobility. The fact that a number of underlying muscles insert directly into the skin contributes also to the mobility of the skin of the face evident in the myriad changes of facial expression.

The facial artery, a branch of the external carotid artery, supplies superficial structures of the face and can be felt pulsating as it crosses bone just anterior to the angle of the mandible. Just below the angle of the mandible, pulsations of the external carotid artery are palpable.

Three divisions of the fifth cranial nerve, the trigeminal nerve, are sensory to skin of the face. The ophthalmic division innervates the forehead, upper eyelids, and medial parts of the nose; the maxillary division, the cheek; and the mandibular division, the lower jaw and chin.

THE SCALP

The scalp consists of five layers of tissue covering the uppermost parts of the skull: skin; dense connective tissue; frontal and occipital scalp muscles connected by an aponeurosis; loose connective tissue; and the periosteal covering of the bones of the skull. Because of the density of the connective tissue comprising the second layer just under the skin, injured blood vessels do not contract readily, hence the profuse bleeding from scalp wounds.

The most prominent region of the forehead, viewed laterally, is called the _____ eminence.	QUESTION 51
frontal	ANSWER
Just above the eyebrows are the _____ ridges.	QUESTION 52
superciliary	ANSWER
The flattened area of the forehead between the eyebrows is the _____.	QUESTION 53
glabella	ANSWER
The depressed area at the root of the nose is the _____.	QUESTION 54
nasion	ANSWER
The partition between the nares is the nasal _____; the winglike areas outlying the nares are the _____.	QUESTION 55
septum . . . alae	ANSWER
The upper lip has a vertical groove called the _____, which terminates at a thickened area of the upper lip called the _____.	QUESTION 56
philtrum . . . tubercle	ANSWER

QUESTION
57

The depression lateral to the angle of the mouth, caused by attachment of converging muscles, is called the _____.

ANSWER

modiolus

QUESTION
58

The groove between the upper lip and cheek is called the _____ sulcus; that between the lower lip and chin the _____ groove.

ANSWER

nasolabial . . . labiomental

QUESTION
59

The anteriormost part of the chin is called the _____ protuberance.

ANSWER

mental

QUESTION
60

Three main parts of the mandible are the _____, the _____, and the _____.

ANSWER

body . . . angle . . . ramus (in any order)

QUESTION
61

The bony prominence of the cheek is the _____.

ANSWER

zygoma

QUESTION
62

The only freely movable joint in the skull is the _____ joint.

ANSWER

temporomandibular

QUESTION
63

An unusual feature of the muscles of the face is that they attach directly to _____.

ANSWER

skin

QUESTION
64

Blood supply to the face is through the _____ artery, a branch of the _____ carotid artery.

facial . . . external   *ANSWER*

Sensory innervation to the face is supplied by the _____ nerve.   QUESTION
65

_____

trigeminal (fifth cranial)   *ANSWER*

The forehead is supplied by the _____ division of the trigeminal (fifth cranial) nerve.   QUESTION
66

_____

ophthalmic   *ANSWER*

The cheek is supplied by the _____ division of the trigeminal nerve (V).   QUESTION
67

_____

maxillary   *ANSWER*

The chin and lower jaw are supplied by the _____ division of the trigeminal nerve (V).   QUESTION
68

_____

mandibular   *ANSWER*

The layer of the scalp just under the skin is composed of _____ _____ tissue.   QUESTION
69

_____

dense connective   *ANSWER*

Profuse bleeding of scalp wounds is due to the fact that the second layer, made up of _____ connective tissue, does not permit blood vessels to _____ _____ readily.   QUESTION
70

_____

dense . . . contract   *ANSWER*

Unit Two ☐ THE SKULL

ITEM
1

THE SKULL: GENERAL CONSIDERATIONS

The skull can be considered as two portions. One portion is primarily involved in housing and protecting the brain and is called the *cranium*. The other is a complex portion supporting visceral structures related to the face. Several bones are shared by both portions of the skull. Some of the bones in each portion are paired; others are single. The bones listed below are major topographical landmarks, or points of reference, for locating the position of numerous structures studied in head and neck anatomy. Do not attempt to memorize the list at this time. It is presented at the outset merely to give a preliminary overview of the bones of the skull to be studied in this unit.

Bones of the Cranium		Bones of the Face	
Single	*Paired*	*Single*	*Paired*
Occipital	Parietal	Mandible	Maxilla
Frontal	Temporal	Vomer	Zygomatic
Sphenoid			Nasal
Ethmoid			Lacrimal
			Palatine

QUESTION
1

The part of the skull which houses the brain is called the _____.

ANSWER

cranium

QUESTION
2

The bones of the skull which do not house the brain support visceral structures of the _____.

ANSWER

face

QUESTION
3

The term which includes both cranium and bones of the face is _____.

20 ANSWER

skull

THE JOINTS OF THE SKULL   ITEM 2

The typical joint between bones of the skull is known as a *suture*. Sutures form jagged lines on exposed surfaces of the skull as a result of the interlacing of many short needle-like projections of the articulating bones. The actual connection between the bones consists of strands of connective tissue fibers passing from one bone across the suture into the opposing bone.

A striking exception to the typical rigid suture is the freely moving *temporomandibular joint* by which the mandible articulates with the base of the skull. Because of its importance in dentistry, the temporomandibular joint is treated in detail later in this unit.

The joints between most bones of the skull are termed _____.

QUESTION 4

_____

sutures

ANSWER

Sutures arc _____ _____ fibers which pass from one bone to the next.

QUESTION 5

connective tissue

ANSWER

The freely movable articulation between the mandible and the base of the skull is called the _____ joint.

QUESTION 6

temporomandibular

ANSWER

THE SUTURES   ITEM 3

Sutures are often spoken of as being immovable, but in fact they do permit a limited amount of movement and provide mechanical protection for the brain by absorbing much of the force of a blow to the head. Sutures are broad and flexible in infants, so that considerable molding of the head can occur during birth. Most adult sutures have reached a state of relative immobility at about 25 to 30 years of age.

The fact that sutures permit a small amount of _____ enables them to absorb part of the force of a blow.

QUESTION 7

ANSWER　　　　　　　　　　　　　　　　movement

QUESTION　　Sutures are wide and flexible in *adults/infants* (circle one), narrow and more
8　　rigid in *adults/infants* (circle one).

_____

ANSWER　　　　　　　　　　　　　　infants . . . adults

ITEM 4　SUPERIOR ASPECT OF THE SKULL: THE BONES

Refer to Figure 2–1 as you read this item. Locate each bone in the illustration
as it is mentioned, then locate the bone with your fingers on your own skull.

When the skull is viewed from above, four bones are visible. At the front of the
skull is the *frontal bone*. At the level of the ears, paired *parietal bones* can be seen.
At the back of the skull is the single *occipital bone*.

QUESTION　　Four bones of the skull are visible from the superior aspect: the anteriormost
9　　_____ bone, the two lateral _____ bones, and the posteriormost
_____ bone.

_____

ANSWER　　　　　　　　frontal . . . parietal . . . occipital

QUESTION　　The four bones seen from the superior aspect form the upper part of the
10　　_____.

_____

ANSWER　　　　　　　　　　　　　　skull

ITEM 5　SUPERIOR ASPECT OF THE SKULL: THE SUTURES

Sutures of the skull are usually named for the bones involved. The sutures seen
in the superior aspect, however, have special names. As you read this item, locate
each suture in Figure 2–2 and then, with your fingers, identify the location of the
suture on your own skull.

The suture extending transversely between the frontal and parietal bones is

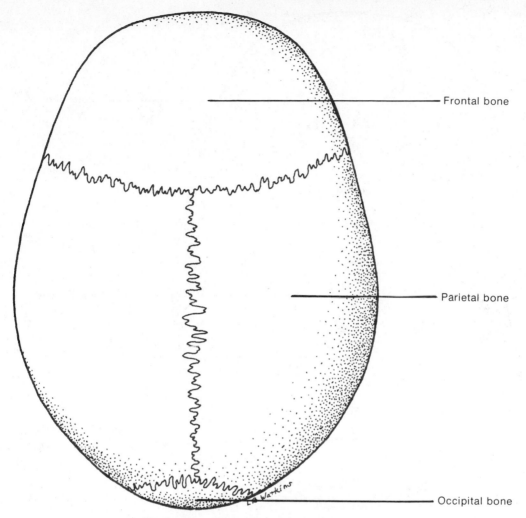

Figure 2–1. Bones of the skull, superior aspect.

known as the *coronal suture*. A second suture, called the *sagittal suture*, extends from front to back between the parietal bones. The third suture, lying between the occipital bone and the two parietal bones, is the *lambdoidal suture*.

Occasionally a fourth suture is observed. The frontal bone develops as two bones, but the suture between these bones normally disappears at about the age of two. In approximately 8 per cent of the population, however, this suture, called the *metopic suture*, persists. It is of little importance except that if seen radiologically, it may be diagnosed erroneously as a fracture line in the skull.

The coronal suture runs between the _____ bone and the _____ bones.

QUESTION
11

frontal . . . parietal

ANSWER

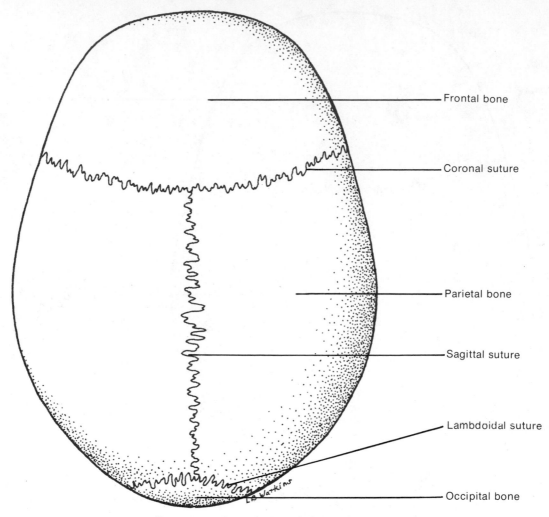

Figure 2-2. Sutures of the skull, superior aspect.

QUESTION
12
    The line of demarcation between the parietal bones is the _____ suture.

_____

ANSWER
                                    sagittal

QUESTION
13
    The lambdoidal suture joins the _____ bone with the _____ bones.

_____

ANSWER
                              occipital . . . parietal

QUESTION
14
    The metopic suture, which persists to adulthood in a few individuals, extends vertically down the _____ bone.

_____

ANSWER
                                    frontal

SUPERIOR ASPECT OF THE SKULL: THE RADIOLOGICAL LANDMARKS

ITEM 6

Examine Figure 2–3. Locate the coronal and sagittal sutures. The intersection of these two sutures is the *bregma*.

Now follow the sagittal suture backward until it intersects the lambdoidal suture. The point of intersection is the *lambda*.

The convex *parietal eminence* is the widest point of the skull. The highest point on the sagittal suture is the *vertex*. The vertex is not visible in the superior aspect, but can be seen from the lateral view.

The bregma is the intersection between the _____ and the _____ sutures.

QUESTION 15

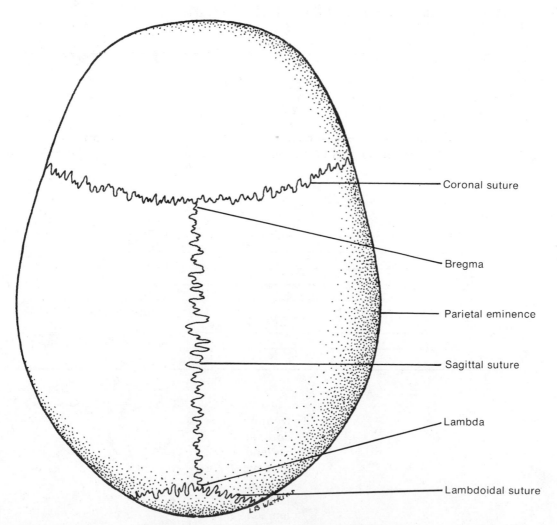

Figure 2–3. Bregma, lambda, and parietal eminence.

ANSWER   coronal . . . sagittal (in either order)

QUESTION   The lambda is the intersection between the _____ and the
16   _____ sutures.

ANSWER   sagittal . . . lambdoidal (in either order)

QUESTION   The highest point of the skull is called the *vertex/parietal eminence* (circle
17   one) and lies behind the *bregma/lambda* (circle one).

ANSWER   vertex . . . bregma

QUESTION   The wide convex area of the parietal bone is the _____
18   _____.

ANSWER   parietal eminence

QUESTION   In the numbered spaces below, write the names of the corresponding
19   numbered bones and sutures in the diagram on the facing page.

Labels
1. _____ bone
2. _____ suture
3. _____ bone
4. _____
5. _____ suture
6. _____ suture
7. _____
8. _____ bone

ANSWER
1. frontal
2. coronal
3. parietal
4. bregma
5. sagittal
6. lambdoidal
7. lambda
8. occipital

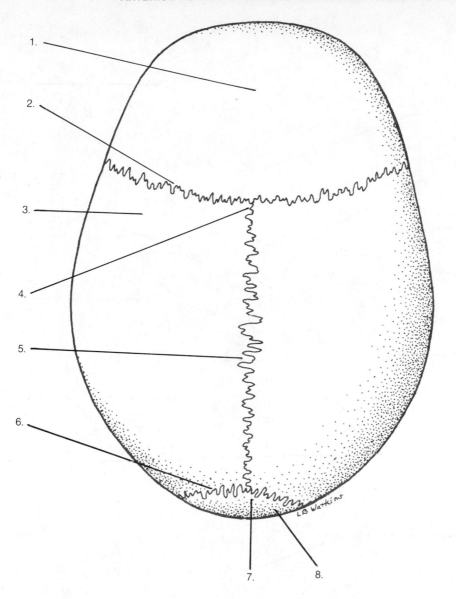

ANTERIOR ASPECT OF THE SKULL: GENERAL CONSIDERATIONS

ITEM 7

    The anterior aspect of the skull reveals most of the bones of the face. Before looking at individual bones, examine the general areas of the face on Figure 2–4. Observe the forehead and its relationship to the two *orbits*, which protect and house the eyeballs. Below the orbits laterally are the bony prominences of the cheek; below the orbits medially are the bony structures associated with the nose. Notice the opening of the nasal cavity, the *piriform aperture*. The lower border of the maxilla is the *alveolar process*, containing the maxillary teeth. The lower jaw consists of a single bone, the *mandible*.

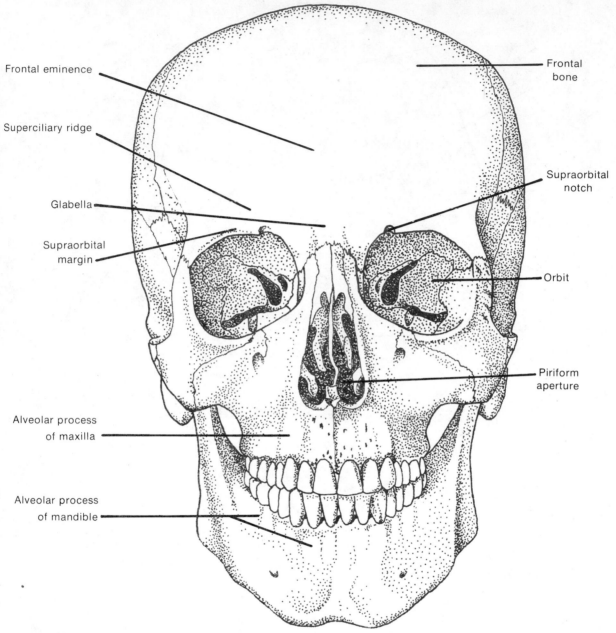

Frontal eminence

Superciliary ridge

Glabella

Supraorbital margin

Alveolar process of maxilla

Alveolar process of mandible

Frontal bone

Supraorbital notch

Orbit

Piriform aperture

Figure 2–4.   Skull, anterior aspect. (Redrawn from Wolf-Heidegger: Atlas of Systematic Human Anatomy. Vol. I. Basel, S. Karger AG.)

Without attempting to go into detail at this point, note that several of the bones of the face are shared by two or more soft tissue compartments of the face. For example, the frontal bone forms the forehead and part of the orbits; the maxilla forms part of the orbits, part of the nasal cavity, and part of the oral cavity. The fact that a single bone may be shared by two or more soft tissue compartments has important clinical significance because the fracture of one facial bone often endangers soft tissues contained within several compartments.

The frontal bone extends inferiorly to form the roof of the _____ .

orbits

The floor of the orbits is formed in large part by the _____.

maxilla

The opening in the skull for the nasal cavity is the _____ aperture.

piriform

The portion of the maxilla which houses the teeth is the _____ process.

alveolar

The maxilla, in addition to being part of the cheek, forms part of each _____, as well as the _____ cavity and the _____ cavity.

orbit . . . nasal . . . oral

The fact that the maxilla forms part of the bony framework of several compartments has clinical significance in cases of _____ of the maxilla.

fractures

ANTERIOR ASPECT OF THE SKULL: THE FOREHEAD
ITEM 8

In this and the following items, identify the bones and landmarks as they are mentioned, first on the diagram in Figure 2–4, then on a skull, and, whenever possible, on yourself. It is helpful to use a mirror while feeling these structures on yourself so that you not only feel but also see where the structures are located.

The forehead is supported by a single bone, the frontal bone, which has several surface landmarks. When you studied Unit One, Item 2, you identified the frontal eminence, the superciliary ridge, and the glabella. Review these markings on the skull itself, then proceed to the additional structures shown in Figure 2–4.

The *supraorbital margin* is the area where the frontal bone turns into the orbits below. On the superior margin of the orbit note the *supraorbital foramen,* which is often present as a notch rather than a foramen. This foramen carries the supraorbital nerve and artery from the orbit to the forehead. Medial to the supraorbital notch one often sees a supratrochlear notch, which transmits the supratrochlear artery and nerve to the medial forehead.

QUESTION
26

Surface landmarks on the frontal bone include the _____ eminence, the _____ ridge, the _____ margin, and the glabella.

ANSWER

frontal . . . superciliary . . . supraorbital

QUESTION
27

The most prominent foramen, or notch, penetrating the upper rim of the orbit is the _____ foramen.

ANSWER

supraorbital

QUESTION
28

The prominent foramen on the upper margin of the orbit transmits an _____ _____ and a _____ having the same name as the foramen itself.

ANSWER

artery . . . nerve

QUESTION
29

A notch sometimes found medial to the supraorbital notch is the _____ _____ notch, which carries the _____ artery and nerve.

ANSWER

supratrochlear . . . supratrochlear

ITEM
9

ANTERIOR ASPECT OF THE SKULL: THE RIM OF THE ORBIT

Examine Figure 2–5. This illustration directs attention to the detailed structure of the orbit. Notice the three bones which make up the orbital margin: the frontal bone, the zygoma, and the maxilla. The upper half of the orbital margin is formed by the *supraorbital margin* of the frontal bone. The lateral margin and part of the inferior margin are formed by the *zygoma,* or zygomatic bone, which

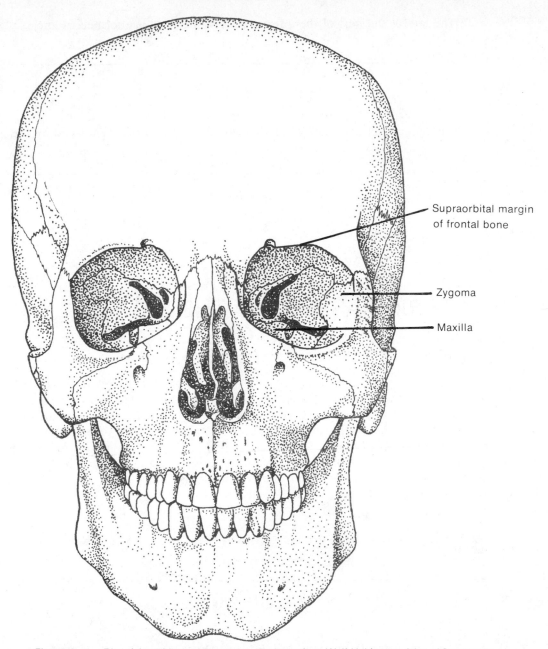

Supraorbital margin of frontal bone

Zygoma

Maxilla

Figure 2–5. Rim of the orbit, anterior aspect. (Redrawn from Wolf-Heidegger: Atlas of Systematic Human Anatomy. Vol. I. Basel, S. Karger AG.)

also forms the bony prominence of the cheek. The *maxilla* forms the medial and inferior parts of the rim of the orbit.

The upper part of the orbital rim is formed by the _____ margin of the _____ bone.

QUESTION 30

_____

supraorbital . . . frontal

ANSWER

QUESTION
31

The lateral and part of the inferior rims of the orbit are formed by the ____ _____ .

ANSWER

zygoma (zygomatic bone)

QUESTION
32

The medial rim and most of the inferior rim of the orbit are formed by the _____ .

ANSWER

maxilla

ITEM 10   ANTERIOR ASPECT OF THE SKULL: THE WALLS OF THE ORBIT

Locate the structures described in this and the next item on Figure 2–6 as well as on a skull, if you have one available. Notice that most of the roof of the orbit is formed by the frontal bone; most of the floor, by the maxilla. Observe on the right side of Figure 2–6 how the anterior portion of the lateral wall is formed by the *orbital process of the zygoma*. The posterior portion of the lateral wall is formed by one surface of the *greater wing of the sphenoid bone*. The sphenoid bone is very complex, some part of it being encountered in almost every significant area of the skull.

QUESTION
33

Most of the roof of the orbit is formed by the _____ bone; most of the floor is formed by the _____ .

ANSWER

frontal . . . maxilla

QUESTION
34

The anterolateral wall of the orbit is formed by the _____ process of the _____ .

ANSWER

orbital . . . zygoma

QUESTION
35

The posterolateral wall of the orbit is formed by the _____ _____ of the _____ bone.

ANSWER

greater wing . . . sphenoid

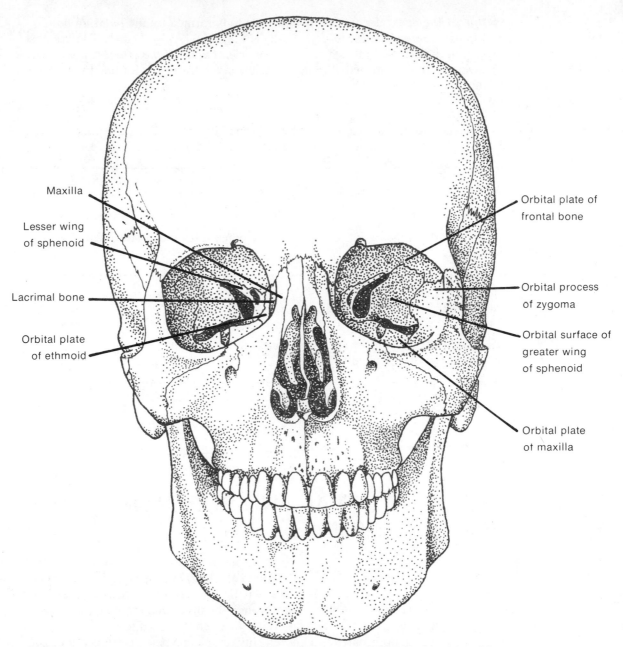

Maxilla

Lesser wing
of sphenoid

Lacrimal bone

Orbital plate
of ethmoid

Orbital plate of
frontal bone

Orbital process
of zygoma

Orbital surface of
greater wing
of sphenoid

Orbital plate
ot maxilla

Figure 2-6.   Walls of the orbit, anterior aspect. (Redrawn from Wolf-Heidegger: Atlas of Systematic Human Anatomy. Vol. I. Basel, S. Karger AG.)

ANTERIOR ASPECT OF THE SKULL: THE MEDIAL WALL OF THE ORBIT

ITEM 11

Refer to Figure 2–6 above and locate the bones of the orbit labeled on the left side of the illustration. The medial wall is formed anteriorly by the maxilla, as it forms part of the rim. At the *apex,* the deepest portion of the orbit, a part of the base of the *lesser wing of the sphenoid bone* may be seen. A small portion at the lower section of the apex, not visible in Figure 2–6, is formed by the *palatine bone*.

Immediately posterior to the maxilla is the small *lacrimal bone*. The greatest portion of the medial wall is formed by the *orbital plate of the ethmoid bone*. The posterior portion of the medial wall, not visible in Figure 2–6, is formed by the *body of the sphenoid bone*.

QUESTION
36

The anteromedial wall of the orbit is formed by the _____, the _____ bone, and the orbital plate of the _____ bone.

ANSWER

maxilla . . . lacrimal . . . ethmoid

QUESTION
37

The body of the _____ bone constitutes the posteromedial wall of the orbit.

ANSWER

sphenoid

QUESTION
38

The lesser wing of the sphenoid bone and the palatine bone form the deepest portion of the orbit, called the _____.

ANSWER

apex

ITEM 12   THE OPTIC CANAL AND SUPERIOR ORBITAL FISSURE

Examine Figure 2–7 and notice the round opening at the apex of the orbit. This opening is the *optic canal,* which lies between the two roots of the lesser wing of the sphenoid bone. The optic nerve passes through the optic canal to reach the brain, and the ophthalmic artery extends anteriorly through the canal to reach the eye.

Lateral to the optic canal is a curved slitlike opening between the greater and lesser wings of the sphenoid bone, the *superior orbital fissure*. The superior orbital fissure transmits nerves to the muscles of the eye and to the ophthalmic vein, which drains the orbit.

QUESTION
39

The round opening at the apex of the orbit is the _____ canal, which contains the _____ nerve and the _____ artery.

ANSWER

optic . . . optic . . . ophthalmic

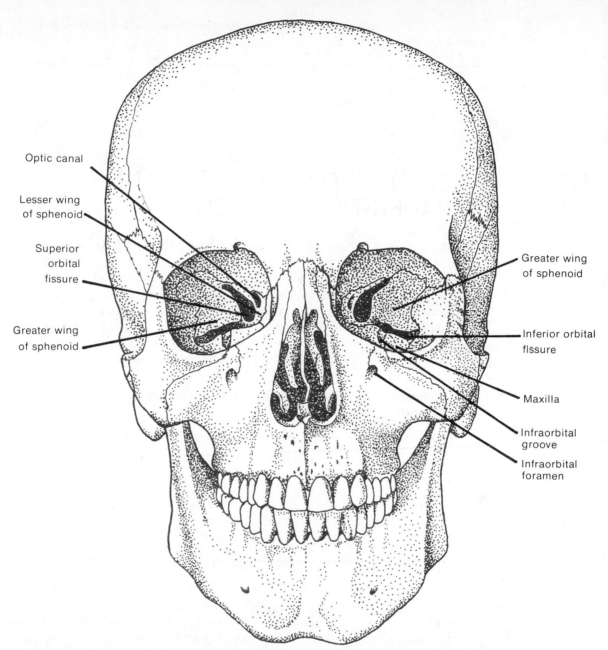

Figure 2-7. Openings into the orbit, anterior aspect. (Redrawn from Wolf-Heidegger: Atlas of Systematic Human Anatomy. Vol. I. Basel, S. Karger AG.)

The slitlike opening lateral to the optic canal is the _____ _____ fissure, which carries nerves and a vein to the muscles of the eye.

QUESTION
40

---

superior orbital

ANSWER

The opening between the roots of the lesser wing of the sphenoid is the _____

QUESTION
41

_____ _____; the opening between the greater and lesser wings of the sphenoid is the _____ _____ _____.

ANSWER   optic canal . . . superior orbital fissure

ITEM 13   INFERIOR ORBITAL FISSURE AND INFRAORBITAL FORAMEN

Refer to Figure 2–7 and note the structures labeled on the right side of the illustration. At the lateral margin of the floor of the orbit, the *inferior orbital fissure* can be seen between the greater wing of the sphenoid bone and the maxilla, extending to the zygoma. The infraorbital nerve, a branch of the maxillary nerve, and the infraorbital artery enter the orbit through this fissure. The infraorbital nerve and artery then lie in the *infraorbital groove* on the posterior part of the floor of the orbit. Anteriorly the infraorbital groove becomes a canal covered by bone, ending as the *infraorbital foramen,* which opens onto the anterior surface of the maxilla.

QUESTION 42

The inferior orbital fissure is located between the greater wing of the _____ _____ and the _____.

ANSWER   sphenoid . . . maxilla

QUESTION 43

The infraorbital nerve and artery enter the orbit through the inferior orbital _____, lie in the infraorbital groove and canal, and pass through the infraorbital _____ to surface just under the eye.

ANSWER   fissure . . . foramen

QUESTION 44

As a review, write in the numbered spaces below the names of the corresponding numbered structures on the accompanying diagram.

Labels

1. _____ bone
2. _____ canal
3. _____ _____ fissure
4. _____ bone
5. _____ bone
6. _____ bone
7. _____
8. _____ _____ fissure
9. _____
10. _____ foramen

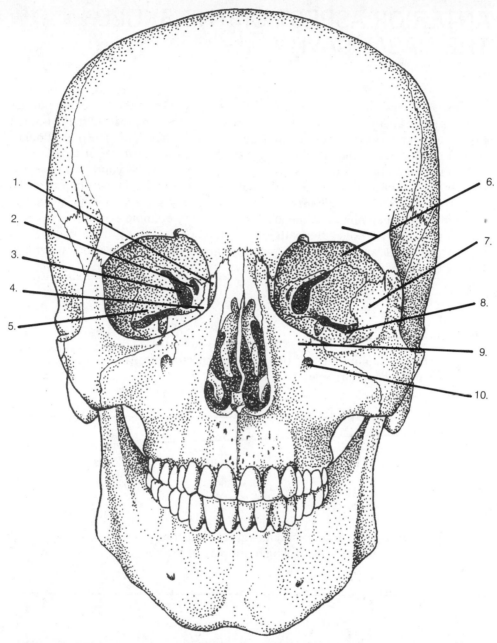

(Redrawn from Wolf-Heidegger: Atlas of Systematic Human Anatomy. Vol. I. Basel, S. Karger AG.)

1. lacrimal
2. optic
3. superior orbital
4. ethmoid
5. sphenoid

6. frontal
7. zygoma
8. inferior orbital
9. maxilla
10. infraorbital

ANSWER

ITEM 14   ANTERIOR ASPECT OF THE SKULL: THE NASAL CAVITY

As you read this item, refer to Figure 2–8. Notice first the boundaries of the piriform aperture, the bony rim of the nasal cavity. Above it are the two small *nasal bones* which form the bridge of the nose in the intact skull. The other boundaries are all formed by the maxillae. Note the protrusion, the *anterior nasal spine*, at the midline on the inferior margin. You can locate this on your own nose.

On the lateral wall of each nasal cavity are three projecting structures called the *nasal conchae*, or *turbinates*, extending scroll-like into the nasal cavity. The superior and middle conchae are formed by the ethmoid bones; the inferior concha is a separate bone. Beneath each of the conchae is a groove known as a *meatus*. Within these meatuses lie openings through which the various paranasal sinuses communicate with the nasal cavity.

QUESTION 45

The superior boundaries of the piriform aperture are the _____ bones; the other boundaries are formed by the _____.

ANSWER

nasal . . . maxillae

QUESTION 46

Each lateral nasal wall contains three projecting structures called nasal _____, the top two of which are part of the _____ bone.

ANSWER

conchae . . . ethmoid

QUESTION 47

The paranasal sinuses communicate with the nasal cavity through openings under the conchae; each of these openings lies in a groove called a _____.

ANSWER

meatus

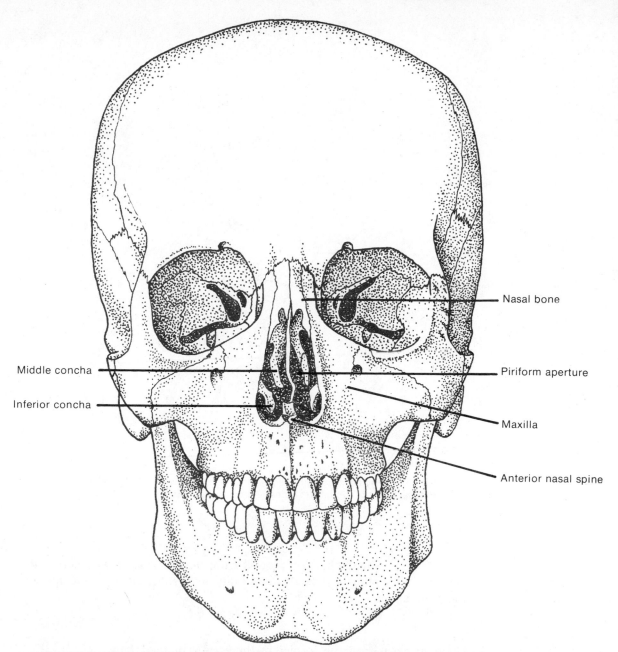

Nasal bone

Middle concha

Piriform aperture

Inferior concha

Maxilla

Anterior nasal spine

Figure 2-8. The nasal cavity, anterior aspect. (Redrawn from Wolf-Heidegger: Atlas of Systematic Human Anatomy. Vol. I. Basel, S. Karger AG.)

THE NASAL SEPTUM   ITEM 15

Looking through the piriform aperture on the skull, one can see a vertical partition dividing the nasal cavity into two halves. In the intact person, this nasal septum is made up anteriorly and superiorly by cartilage and the *vertical plate of the ethmoid bone*. The posterior, inferior portion is formed mainly by bone, the *vomer*. Figure 2–9 shows the relationship between the vertical plate of the ethmoid and

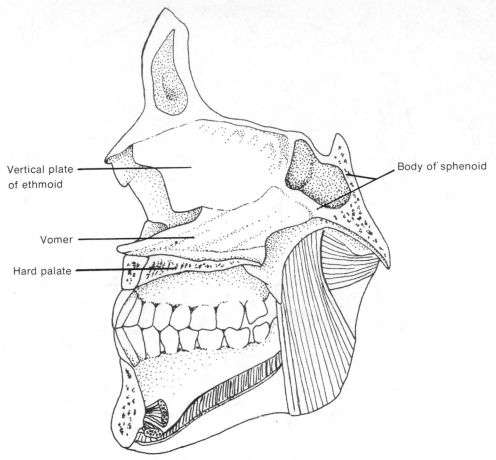

Figure 2-9.   The bony nasal septum, parasagittal section, viewed from the left side. (Redrawn from Wolf-Heidegger: Atlas of Systematic Human Anatomy. Vol. I. Basel, S. Karger AG.)

the vomer in a parasagittal section viewed from the left side. It also shows the relationship of the septum posteriorly to the body of the sphenoid bone and inferiorly to the hard palate.

QUESTION 48   The bony nasal septum is formed by the vertical plate of the _____ bone and by the _____ .

ANSWER   ethmoid . . . vomer

QUESTION 49   The movable part of the nasal septum is composed of _____ .

ANSWER   cartilage

Posterior and superior to the vomer is the body of the _____ bone.

sphenoid

Inferior to the vomer is the _____ _____.

hard palate

ANTERIOR ASPECT OF THE SKULL: THE ZYGOMA

ITEM 16

The zygomatic bone, or zygoma, articulates with the frontal, maxillary, sphenoid, and temporal bones. In Figure 2–10, notice the articulations at the *zygomatic process of the frontal bone*, the *zygomatic process of the temporal bone*, and the *zygomatic process of the maxilla*. The zygomatic arch, shown from the lateral aspect in Figure 2–15, is formed by the zygoma together with the zygomatic processes of the temporal bone and maxilla.

The zygoma has three small foramina. On the orbital surface is the *zygomatico-orbital foramen*, through which the zygomatic nerve, a branch of the maxillary nerve, enters the zygoma. The zygomatic nerve divides within the bone into two cutaneous nerves of the face, the zygomaticotemporal nerve and the zygomatico-facial nerve. The zygomaticotemporal nerve passes through one or two very small foramina on the posterior surface of the bone at the *zygomaticofrontal suture* to reach skin lateral to the eye. The zygomaticofacial nerve passes out through a foramen of the same name on the facial surface of the zygoma.

The bones with which the zygoma articulates include the _____, the _____, the _____, and the _____.

frontal . . . maxillary . . . sphenoid . . . temporal (any order)

Foramina of the zygoma transmit the _____ nerve and two of its cutaneous branches, the _____ and _____ nerves.

zygomatic . . . zygomaticotemporal . . . zygomaticofacial

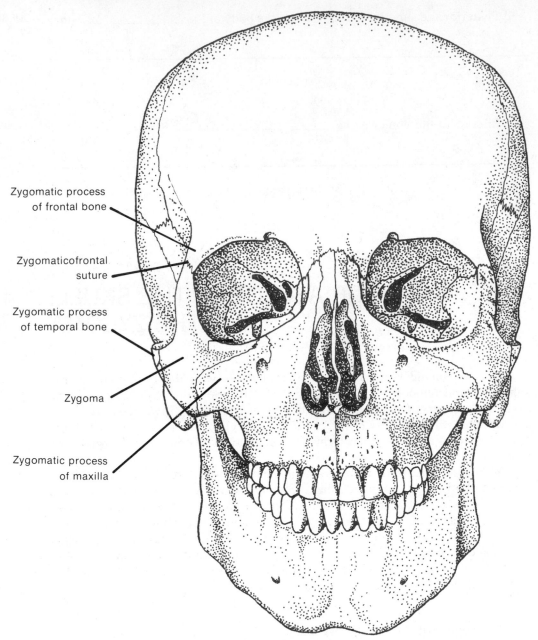

Zygomatic process
of frontal bone

Zygomaticofrontal
suture

Zygomatic process
of temporal bone

Zygoma

Zygomatic process
of maxilla

Figure 2-10. Zygoma, anterior aspect. (Redrawn from Wolf-Heidegger: Atlas of Systematic Human Anatomy. Vol. I. Basel, S. Karger AG.)

ITEM 17   ANTERIOR ASPECT OF THE SKULL: THE MAXILLA

As pointed out in Item 10, much of the floor of the orbit is formed by the *orbital plate of the maxilla*. Examine Figure 2–11 and notice how the orbital plate of the maxilla is continuous at the rim of the orbit with the *frontal process of the maxilla*. The frontal process extends upward to articulate with the nasal and frontal bones.

The inferior portion of the maxilla, as seen from the external surface, is the

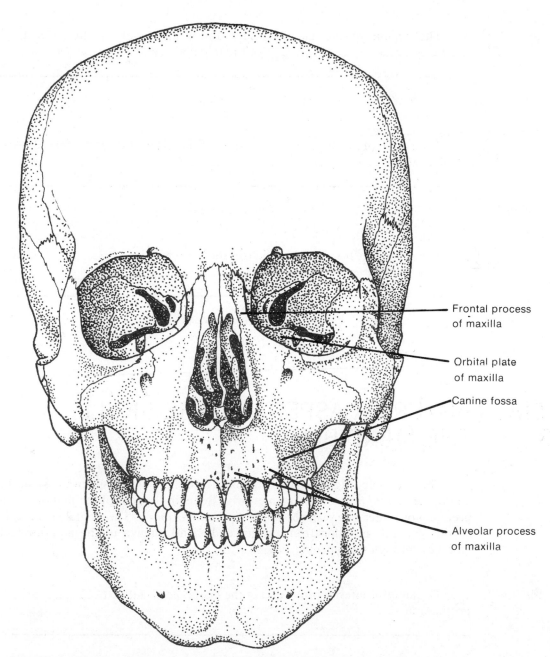

Frontal process
of maxilla

Orbital plate
of maxilla

Canine fossa

Alveolar process
of maxilla

Figure 2-11. Maxilla, anterior aspect. (Redrawn from Wolf-Heidegger: Atlas of Systematic Human Anatomy. Vol. I. Basel, S. Karger AG.)

alveolar process, containing the maxillary teeth. Just lateral to the long root of each canine tooth is a small depression, the *canine fossa*. Bone covering the anterior teeth is extremely thin, and usually the roots of the anterior teeth can be seen in the skull.

QUESTION
54

The region of the maxilla which forms the floor of the orbit is the _____ _____ of the maxilla.

ANSWER

orbital plate

QUESTION
55

The region of the maxilla which forms the medial portion of the orbital margin is called the _____ _____.

ANSWER

frontal process

QUESTION
56

The part of the maxilla which houses the teeth is the _____ _____.

ANSWER

alveolar process

ITEM
18
ANTERIOR ASPECT OF THE SKULL:
THE MANDIBLE

The mandible, Figure 2–12, is the only freely movable bone of the skull. Examine the *mental protuberance* anteriorly. Beneath the root of the first or second premolar on either side is an opening, the *mental foramen*. The mental nerve which carries general sensation from the lower lip and gingiva of the anterior teeth emerges through this opening.

QUESTION
57

The anterior inferior projection of the mandible is called the _____ protuberance.

ANSWER

mental

QUESTION
58

The mental nerve provides sensory input from the lower _____ and lower anterior _____.

ANSWER

lip . . . gingiva

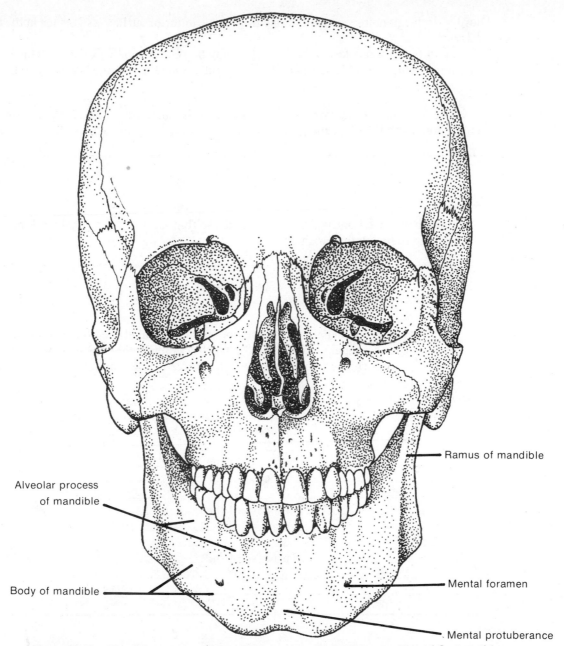

Figure 2-12. Mandible, anterior aspect. (Redrawn from Wolf-Heidegger: Atlas of Systematic Human Anatomy. Vol. I. Basel, S. Karger AG.)

THE BODY OF THE MANDIBLE ITEM 19

Refer to Figure 2–12 for this item.

The heavy, horizontal portion of the mandible below the mental foramen is called the *body of the mandible*. That portion which holds the teeth is the *alveolar process*. Upon loss of the mandibular teeth, the alveolar process may be resorbed to such an extent that the mental foramen is virtually transposed to the superior border of the mandible, instead of opening on the anterior surface as you see in the diagram.

Posteriorly, a portion of the mandible may be seen extending upward. This is the *ramus*, which will be discussed when the skull is studied from the lateral aspect.

QUESTION
59
The main horizontal portion of the mandible is called the _____; the region which houses the teeth is the _____ _____.

ANSWER
body . . . alveolar process

QUESTION
60
If teeth are lost, bone is _____, so that some of the normal markings may change their relative position.

ANSWER
resorbed

QUESTION
61
As a review of the zygoma, maxilla, and mandible, label the bones and bone markings on the accompanying diagram by writing in the numbered spaces below the names of the corresponding numbered structures in the diagram.

Labels

1. _____ process of the _____ bone
2. _____ process of the _____ bone
3. _____
4. _____ process of the _____
5. _____ process of the _____
6. _____ of _____
7. _____ process of the _____
8. _____ plate of the _____
9. _____ _____
10. _____ process of the _____
11. _____ _____
12. _____ _____

ANSWER
1. zygomatic . . . frontal
2. zygomatic . . . temporal
3. zygoma
4. zygomatic . . . maxilla
5. alveolar . . . mandible
6. body . . . mandible
7. frontal . . . maxilla
8. orbital . . . maxilla
9. canine fossa
10. alveolar . . . maxilla
11. mental foramen
12. mental protuberance

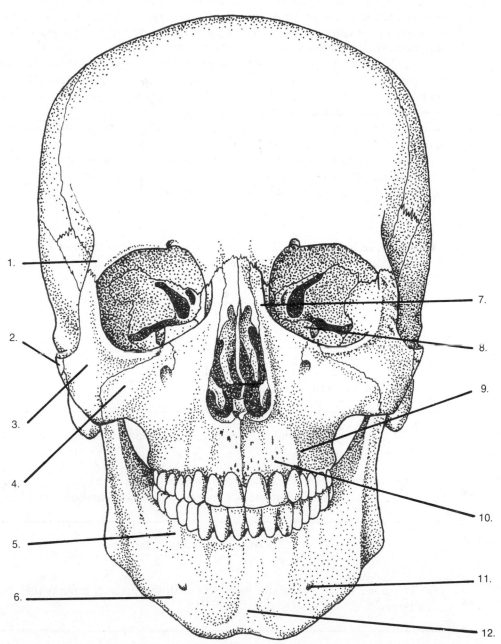

(Redrawn from Wolf-Heidegger: Atlas of Systematic Human Anatomy. Vol. I. Basel, S. Karger AG.)

ITEM 20

LATERAL ASPECT OF THE SKULL: GENERAL CONSIDERATIONS

When the skull is viewed from the lateral aspect, as shown in Figure 2–13, an approximation of the division of the skull into cranium and bones of the face can be made by imagining a diagonal line passing downward and backward from the superior orbital margin to the tip of the mastoid process.

Visible in the lateral view of the skull, shown in Figure 2–13, are the bones of the upper part of the cranium which were seen in the superior aspect: the frontal, occipital, and parietal bones. Also two of the sutures previously seen in the superior aspect, the coronal and lambdoidal sutures, appear in the lateral view. Figure 2–13 also shows two additional bones not seen in the superior view, the *temporal bone* and the *greater wing of the sphenoid bone.*

The temporal bone articulates superiorly and posteriorly with the parietal and occipital bones. Anterior to the temporal bone is an essentially quadrangular surface formed by the greater wing of the sphenoid bone.

QUESTION
62

From the lateral view, the cranium and the bones of the face can be roughly demarcated by an imaginary line passing from the _____ _____ margin to the _____ process.

ANSWER

superior orbital . . . mastoid

QUESTION
63

Bones of the cranium include the _____, _____, _____, and _____.

ANSWER

frontal . . . parietal . . . temporal . . . occipital (in any order)

QUESTION
64

The suture between the frontal and parietal bones is the _____ suture; the _____ suture is between the parietal and occipital bones.

ANSWER

coronal . . . lambdoidal

QUESTION
65

The bone which articulates inferiorly with the parietal bone is the _____ bone.

ANSWER

temporal

QUESTION
66

The bone which articulates anteriorly with the temporal bone is the _____ _____ of the _____.

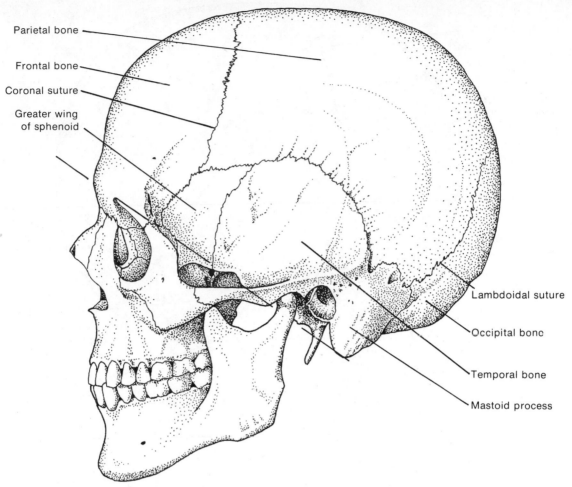

Figure 2-13. Skull, lateral aspect. (Redrawn from Wolf-Heidegger: Atlas of Systematic Human Anatomy. Vol. I. Basel, S. Karger AG.)

greater wing . . . sphenoid   *ANSWER*

LATERAL ASPECT OF THE SKULL: THE TEMPORAL BONE
ITEM 21

Examine the temporal bone shown in Figure 2–14. The temporal bone consists of three parts: the *squamous, tympanic,* and *petrous portions*. The squamous portion of the temporal bone is the fanshaped flattened part articulating with the sphenoid, parietal, and occipital bones. The tympanic portion is the region associated with the ear. The petrous portion, because it is part of the floor of the cranium, is not visible in the lateral aspect.

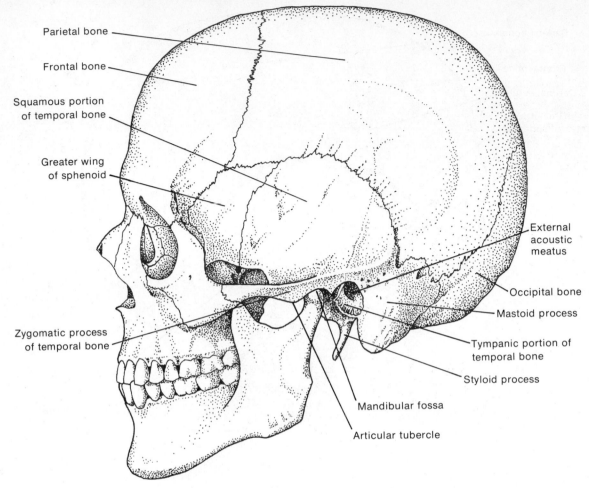

Figure 2-14. Skull, lateral aspect, showing the temporal bone. (Redrawn from Wolf-Heidegger: Atlas of Systematic Human Anatomy. Vol. I. Basel, S. Karger AG.)

QUESTION
67

The three parts of the temporal bone are the _____, the _____, and the _____ portions.

ANSWER

squamous . . . tympanic . . . petrous (in any order)

QUESTION
68

The flattened squamous portion of the temporal bone articulates anteriorly with the _____ bone; superiorly with the _____ bone; and posteriorly with the _____ bone.

ANSWER

sphenoid . . . parietal . . . occipital

THE TEMPORAL BONE: ZYGOMATIC PROCESS

ITEM
22

At the inferior part of the squamous portion of the temporal bone is a bony projection, the *zygomatic process,* which articulates with the zygoma to form the *zygomatic arch*. This arch can be seen in Figure 2–14. You palpated the zygomatic arch earlier. At the base of the zygomatic process, on its inferior surface, note the *mandibular fossa,* with the *articular tubercle* anterior to the fossa. These structures are important components of the temporomandibular articulation.

The articulation of the temporal bone with the zygoma is by way of the _____ process.

QUESTION
69

---

zygomatic

ANSWER

Inferior to the temporal part of the zygomatic process is the point of articulation of the temporal bone with the mandible, the _____ fossa.

QUESTION
70

---

mandibular

ANSWER

A projection on the base of the zygomatic process anterior to the mandibular fossa is the _____ tubercle.

QUESTION
71

---

articular

ANSWER

THE TEMPORAL BONE: TYMPANIC AND PETROUS PORTIONS

ITEM
23

The tympanic portion of the temporal bone, seen in Figure 2–14, is a small, irregularly shaped structure forming the anterior and inferior walls of the *external acoustic meatus* as well as part of the posterior wall.

The petrous portion of the temporal bone will be seen more fully from the internal aspect. However, it is well to mention at this point that the petrous portion extends to the surface to form the posterior part of the external acoustic meatus. The petrous portion projects inferiorly, forming the *mastoid process,* which can be palpated behind the ear.

Just beneath the external acoustic meatus, at the anteromedial border of the mastoid process, is a long, slender bony extension called the *styloid process*. This process, directed forward and downward, is a point of attachment for ligaments and muscles.

QUESTION
72

The anterior and inferior walls of the external acoustic meatus are formed by the _____ portion of the temporal bone.

ANSWER

tympanic

QUESTION
73

The location of the temporomandibular joint is _____ to the external acoustic meatus.

ANSWER

anterior

QUESTION
74

The petrous part of the temporal bone is found on the lateral surface of the skull posterior to the external _____ meatus.

ANSWER

acoustic

QUESTION
75

The extension of the petrous part of the temporal bone that is located inferiorly behind the ear is the _____ process.

ANSWER

mastoid

QUESTION
76

Anteromedial to the mastoid process is the long, slender _____ process.

ANSWER

styloid

ITEM 24   LATERAL ASPECT OF THE SKULL: THE TEMPORAL FOSSA

Examine the location of the *temporal fossa* in Figure 2–15. The temporal fossa is classically described as a delimited space, but its only clear boundaries on the skull are the anterior and medial walls. The anterior wall is formed by the *zygomatic process of the frontal bone* and the *frontal process of the zygomatic bone*. The medial wall is formed by the temporal surface of the greater wing of the sphenoid bone, the squamous portion of the temporal bone, and adjacent portions of the frontal and

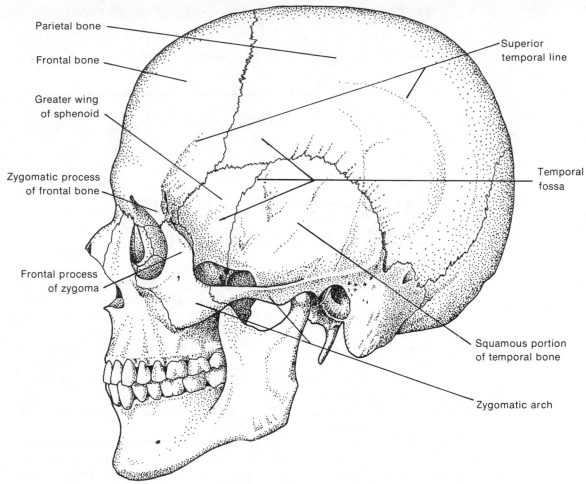

Parietal bone

Frontal bone

Greater wing
of sphenoid

Zygomatic process
of frontal bone

Frontal process
of zygoma

Superior
temporal line

Temporal
fossa

Squamous portion
of temporal bone

Zygomatic arch

Figure 2-15. The temporal fossa. (Redrawn from Wolf-Heidegger: Atlas of Systematic Human Anatomy. Vol. I. Basel, S. Karger AG.)

parietal bones. The superior margin of the temporal fossa is the *superior temporal line*. The superior temporal line arches from the zygomatic process of the frontal bone in a line nearly parallel to the curved border of the squamous portion of the temporal bone. As this line is followed posteriorly, it becomes more and more vague.

The anterior border of the temporal fossa is the zygomatic process of the _____ bone and the frontal process of the _____ bone.

QUESTION
77

---

frontal . . . zygomatic

ANSWER

Portions of four bones form the medial wall of the temporal fossa: the _____ bone, the _____ bone, the _____ bone, and the _____ bone.

QUESTION
78

ANSWER

sphenoid . . . temporal . . . frontal . . . parietal (in any order)

QUESTION
79

The upper boundary of the temporal fossa is the superior _____ line.

ANSWER

temporal

ITEM 25   LATERAL ASPECT OF THE SKULL: THE RAMUS OF THE MANDIBLE

Refer to Figure 2–16 as you work through this item. Note the broad, flattened quadrilateral portion extending upward and backward from the body of the mandible. This portion is called the *ramus of the mandible*, and it is the primary area for attachment of muscles of mastication.

The anterior border of the ramus is a thin, sharp margin. Superiorly, the anterior border terminates in the *coronoid process*. The main portion of the anterior border forms a concave forward curve, called the *coronoid notch*. Inferiorly this margin ends as an *oblique line*, or *external oblique line*, which becomes nearly horizontal on the body of the mandible, terminating near the *mental foramen*. The anteriormost part of the mandible is the *mental p................e*.

The posterior border of the ramus is thickened ... and extends from the *angle* to a projection which forms the mandibular portion of the temporomandibular joint. This projection is the *condylar process*, or *condyle*. Between the coronoid process and the condyle a concave margin forms the *mandibular notch*.

QUESTION
80

The principal area of attachment of the muscles of mastication to the mandible is the _____.

ANSWER

ramus

QUESTION
81

The anterior superior part of the ramus of the mandible is the _____ process.

ANSWER

coronoid

QUESTION
82

The concave anterior margin of the ramus of the mandible is the _____ _____ notch.

ANSWER

coronoid

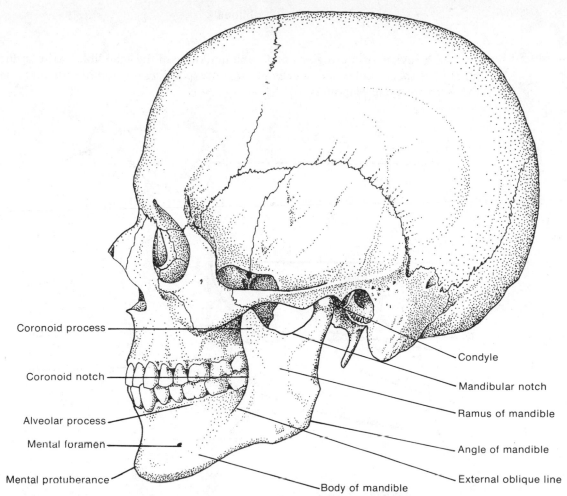

Coronoid process

Coronoid notch

Alveolar process

Mental foramen

Mental protuberance

Condyle

Mandibular notch

Ramus of mandible

Angle of mandible

External oblique line

Body of mandible

Figure 2-16. Skull, lateral aspect, showing the ramus of the mandible. (Redrawn from Wolf-Heidegger: Atlas of Systematic Human Anatomy. Vol. I. Basel, S. Karger AG.)

The posterior superior projection from the ramus of the mandible is the _____.

QUESTION **83**

condyle (condylar process)

ANSWER

The concave region between the coronoid process and the condyle is the _____ notch.

QUESTION **84**

mandibular

ANSWER

The anterior border of the ramus of the mandible ends inferiorly as an external _____ line which continues to the body of the mandible.

QUESTION **85**

ANSWER   oblique

QUESTION   As a review of the regions and bone markings of the mandible, write in the
86   numbered spaces below the names of the corresponding numbered structures on
the accompanying diagram.

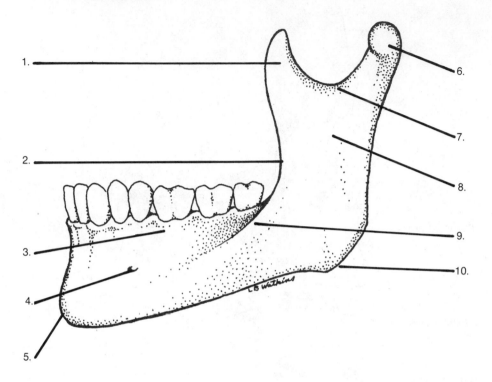

Labels

1. _____ process
2. _____ notch
3. _____ process
4. _____ foramen
5. _____ protuberance
6. _____
7. _____ notch
8. _____
9. _____ line
10. _____ of the mandible

ANSWER

1. coronoid	6. condyle
2. coronoid	7. mandibular
3. alveolar	8. ramus
4. mental	9. external oblique
5. mental	10. angle

LATERAL ASPECT OF THE SKULL: THE INFRATEMPORAL FOSSA

ITEM 26

If you have a skull available, insert your index finger behind the ramus of the mandible, angling upward and forward toward the orbit. Your finger is in the *infratemporal fossa*. This space is closely confined by bony structures, but is crowded with arteries and nerves which are important in relationship to the oral cavity. Some of the muscles of mastication are also found in the infratemporal fossa.

The tip of your finger can be seen in the orbit through the inferior orbital fissure. Some important structures pass from the infratemporal fossa into the orbit through this fissure. Just below the tip of your finger is the bulge of the posterior surface of the maxilla, the *maxillary tuberosity*. The anterior boundary of the infratemporal fossa is formed by the maxillary tuberosity and by that portion of the maxillary alveolar crest which supports the posterior teeth. The lateral wall of the infratemporal fossa is formed by the upper portion of the ramus of the mandible.

The infratemporal fossa is important in the study of dentistry because it contains _____ and _____ related to the oral cavity as well as some muscles of _____.

QUESTION 87

---

nerves . . . arteries . . . mastication

ANSWER

The word *infratemporal* indicates that the infratemporal fossa is located _____ the temporal fossa.

QUESTION 88

---

below

ANSWER

The anterior boundary of the infratemporal fossa is the posterior border of the _____.

QUESTION 89

---

maxilla

ANSWER

The lateral boundary of the infratemporal fossa is the _____ of the _____.

QUESTION 90

---

ramus . . . mandible

ANSWER

ITEM 27   LATERAL ASPECT OF THE SKULL: THE PTERYGOID PROCESS

If possible, continue to use a skull while studying this item. Notice that there is no clear bony posterior wall of the infratemporal fossa. The medial wall can be identified, although it is not complete. The superior wall is formed by the *infratemporal surface* of the greater wing of the sphenoid bone. Continuous with the superior surface is the lateral surface of a sheet of bone called the *pterygoid process*, which projects downward from the sphenoid bone. The pterygoid process enters into a suture with the maxilla, just behind the most posterior tooth. A V-shaped slit between the maxilla and the pterygoid process is known as the *pterygomaxillary fissure*. The surface of the pterygoid process seen from this aspect is the *lateral plate* of the pterygoid process.

QUESTION 91

The superior wall of the infratemporal fossa is formed by the _____ _____ surface of the _____ wing of the sphenoid bone.

ANSWER

infratemporal . . . greater

QUESTION 92

The downward projection of bone continuous with the superior surface of the infratemporal fossa is called the _____ process.

ANSWER

pterygoid

QUESTION 93

The slit between the pterygoid process and the maxilla is the _____ _____ fissure.

ANSWER

pterygomaxillary

QUESTION 94

The fossa below the temporal fossa is the _____ fossa.

ANSWER

infratemporal

THE PTERYGOPALATINE FOSSA

Continue to use a skull (if available) to help you study this item. Locate the pterygomaxillary fissure again. Looking through this fissure, one can see a space, the *pterygopalatine fossa*. On the deep surface of this fossa, another opening can be seen, the *sphenopalatine foramen,* which provides a communication between the pterygopalatine fossa and the nasal cavity. If you run a wire medially from the pterygopalatine fossa, you will see the wire appearing in the nasal cavity. Like the infratemporal fossa, the pterygopalatine fossa is crowded with arteries and nerves.

Extending inward from the pterygomaxillary fissure is the _____ _____ fossa.

QUESTION
95

---

pterygopalatine

ANSWER

An opening in the medial wall of the pterygopalatine fossa which contains nerves and arteries to the nose is the _____ foramen.

QUESTION
96

---

sphenopalatine

ANSWER

INFERIOR ASPECT OF THE SKULL: GENERAL CONSIDERATIONS

The inferior aspect of the skull shows a large number of important bony structures and openings. These openings provide entrance for the arteries and veins supplying the brain and some of the facial viscera. They are also the means whereby cranial nerves leave the cranial vault. These structures are most easily considered if this aspect of the skull is studied with the mandible removed.

Openings in the base of the skull contain arteries and veins to the _____ _____ and to some of the _____ viscera.

QUESTION
97

---

brain . . . facial

ANSWER

Besides transmitting arteries and veins, foramina in the base of the skull are also the openings through which _____ nerves leave the cranial vault.

QUESTION
98

---

cranial

ANSWER

ITEM 30   INFERIOR ASPECT OF THE SKULL: THE HARD PALATE

Refer to Figure 2–17 for this item, and also use a skull, if you have one available. The anterior part of the inferior aspect of the skull, bounded by the maxillary teeth, is the bony *hard palate*. The hard palate is formed by the *palatine processes* of the maxillae and by the *horizontal plates* of the palatine bones. The right and left sides of the maxillary portion of the hard palate are united in the midline by the *median palatine suture*. The *transverse palatine suture* delimits the maxillary portion of the hard palate from the horizontal plates of the palatine bones.

In the midline anteriorly is the *incisive foramen,* which transmits blood vessels and nerves supplying the anterior region of the hard palate. The *greater palatine foramen,* located in the posterolateral region of the hard palate, transmits vessels

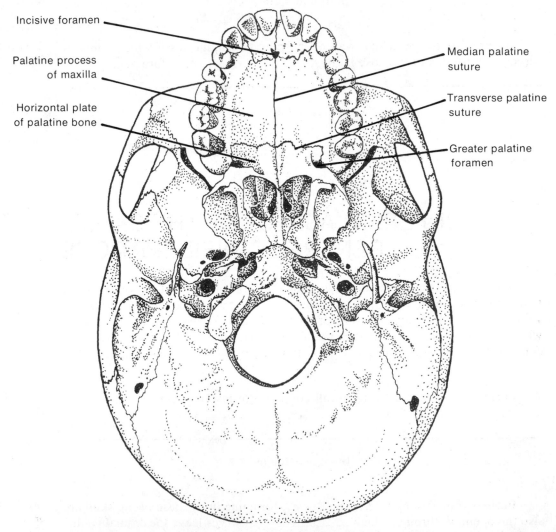

Figure 2-17. Skull, inferior aspect, showing the hard palate. (Redrawn from Wolf-Heidegger: Atlas of Systematic Human Anatomy. Vol. I. Basel, S. Karger AG.)

and nerves from the pterygopalatine fossa to the roof of the mouth. The smaller *lesser palatine foramen,* not visible in Figure 2–17, transmits nerves and arteries to the soft palate.

The hard palate is formed by the palatine processes of the two _____ and by the horizontal plates of the _____ bones.

QUESTION
99

_____

maxillae . . . palatine

ANSWER

Located between the two plates of the maxillary portion of the hard palate is the _____ palatine suture.

QUESTION
100

median

ANSWER

The suture which delimits the maxillae and the palatine bones in the hard palate is the _____ _____ suture.

QUESTION
101

transverse palatine

ANSWER

Nerves and vessels are transmitted to the anterior region of the hard palate through the _____ foramen.

QUESTION
102

incisive

ANSWER

The largest foramen located in the posterolateral region of the hard palate is called the _____ _____ foramen.

QUESTION
103

greater palatine

ANSWER

INFERIOR ASPECT OF THE SKULL: THE POSTERIOR NASAL APERTURES

ITEM 31

Examine Figure 2–18, and notice the posterior edge of the hard palate. This edge forms the lower border of the *posterior nasal apertures,* or *choanae.* The medial border of each aperture is formed by the posterior edge of the *vomer,* which runs vertically from the palatine bones to the body of the sphenoid bone. The superior border of each aperture is formed by extensions of the vomer and the

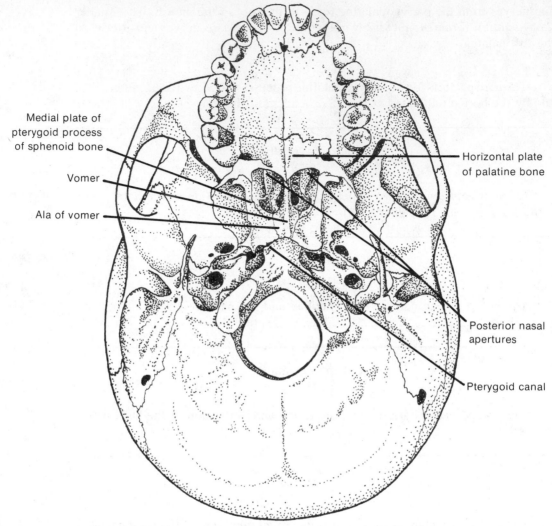

Medial plate of
pterygoid process
of sphenoid bone

Vomer

Ala of vomer

Horizontal plate
of palatine bone

Posterior nasal
apertures

Pterygoid canal

Figure 2-18.   Skull, inferior aspect, showing posterior nasal apertures. (Redrawn from Wolf-Heidegger: Atlas of Systematic Human Anatomy. Vol. I. Basel, S. Karger AG.)

pterygoid plates. At the posterolateral end of these superior borders is a small canal, the *pterygoid canal,* which extends forward to open into the pterygopalatine fossa. The lateral borders of the posterior nasal apertures are formed by *medial plates* of the pterygoid processes of the sphenoid.

QUESTION
104

Superior to the posterior border of the horizontal plate of the palatine bones are the posterior nasal _____.

ANSWER

apertures (choanae)

QUESTION
105

The bone forming the posterior part of the nasal septum is the _____.

ANSWER

vomer

The canal located at the posterolateral border of the base of the pterygoid plates is the _____ canal.

QUESTION
106

pterygoid

ANSWER

The medial pterygoid plate forms the _____ border of the posterior nasal apertures.

QUESTION
107

lateral

ANSWER

INFERIOR ASPECT OF THE SKULL: ITEM
THE PTERYGOID PROCESSES   32

In Figure 2–19, notice the *pterygoid processes* of the sphenoid bone. These processes serve as areas for attachment of the muscles of mastication, and also form pillars supporting the posterior maxillary teeth. You have already seen parts of the pterygoid processes, but they should be reviewed at this time. Each pterygoid process consists of a flattened *lateral plate* and a thinner *medial plate*. The depression between the medial and lateral pterygoid plates is the *scaphoid fossa*. At the lower end of the medial plate is a pointed process directed posteriorly and then laterally. This process, the *pterygoid hamulus,* serves as a pulley for a muscle tendon.

In this and the next several items you are dealing with a number of markings and foramina which occupy a relatively small area on the base of the skull. The relationships of these structures to each other will be discussed in terms such as medial and posterolateral. To avoid feeling lost in a maze of description, start the practice of making line diagrams of the relationships of these structures as they are described. Most of the structures will be talked about in terms of their relationship to the groove for the auditory tube (see in Item 33), and the mandibular fossa (see in Item 35).

QUESTION
108

These line drawings (straight lines and circles will do fine) will not be done for you; you should do them yourself. Refer to Figure 2–19 to get started. Locate the medial and lateral pterygoid plates. In the space on the following page, draw two vertical lines in the approximate relationship of the medial plates. On each side draw two oblique lines representing the lateral plates. Put a hook on the anterior (top) of the medial plate for the hamulus. Shade in the scaphoid fossa between the plates.

Label the following parts of your drawing: medial pterygoid plate, lateral pterygoid plate, scaphoid fossa, and pterygoid hamulus.

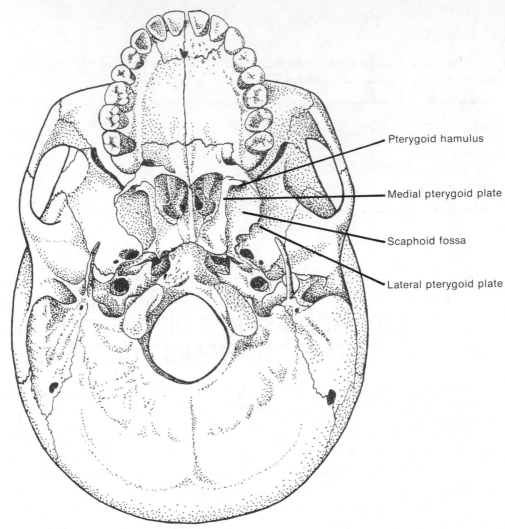

Pterygoid hamulus

Medial pterygoid plate

Scaphoid fossa

Lateral pterygoid plate

Figure 2-19. Pterygoid processes of the sphenoid bone, inferior aspect. (Redrawn from Wolf-Heidegger: Atlas of Systematic Human Anatomy. Vol. I. Basel, S. Karger AG.)

ANSWER   Use the space below to draw your sketch.

The posterior extensions from the pterygoid process are called the _____ _____ and _____ pterygoid plates.

medial . . . lateral (in either order)

Two functions of the pterygoid plates are attachment for the muscles of _____ and support for the posterior maxillary _____.

mastication . . . teeth

The depression between the pterygoid plates is the _____ fossa.

scaphoid

The pointed lower end of the medial pterygoid plate is the _____.

hamulus

The pterygoid hamulus functions as a _____ for a muscle tendon.

pulley

INFERIOR ASPECT OF THE SKULL: THE FORAMINA   ITEM 33

In Figure 2–20, notice how the base of the scaphoid fossa is continuous with a groove which arches posteriorly and laterally toward the medial border of the *mandibular fossa*. This groove is known as the *groove for the auditory tube,* the tube which equalizes air pressure in the middle ear. Situated lateral to the groove for the auditory tube are two foramina. The anterior one is larger, and is oval in shape, from which it derives its name, the *foramen ovale*. The mandibular division of the trigeminal nerve leaves the skull through the foramen ovale. Posterior to the foramen ovale is a smaller foramen, the *foramen spinosum,* which transmits an artery to the meninges.

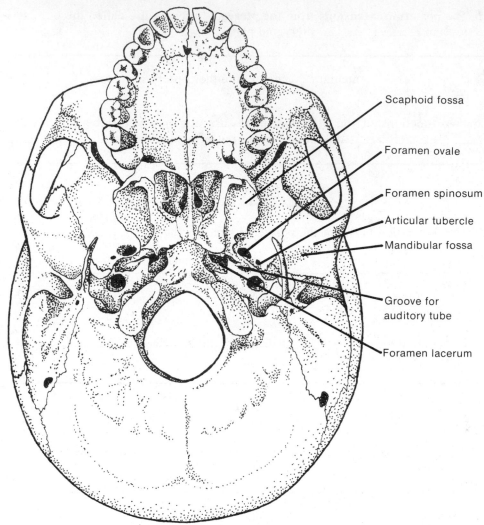

Figure 2-20. Skull, inferior aspect, showing foramina. (Redrawn from Wolf-Heidegger: Atlas of Systematic Human Anatomy. Vol. I. Basel, S. Karger AG.)

QUESTION
114

The auditory tube runs posterolaterally from the base of the _____ fossa toward the _____ fossa.

ANSWER

scaphoid . . . mandibular

QUESTION
115

The two foramina anterolateral to the groove for the auditory tube are: (1) the larger foramen _____, and (2) the smaller foramen _____.

ANSWER

ovale . . . spinosum

The foramen ovale transmits the _____ division of the trigeminal (fifth cranial) nerve

---

mandibular

The foramen spinosum transmits an _____ to the meninges.

---

artery

INFERIOR ASPECT OF THE SKULL: THE FORAMEN LACERUM

ITEM 34

Medial to the groove for the auditory tube, usually opposite the foramen ovale, is the large, irregularly shaped *foramen lacerum*. The foramen lacerum, closed in the intact skull by a layer of fibrocartilage on its outer aspect, serves as the lower medial border of a channel containing the internal carotid artery. The foramen lacerum can be seen on Figure 2–20, posteromedial to the foramen ovale.

Medial to the foramen ovale and the groove for the auditory tube is the foramen _____.

---

lacerum

The foramen lacerum is located at the lower border of the route for the _____ _____ artery.

---

internal carotid

Refer again to Figure 2–20 to see the scaphoid fossa extending into the groove for the auditory tube. Reproduce your first drawing of the pterygoid plates (abbreviating labels with initials, if you wish), and add two oblique lines directed posterolaterally to represent the groove for the auditory tube. Now draw circles in the positions for the foramen ovale, the foramen spinosum, and the foramen lacerum. If you do not know where to put these foramina, reread the item, observe the shape and positions of these features on Figure 2–20, and refer to a skull, if possible. Label all the new structures in full.

ANSWER

Use this space to draw your sketch.

ITEM 35   INFERIOR ASPECT OF THE SKULL: THE MANDIBULAR FOSSA

A large depression lateral to the end of the groove for the auditory tube is the *mandibular fossa,* shown in Figure 2–20. The anterior border of the mandibular fossa constitutes the *articular tubercle,* a transverse bony ridge which ends antero-laterally in the zygomatic process of the temporal bone. The entire lateral half of the mandibular fossa, and the superior and anterior portions of the medial half of the fossa, are formed by the squamous part of the temporal bone. The posterior medial part of the fossa is formed by the tympanic part of the temporal bone.

QUESTION
121

Refer to Figure 2–20 and locate the structures described in this item. Reproduce the drawing you made in Question 120, including the pterygoid plates and the groove for the auditory tube. Redraw these lines and the three foramina you drew in answering the preceding question. Now, looking back to Figure 2–20, add laterally two oblique lines representing the mandibular fossae. These lines should be directed medially and slightly toward the bottom of the page. Add the articular tubercle. Label all structures.

Use this space to draw your sketch.

The mandibular fossa is located ＿＿＿＿＿＿＿ to the groove for the auditory tube.

QUESTION
122

lateral

ANSWER

The projection anterior to the mandibular fossa is the ＿＿＿＿＿＿＿ ＿＿＿＿＿＿＿.

QUESTION
123

articular tubercle

ANSWER

The projection anterior to the mandibular fossa is continuous with the ＿＿＿＿＿＿＿ process of the temporal bone.

QUESTION
124

zygomatic

ANSWER

The lateral and anteromedial part of the mandibular fossa is part of the ＿＿＿＿＿＿＿ portion of the temporal bone.

QUESTION
125

squamous

ANSWER

The posterior and posteromedial areas of the mandibular fossa are parts of the ＿＿＿＿＿＿＿ portion of the temporal bone.

QUESTION
126

tympanic

ANSWER

ITEM 36   INFERIOR ASPECT OF THE SKULL: THE TEGMEN TYMPANI

Refer to a skull as you study this item. The greatest dimension of the mandibular fossa is from side to side. It is inclined so that a line through the fossa, if extended, would pass through the foramen magnum.

The *tympanosquamous fissure,* which actually looks like a crack, runs diagonally across the posterior portion of the mandibular fossa. A small, sharp, bony structure projecting downward into the medial portion of this fissure is the *tegmen tympani,* a part of the petrous portion of the temporal bone. The projection of the tegmen tympani into the fissure line causes three distinct fissures to be formed at this point. These three fissures will be discussed in the next item.

QUESTION 127

The mandibular fossa is slanted from the anterolateral end to the posteromedial end, so that an extended line through the fossa would pass through the foramen _____.

ANSWER

magnum

QUESTION 128

The projection of bone which extends into the tympanosquamous fissure is the _____ _____.

ANSWER

tegmen tympani

QUESTION 129

The bony projection extending into the tympanosquamous fissure is part of the _____ portion of the temporal bone.

ANSWER

petrous

ITEM 37   INFERIOR ASPECT OF THE SKULL: THE FISSURES

The single lateral fissure between the tympanic and squamous portions of the temporal bone is called the *tympanosquamous fissure*. If the tegmen tympani does not appear in the medial portion, then the whole fissure is called *tympanosquamous*. When the tegmen tympani is visible, two additional fissures are formed medially, one anterior and one posterior to the wedge of bone. The anterior fissure is between the petrous and squamous parts of the temporal bone and is termed the *petrosquamous fissure*. The posterior fissure is between the petrous and tympanic parts of the temporal bone and is called the *petrotympanic fissure*.

The fissure which runs laterally across the mandibular fossa is called the _____ fissure.

---

tympanosquamous

The fissure between the tegmen tympani and the anterior squamous portion of the temporal bone is the _____ fissure.

---

petrosquamous

The fissure between the tegmen tympani and the posterior tympanic portion of the temporal bone is the _____ fissure.

---

petrotympanic

Draw two Y-shaped lines directed so that the stems of the Y's are pointing toward the sides of the page and the forked tops of the Y's are facing each other. These lines represent the fissures which have just been described, one on each mandibular fossa.

The tegmen tympani is in the space between the arms of the Y; it is an extension of the petrous portion of the temporal bone. The squamous portion of the temporal bone is anterior (toward top of the page); the tympanic portion of the temporal bone is posterior. Write in these names around the Y's. Notice how the suture names were derived from adjacent bones.

Use this space to draw your sketch.

ITEM 38   THE SPINE OF THE SPHENOID AND THE CAROTID CANAL

At the lateral end of the groove for the auditory tube, a small spine can be seen medial to the mandibular fossa. This bony projection, the *spine of the sphenoid bone,* appears between the end of the groove for the auditory tube and foramen spinosum. It serves as a point of attachment for a ligament which extends the mandible. Locate the spine on Figure 2–21.

Just posterior to the end of the groove for the auditory tube is the round opening of the *carotid canal.* On the skull, the carotid canal can be seen to arch toward the foramen lacerum. The *styloid process,* already seen from the lateral aspect, can again be seen lateral and posterior to the carotid canal.

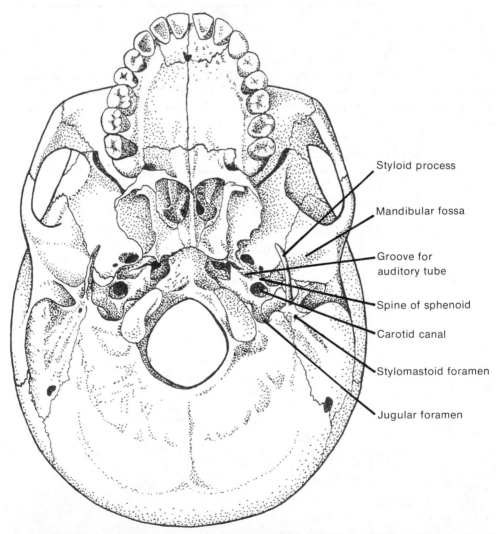

Figure 2-21. Spine of sphenoid, carotid canal, styloid process, and foramina, inferior aspect. (Redrawn from Wolf-Heidegger: Atlas of Systematic Human Anatomy. Vol. I. Basel, S. Karger AG.)

Redraw lines to represent the auditory groove. Put in lines to show the mandibular fossa. Now add circles for the foramen ovale, foramen spinosum, and foramen lacerum. Examine Figures 2–20 and 2–21 again if necessary. Now add lines for the spine of the sphenoid, a circle for the entrance of the carotid canal, and a spike for the styloid process.

QUESTION 134

Use this space to draw your sketch.

ANSWER

The projection seen between the posterolateral end of the groove for the auditory tube and the mandibular fossa is the _____ of the _____ bone.

QUESTION 135

spine . . . sphenoid

ANSWER

The canal which lies posterior to the groove for the auditory tube is the _____ canal.

QUESTION 136

carotid

ANSWER

The canal for the carotid artery runs anteromedially toward the foramen _____.

QUESTION 137

lacerum

ANSWER

A long, sharp process posterolateral to the carotid canal is the _____ process.

QUESTION 138

styloid

ANSWER

ITEM 39   THE STYLOMASTOID AND JUGULAR FORAMINA

Refer to Figure 2–21 and locate the *stylomastoid foramen*. This foramen is situated in the suture between the occipital bone and the mastoid process, immediately posterolateral to the styloid process. The stylomastoid foramen is the opening through which branches of the facial nerve exit from the skull.

Look at Figure 2–21 again and find the *jugular foramen,* the large opening medial to the base of the styloid process. If you are using a skull, tilt it somewhat; the jugular foramen will be more clearly visible. The jugular foramen is the opening through which the internal jugular vein and the three cranial nerves called the glossopharyngeal (IX), vagus (X), and spinal accessory (XI) nerves leave the skull.

QUESTION
139

Sketch from memory, if you can, the structures in your previous drawing. Then add the stylomastoid and jugular foramina. Check your drawing with Figure 2–21 after you have sketched it from memory.

ANSWER

Use this space to draw your sketch.

QUESTION
140

The foramen between the styloid process and the mastoid process is appropriately named the _____ foramen.

ANSWER

stylomastoid

QUESTION
141

The stylomastoid foramen is the point of exit of branches of the _____ nerve.

ANSWER

facial

The large opening medial to the styloid process is the _____ foramen.

---

jugular

Besides transmitting the internal jugular vein, the jugular foramen also transmits three _____ _____.

---

cranial nerves

THE FORAMEN MAGNUM AND OCCIPITAL CONDYLES

ITEM 40

In the center of the posterior part of the skull, Figure 2–22, is the large *foramen magnum,* through which passes the spinal cord. On the anterolateral borders of the foramen magnum are two curving, smooth areas called the *occipital condyles.* These condyles form part of the articulation of the skull with the first cervical vertebra.

Redraw your previous sketch and add to it the foramen magnum.

Use this space to draw your sketch.

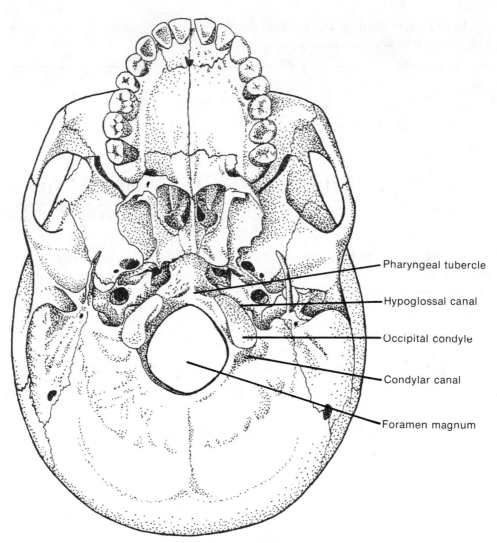

Figure 2-22.   Foramen magnum, occipital condyles, and canals, inferior aspect. (Redrawn from Wolf-Heidegger: Atlas of Systematic Human Anatomy. Vol. I. Basel, S. Karger AG.)

In relationship to the foramen magnum, the occipital condyles are (circle one) *anterolateral/posterolateral*.

anterolateral

THE CONDYLAR AND HYPOGLOSSAL CANALS

Refer to Figure 2–22 as you study this item. The *condylar canal*, an opening at the posterior border of the occipital condyle, is a point of exit for an emissary vein. Passing horizontally beneath the anterior portion of each occipital condyle is another opening, the *hypoglossal canal*, which transmits the hypoglossal (twelfth cranial) nerve. The hypoglossal canal is not visible unless you tilt the skull; the label on Figure 2–22 shows the area of the occipital condyle beneath which the canal lies.

In the midline, about one half inch from the anterior margin of the foramen magnum, is a small elevation of the bony surface. This elevation is the *pharyngeal tubercle*, which provides attachment for a muscle of the pharynx. The roughened area posterior to the foramen magnum is primarily an area of attachment for muscles of the neck and shoulder.

Openings on the posterior wall of the occipital condyles which transmit veins are the _____ canals; openings under the anterior part of the condyles transmit the _____ nerve and are called the _____ canals.

condylar . . . hypoglossal (fifth cranial) . . . hypoglossal

The elevation of bone near the anterior margin of the foramen magnum is the _____ tubercle, a point of attachment for a muscle of the _____.

pharyngeal . . . pharynx

QUESTION
148

The roughened surface posterior to the foramen magnum serves as a point of attachment for muscles of the _____ and _____.

ANSWER

neck . . . shoulder (in either order)

ITEM 42 MEDIAL ASPECT OF THE MANDIBLE

Figure 2–23 shows the medial aspect of the mandible. Notice the following basic structures: the *body, alveolar crest,* and *ramus* of the mandible.

At the midline, near the lower border of the body of the mandible, is seen a cluster of small projections called *genial tubercles,* referred to collectively as the *mental spine.* The genial tubercles serve as attachments for certain muscles to be studied later.

QUESTION
149

Projections on the inferomedial aspect of the mandible are the _____ tubercles, which together are termed the _____ spine.

ANSWER

genial . . . mental

QUESTION
150

The projections on the inferomedial aspect of the mandible serve as _____ attachments.

ANSWER

muscle

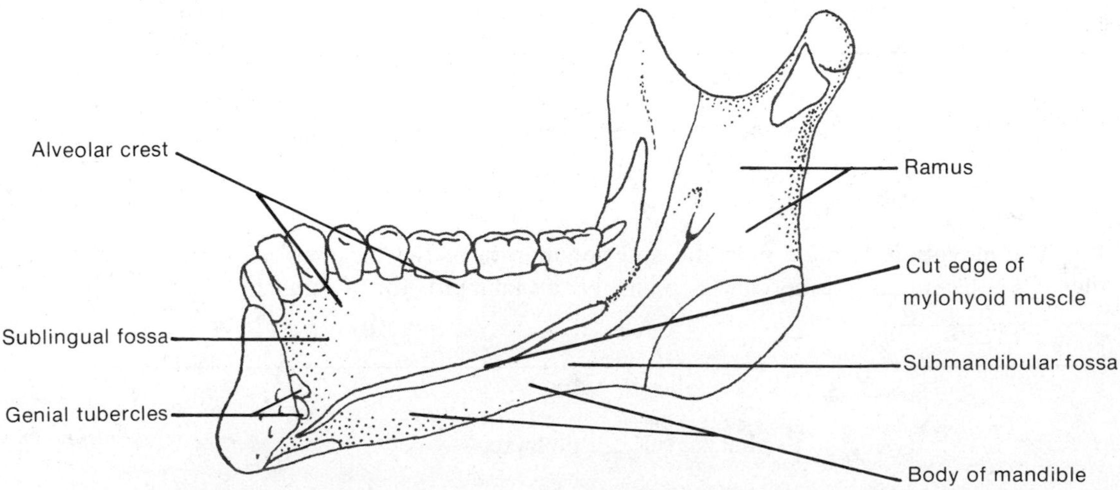

Figure 2-23. Right half of the mandible, medial aspect. (Redrawn from Wolf-Heidegger: Atlas of Systematic Human Anatomy. Vol. I. Basel, S. Karger AG.)

MEDIAL ASPECT OF THE MANDIBLE: THE MYLOHYOID LINE AND MUSCLE

ITEM 43

Re-examine Figure 2–23 and notice the location of the *mylohyoid muscle,* which forms part of the floor of the oral cavity. Beginning near the mental spine is a line which extends posteriorly and superiorly, becoming more prominent as it ascends. This line, called the *mylohyoid line,* is the point of attachment for the mylohyoid muscle. The roots of the mandibular molar and premolar teeth extend below the mylohyoid line, a fact which is clinically significant, as will be seen later.

The oblique line running posteriorly and superiorly across the inner surface of the body of the mandible is the _____ line.

QUESTION 151

---

mylohyoid

ANSWER

Roots of the mandibular molars and premolars extend _____ the mylohyoid line.

QUESTION 152

---

below

ANSWER

MEDIAL ASPECT OF THE MANDIBLE: THE SUBLINGUAL AND SUBMANDIBULAR FOSSAE

ITEM 44

A vague depression, seen bilaterally above the anterior portion of the mylohyoid line, is known as the *sublingual fossa.* Below the posterior portion of the mylohyoid line and below the distal teeth is a larger, more prominent fossa, the *submandibular fossa.* The sublingual and submandibular fossae contain salivary glands of the same names. Both these areas can be seen in Figure 2–23.

The fossa located superior to the anterior part of the mylohyoid line is the _____ fossa; that located inferior to the posterior part of the line is the _____ fossa.

QUESTION 153

---

sublingual . . . submandibular

ANSWER

ITEM 45   THE MANDIBULAR FORAMEN AND ADJACENT STRUCTURES

Examine Figure 2–24 and observe the location of the *mandibular foramen,* located near the middle of the internal surface of the ramus. This foramen is the opening of the mandibular canal, through which vessels and a nerve pass into the mandible. The region around the mandibular foramen is clinically important because it is the area which is infiltrated with anesthesia in an inferior alveolar nerve block.

Overhanging the mandibular foramen is a bony spine, the *lingula.* A small groove, the *mylohyoid groove,* can be seen passing forward and downward from the mandibular foramen.

QUESTION
154

The mandibular foramen is the opening of the _____ _____ located on the inner surface of the _____ of the mandible.

ANSWER

mandibular canal . . . ramus

QUESTION
155

The flange of bone which overhangs the mandibular foramen is called the _____; the groove passing anteriorly and inferiorly from the foramen is called the _____ groove.

ANSWER

lingula . . . mylohyoid

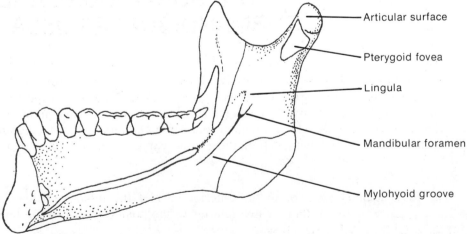

Figure 2-24. Right half of mandible, medial aspect, showing the mandibular foramen and adjacent structures. (Redrawn from Wolf-Heidegger: Atlas of Systematic Human Anatomy. Vol. I. Basel, S. Karger AG.)

MEDIAL ASPECT OF THE MANDIBLE: THE ARTICULAR SURFACE AND PTERYGOID FOVEA

ITEM 46

Look back to Figure 2–24 and notice the roughened area on the upper anterior surface of the condyle of the mandible. This area is the *articular surface*. Just below the articular surface, anteriorly, is a triangular depression called the *pterygoid fovea*. Other important features of the condyle will be discussed in later items concerned with the temporomandibular joint.

The articular surface is a somewhat roughened area on the upper anterior part of the _____ of the mandible.

QUESTION 156

condyle

ANSWER

The depressed area anterior and inferior to the condyle of the mandible is called the _____ fovea.

QUESTION 157

pterygoid

ANSWER

Write in the numbered spaces below the names of the corresponding numbered structures on the accompanying diagram.

QUESTION 158

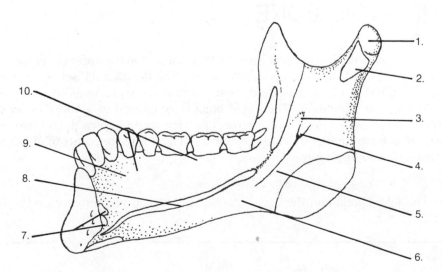

(Redrawn from Wolf-Heidegger: Atlas of Systematic Human Anatomy. Vol. I. Basel, S. Karger AG.)

Labels

1. _____ surface of the condyle
2. _____ _____
3. _____
4. _____ foramen
5. _____ groove
6. _____ fossa
7. _____ tubercles
8. _____ muscle
9. _____ fossa
10. _____ crest

ANSWER

1. articular
2. pterygoid fovea
3. lingula
4. mandibular
5. mylohyoid
6. submandibular
7. genial
8. mylohyoid
9. sublingual
10. alveolar

ITEM 47   THE HYOID BONE

The *hyoid bone,* shown in Figure 2–25, is located in the anterior region of the neck at the level of the third cervical vertebra. The fact that it does not articulate with other bones gives the hyoid bone its characteristic mobility, needed in swallowing and phonation. The hyoid bone is composed of a *body,* or anterior portion; two *greater horns,* which project posteriorly and upward; and two *lesser horns,* which are smaller upward projections. The horns are points of attachment for muscles and ligaments.

QUESTION 159

The hyoid bone and the _____ cervical vertebra are on the same level.

ANSWER

third

QUESTION 160

The greater and lesser horns of the hyoid bone are points for attachment of _____ and _____.

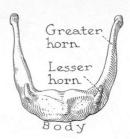

Greater
horn

Lesser
horn

Body

Figure 2–25. The hyoid bone, front view. (From King and Showers: Human Anatomy and Physiology. 6th Ed. Philadelphia, W. B. Saunders Co.)

muscles . . . ligaments (in either order)   *ANSWER*

The fact that the hyoid bone does not articulate with other bones permits the great _____ required for swallowing and phonation.   QUESTION
161

mobility   *ANSWER*

THE CRANIAL CAVITY: THE CRANIAL FOSSAE   ITEM 48

From your study of general anatomy you will remember the lobes of the cerebrum: frontal, parietal, temporal, occipital, and insula. The first four of these lobes correspond spatially to the overlying skull bones of the same names. The cerebellum is posterior and inferior to the cerebrum. You should remember that the midbrain is inferior to the cerebrum and anterior to the cerebellum, and is partially hidden by the cerebrum.

The cranial cavity as viewed from the top presents three levels which correspond to the lobes of the cerebrum, as Figure 2–26 shows. The first and highest level is the *anterior cranial fossa,* which lodges the frontal lobes. The second level, the *middle cranial fossa,* contains the temporal lobes and the midbrain. The third and lowest level, the *posterior cranial fossa,* houses the cerebellum, pons, and medulla.

The bony division between the anterior and middle fossae is the posterior border of the lesser wings of the sphenoid bone. The boundary between middle and posterior fossae is the petrous part of the temporal bone.

The three subdivisions of the cranial cavity, as viewed from above, are the anterior, middle, and posterior _____ _____.   QUESTION
162

cranial fossae   *ANSWER*

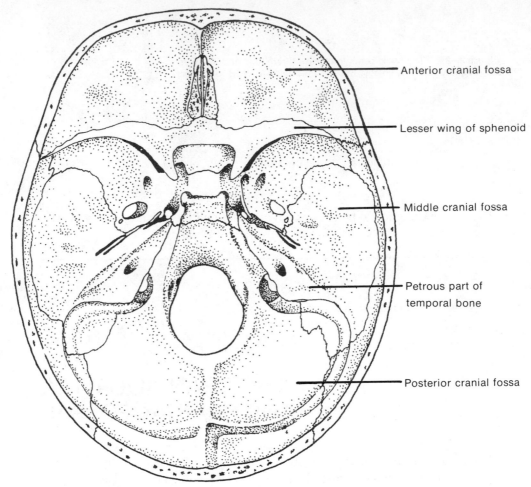

Figure 2-26. Anterior, middle, and posterior cranial fossae, internal aspect. (Redrawn from Wolf-Heidegger: Atlas of Systematic Human Anatomy. Vol. I. Basel, S. Karger AG.)

QUESTION
163   The anterior cranial fossa lodges the _____ lobes of the brain.

ANSWER   frontal

QUESTION
164   The middle cranial fossa lodges the _____ lobes and the
_____.

ANSWER   temporal . . . midbrain

The posterior cranial fossa lodges the _____, the _____, and the _____.

---

cerebellum . . . pons . . . medulla (in any order)

The bony division between anterior and middle cranial fossae is composed of the _____ wings of the _____ bone.

---

lesser . . . sphenoid

The bony division between middle and posterior cranial fossae is the superior edge of the _____ portion of the temporal bone.

---

petrous

THE ANTERIOR CRANIAL FOSSA: THE CRISTA GALLI

ITEM 49

The anterior cranial fossa, Figure 2–27, extends from the frontal bone to the lesser wings of the sphenoid bone. Most of the floor is formed by the oribital plates of the frontal bone. In the anterior midline is the *crista galli,* which gives rise to the *falx cerebri.* The falx cerebri, as you learned in your study of general anatomy, is the partition of dura which extends down between the two cerebral hemispheres.

The anterior cranial fossa extends from the vertical boundary of the frontal bone to the _____ wings of the sphenoid bone.

---

lesser

The vertical projection in the anterior midline of the anterior cranial fossa is the _____ _____, the attachment of the falx cerebri.

---

crista galli

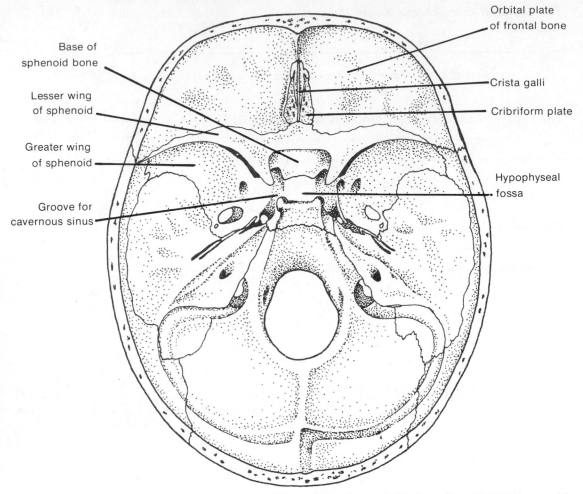

Figure 2-27. Anterior cranial fossa, internal aspect. (Redrawn from Wolf-Heidegger: Atlas of Systematic Human Anatomy. Vol. I. Basel, S. Karger AG.)

ITEM 50   THE ANTERIOR CRANIAL FOSSA: THE CRIBRIFORM PLATE

Posterolateral to the crista galli, the perforated *cribriform plate* transmits branches of the olfactory nerve from the nasal cavity to the olfactory bulbs. The olfactory nerve (I) is the first of the 12 cranial nerves. Both crista galli and cribriform plate are parts of the ethmoid bone. Look at Figure 2–27 above to see the location of the cribriform plate.

QUESTION
170

The horizontal perforated plate on each side of the crista galli is the _____ plate of the _____ bone.

cribriform . . . ethmoid   *ANSWER*

Perforations in the cribriform plate provide sites of entry of the _____   QUESTION
nerve, which transmits the sense of smell.   **171**

_____

olfactory   *ANSWER*

THE MIDDLE CRANIAL FOSSA: THE SELLA TURCICA AND HYPOPHYSEAL FOSSA

ITEM 51

The base of the sphenoid, at the midline, is continuous laterally as the greater wings of the sphenoid bone. Viewed from the top, the base of the sphenoid forms a base for the pons and midbrain, with the hypophysis (pituitary gland) resting in a fossa, the *hypophyseal fossa,* within the *sella turcica.* These can be seen in Figure 2–27.

Lateral to the base of the sphenoid is a groove for the cavernous sinus. The cavernous sinus will be discussed in later items.

Extending laterally from the base of the sphenoid bone are the _____   QUESTION
wings.   **172**

_____

greater   *ANSWER*

Viewed from the top, the base of the sphenoid forms a base for the   QUESTION
_____, the _____, and the _____.   **173**

_____

midbrain . . . pons . . . hypophysis (in any order)   *ANSWER*

Lateral to the base of the sphenoid, on the inner surface of the skull, is the   QUESTION
_____ sinus.   **174**

_____

cavernous   *ANSWER*

ITEM 52
THE MIDDLE CRANIAL FOSSA: THE FORAMINA

Lateral to the groove for the cavernous sinus are several openings, seen in Figure 2–28. Reading from anterior to posterior, these openings include: the *superior orbital fissure* under the *anterior clinoid process;* the *foramen rotundum*, which transmits the maxillary division of the trigeminal nerve (V); the *foramen ovale* for the mandibular division of the trigeminal nerve (V); and the *foramen spinosum* for the middle meningeal vessels. Medial to the foramen ovale is the *foramen lacerum*, marking the site where the internal carotid artery turns upward to enter the cavernous sinus.

QUESTION 175

Foramina which open into the middle cranial fossa include the superior _____ fissure, the foramen _____, the foramen _____, the foramen _____, and the foramen _____.

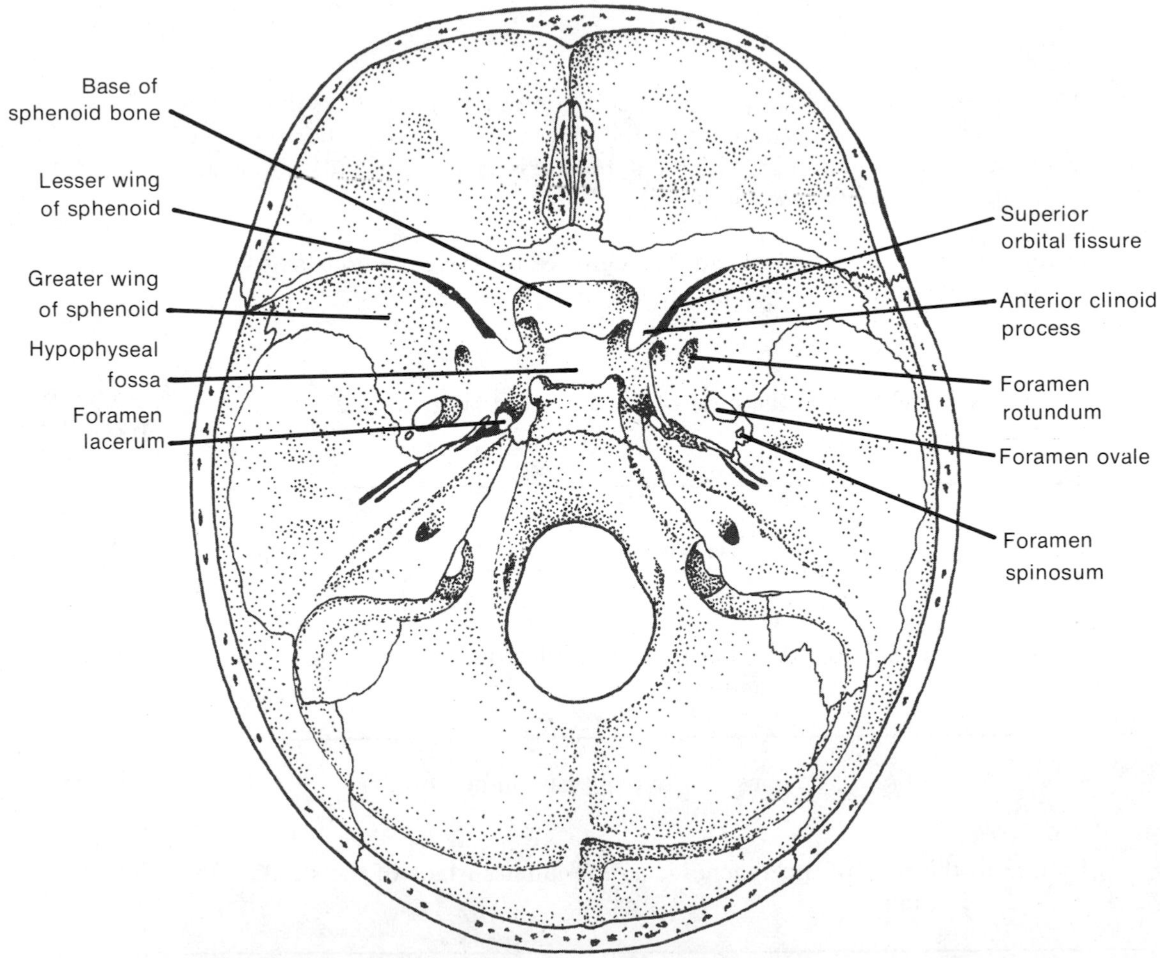

Figure 2-28. Middle cranial fossa, internal aspect. (Redrawn from Wolf-Heidegger: Atlas of Systematic Human Anatomy. Vol. I. Basel, S. Karger AG.)

orbital . . . rotundum . . . ovale . . . spinosum . . . lacerum   *ANSWER*

The foramen rotundum is the exit from the cranium for the _____ division of the trigeminal nerve (V).   *QUESTION* **176**

---

maxillary   *ANSWER*

The mandibular division of the trigeminal nerve (V) leaves the cranium through foramen _____.   *QUESTION* **177**

---

ovale   *ANSWER*

THE MIDDLE CRANIAL FOSSA: EXTENT OF THE SPHENOID BONE   ITEM 53

Refer to Figure 2–28 and, if possible, to a skull to review the extent of the sphenoid bone. Remember that the greater wing of the sphenoid bone is seen from several aspects. The superior surface can be located inside the skull as the anterior wall and part of the floor of the middle cranial fossa. In Figure 2–6, Item 10, the outside surface of the greater wing was seen as the posterolateral wall of the orbit. In Figure 2–15, Item 24, the greater wing was seen to form part of the floor of the temporal and infratemporal fossae.

The lesser wing of the sphenoid, Figure 2–28, is situated above the greater wing and is separated from the latter by the superior orbital fissure. The base of the sphenoid is the plate of bone between the two greater wings. The base contains the hypophyseal fossa, which lodges the hypophysis (pituitary gland).

The greater wing of the sphenoid bone, viewed from above, forms the anterior wall and part of the floor of the _____ _____ fossa.   *QUESTION* **178**

---

middle cranial   *ANSWER*

The outer and inferior surface of the greater wings enter into the formation of the orbit, the _____ fossa, and the _____ fossa.   *QUESTION* **179**

---

temporal . . . infratemporal   *ANSWER*

QUESTION
180

The lesser wings of the sphenoid are *superior to/inferior to* (circle one) the greater wings.

ANSWER

superior to

QUESTION
181

Between the lesser and greater wings of the sphenoid, viewed from the orbit, is the _____ orbital fissure.

ANSWER

superior

QUESTION
182

Located in the body of the sphenoid bone is a depression, called the _____ fossa, which lodges the _____.

ANSWER

hypophyseal . . . hypophysis (pituitary gland)

ITEM 54   THE MIDDLE CRANIAL FOSSA: SQUAMOUS AND PETROUS PORTIONS OF THE TEMPORAL BONE

Look at the superior view of the three cranial fossae in Figure 2–29, and notice the parts of the middle cranial fossa formed by the squamous and petrous portions of the temporal bone. The flattened squamous portion makes up most of the side wall of the middle cranial fossa; the petrous portion makes up the back wall. The anterior surface of the petrous bone presents several surface markings. An impression for the trigeminal ganglion is located at the anteromedial surface of the ridge. A bulge on the anterior surface, the *arcuate eminence,* marks the site of the underlying *anterior semicircular canal.* Small foramina are also present for branches of various cranial nerves.

QUESTION
183

The squamous and petrous parts of the _____ bone make up the lateral and posterior walls of the _____ cranial fossa.

ANSWER

temporal . . . middle

QUESTION
184

The bony ridge which marks the boundary between middle and posterior fossae is the _____ part of the _____ bone.

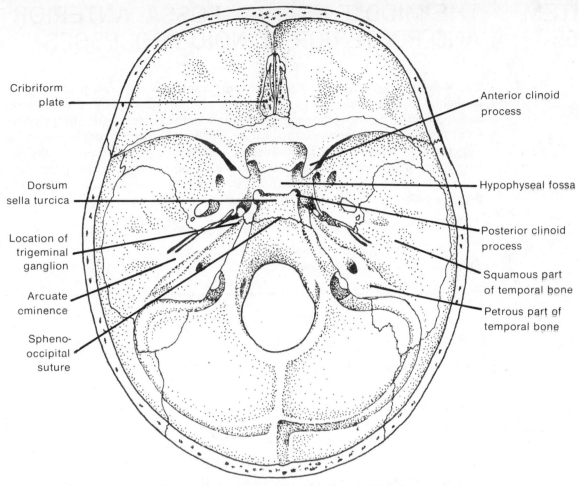

Figure 2-29. Base of the skull, internal aspect, showing structures of the middle cranial fossa. (Redrawn from Wolf-Heidegger: Atlas of Systematic Human Anatomy. Vol. I. Basel, S. Karger AG.)

petrous . . . temporal

ANSWER

A depression at the anteromedial end of the ridge of the petrous bone marks the site of the _____ ganglion of the trigeminal nerve (V).

QUESTION **185**

trigeminal

ANSWER

The bulge which accommodates the anterior semicircular canal is called the _____ eminence.

QUESTION **186**

arcuate

ANSWER

ITEM 55　THE MIDDLE CRANIAL FOSSA: ANTERIOR AND POSTERIOR CLINOID PROCESSES

Refer to Figure 2–29 as you follow the descriptive material of this item. If available, a skull should be examined as you read the description. First note the anteroposterior extent of the sphenoid bone, from the posterior edge of the cribriform plate to the *spheno-occipital suture*. Notice the deep hypophyseal fossa. Superior and lateral to the hypophyseal fossa are the posteromedially directed extensions of the lesser wings, the *anterior clinoid processes*. The transverse ridge posterior to the hypophyseal fossa is the *dorsum sella turcica*. Knoblike projections on this ridge are called the *posterior clinoid processes*.

QUESTION 187

The sphenoid bone extends from the _____ plate anteriorly to the _____ suture.

ANSWER

cribriform . . . spheno-occipital

QUESTION 188

The fossa which houses the hypophysis is the _____ _____.

ANSWER

hypophyseal fossa

QUESTION 189

Posteromedially directed extensions of the lesser wings are the anterior _____ processes.

ANSWER

clinoid

QUESTION 190

The transverse ridge posterior to the hypophyseal fossa is the _____ sella turcica.

ANSWER

dorsum

QUESTION 191

Tubercles on the superior and lateral parts of the dorsum sella turcica are posterior _____ processes.

ANSWER

clinoid

THE CRANIAL CAVITY: THE POSTERIOR CRANIAL FOSSA

The posterior cranial fossa, Figure 2–30, is formed principally by the *occipital bone* and the posterior wall of the petrous part of the temporal bone. This fossa lodges the pons and medulla, which rest on the base of the occipital bone. This flattened base, directed anteriorly and superiorly, is called the *clivus*. The posterior cranial fossa also lodges the cerebellum, which occupies the inferior depression in the squamous part of the occipital bone.

The two bones which make up the posterior cranial fossa are the _____ bone and the _____ portion of the temporal bone.

QUESTION
192

---

occipital . . . petrous

ANSWER

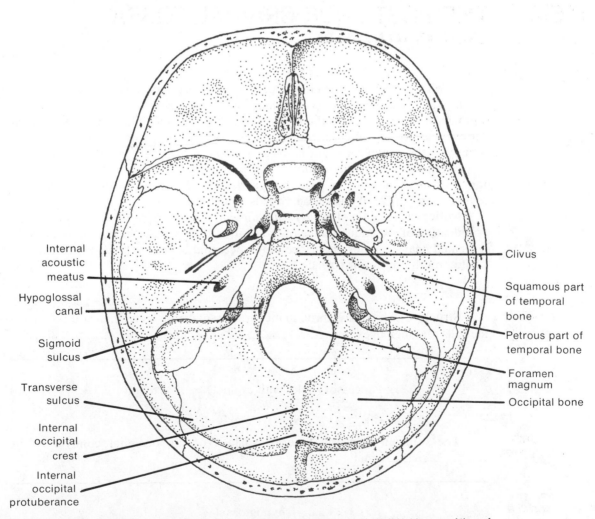

Figure 2-30. Posterior cranial fossa, internal aspect. (Redrawn from Wolf-Heidegger: Atlas of Systematic Human Anatomy. Vol. I. Basel, S. Karger AG.)

QUESTION
193

The flattened shelf of bone leading upward from the foramen magnum is called the _____.

ANSWER

clivus

QUESTION
194

The posterior cranial fossa lodges the _____, the _____, and the _____.

ANSWER

pons . . . medulla . . . cerebellum (in any order)

ITEM 57   THE POSTERIOR CRANIAL FOSSA: THE FORAMINA

Two important foramina in the posterior cranial fossa can be seen in Figure 2–30. These are the *foramen magnum* and the *internal acoustic meatus*. The foramen magnum transmits the lowermost part of the medulla as it becomes continuous with the spinal cord. Also contained within the foramen magnum are the meninges, the *spinal roots* of the *accessory nerve (XI),* and *vertebral arteries.*

The internal acoustic meatus is located on the posterior wall of the petrous bone. Through this meatus pass the *facial nerve (VII),* the *vestibulocochlear* or *acoustic nerve (VIII),* and blood vessels to the inner ear.

Notice the location of the *hypoglossal canal* in Figure 2–30. Recall from your examination of the undersurface of the skull in Item 41 that the hypoglossal canal is located near the anterior surface of the occipital condyle; the condylar canal is located on the posterior surface.

QUESTION
195

Structures which pass through the foramen magnum include, in addition to the medulla and meninges, the _____ nerve and _____ arteries.

ANSWER

accessory (eleventh cranial) . . . vertebral

QUESTION
196

The foramen near the anterior surface of the occipital condyle is the _____ canal.

ANSWER

hypoglossal

The foramen on the posterior slope of the petrous bone is the internal _____ meatus.

___

acoustic

The vestibulocochlear (VIII) and facial (VII) nerves and blood vessels to the inner ear are transmitted by the _____ _____ meatus.

___

internal acoustic

THE CRANIAL CAVITY:
THE POSTERIOR CRANIAL FOSSA

Posterior to the foramen magnum, Figure 2–30, the _internal occipital crest_ leads upward to the _internal occipital protuberance_. Leading medially in to the internal occipital crest is a transverse groove, the _transverse sulcus,_ which lodges a large vein. Note that the transverse sulcus is continuous with the S-shaped _sigmoid sulcus,_ which extends down to the jugular foramen. These channels are part of the venous drainage of the brain.

Extending posteriorly and upward from the foramen magnum is the internal occipital _____, which leads to the internal occipital _____.

___

crest . . . protuberance

The transverse sulcus, a groove lodging a large vein, extends laterally from the internal occipital _crest/protuberance_ (circle one).

___

protuberance

The continuation of the transverse sulcus is the _____ sulcus, which leads to the _____ foramen.

___

sigmoid . . . jugular

ITEM 59   TEMPOROMANDIBULAR JOINT: GENERAL CONFIGURATION

The *temporomandibular joint*, shown in Figure 2–31, is the articulation of the mandibular condyle with the temporal bone. Use a skull, if you have one available, to observe the structures involved in this articulation.

Notice in Figure 2–31, and on the skull, the configuration of the condyle and of the articular surface of the temporal bone. The condyle is rounded anteroposteriorly, with its long, wider axis directed obliquely backward and medially.

The articular surface of the temporal bone includes the *articular tubercle* and the *mandibular fossa*. Notice how this articular surface is first convex downward in the area of the articular tubercle, then concave downward in the area of the mandibular fossa. This general configuration of condyle and articular surface of the temporal bone allows a combination hinge and gliding action as the jaw is opened.

An unusual feature of the temporomandibular joint is that the articular surfaces are covered by fibrocartilage, in contrast to the usual hyaline covering of articular surfaces of most other joints of the body.

QUESTION
202

The temporomandibular joint is the articulation between the mandible and the _____ bone.

ANSWER

temporal

QUESTION
203

Articular surfaces on the temporal bone are the convex _____ tubercle and the concave _____ fossa.

ANSWER

articular . . . mandibular

QUESTION
204

The articular surface of the mandible is the posterior superior projection called the _____ of the mandible.

ANSWER

condyle

QUESTION
205

The configuration of the temporomandibular joint is designed for a combination of _____ and _____ action.

ANSWER

hinge . . . gliding

QUESTION
206

Although the articular surfaces of most joints are covered by hyaline cartilage, the articular surfaces of the temporomandibular joint are covered by _____ _____ .

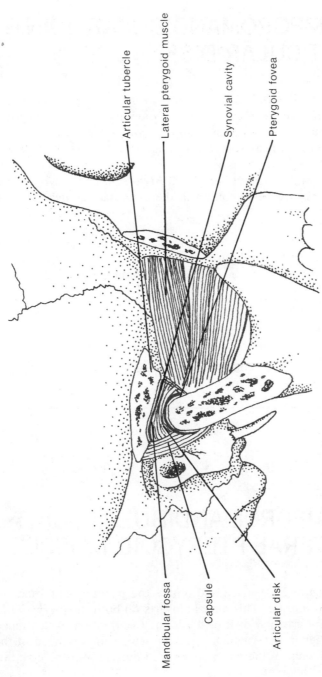

Articular tubercle

Lateral pterygoid muscle

Synovial cavity

Pterygoid fovea

Mandibular fossa

Capsule

Articular disk

Figure 2-31. Right temporomandibular joint, sagittal section. (Redrawn from Wolf-Heidegger: Atlas of Systematic Human Anatomy. Vol. I. Basel, S. Karger AG.)

ANSWER   fibrocartilage

ITEM 60   THE TEMPOROMANDIBULAR JOINT: THE ARTICULAR DISK

Look back to Figure 2–31 and locate the *articular disk,* a dense fibrous connective tissue disk between the two bony components of the temporomandibular joint. The articular disk is concave on its mandibular surface. On the temporal surface, the disk is concavoconvex from anterior to posterior, thus conforming to the shape of the adjacent bone.

Enclosed within the joint *capsule* are two *synovial cavities,* one above the articular disk and one below. Fluid in the synovial cavities reduces friction at the joint.

QUESTION
207

The articular disk is composed of fibrous _____ _____
between the two bony surfaces of the temporomandibular joint.

ANSWER   connective tissue

QUESTION
208

The synovial cavities contain _____ which reduces _____
at the temporomandibular joint.

ANSWER   fluid . . . friction

ITEM 61   THE TEMPOROMANDIBULAR JOINT: THE LATERAL PTERYGOID MUSCLE

Look at Figure 2–31 again and notice the position and attachments of the *lateral pterygoid muscle*. This muscle inserts on both the *pterygoid fovea* of the mandible and the articular disk of the joint. Contraction of this muscle, in synchrony with other muscles which open the jaw, pulls the head of the mandible forward. Attachment of the lateral pterygoid muscle into the disk facilitates the gliding action of the joint.

QUESTION
209

The lateral pterygoid muscle inserts on the pterygoid _____ of the
mandible and on the _____ disk.

---

fovea . . . articular

The gliding action of the temporomandibular joint is facilitated by insertion of the lateral pterygoid muscle into the _____ _____.   QUESTION
210

articular disk   *ANSWER*

THE TEMPOROMANDIBULAR JOINT: THE ARTICULAR CAPSULE

ITEM
62

The lateral aspect of the temporomandibular joint, depicted in Figure 2–32, shows a loose articular capsule enclosing the articular surfaces, articular disk, and synovial cavities. The capsule is attached above to the circumference of the mandibular fossa and to the articular tubercle. It is attached below to the neck of the mandible underneath the condyle.

A thickened band in the lateral wall of the capsule forms the *lateral ligament*. This ligament is attached to the lower edge of the zygoma and the articular tubercle

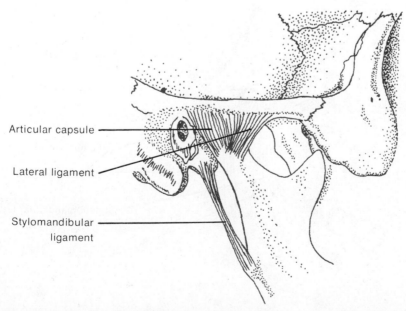

Articular capsule

Lateral ligament

Stylomandibular
ligament

Figure 2-32. Temporomandibular joint, lateral aspect. (Redrawn from Wolf-Heidegger: Atlas of Systematic Human Anatomy. Vol. I. Basel, S. Karger AG.)

above, and to the lateral surface of the neck of the mandible below. Note the *stylomandibular ligament* extending from the styloid process to the posterior border of the ramus near the angle of the mandible.

QUESTION
211

The articular surfaces, disk, and synovial cavities are enclosed in the _____ _____.

ANSWER

articular capsule

QUESTION
212

The thickened band of fibers in the temporomandibular capsule is the _____ ligament.

ANSWER

lateral

QUESTION
213

The stylomandibular ligament extends from the _____ process to the posterior border of the _____ of the mandible.

ANSWER

styloid . . . ramus

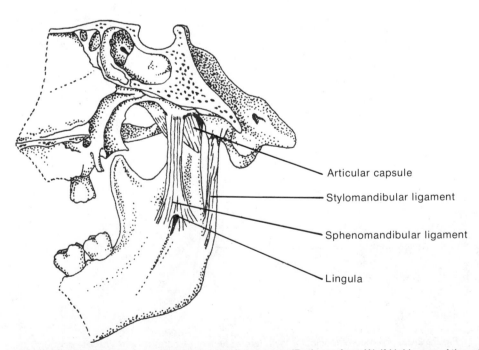

— Articular capsule

— Stylomandibular ligament

— Sphenomandibular ligament

— Lingula

Figure 2-33. Temporomandibular joint, medial aspect. (Redrawn from Wolf-Heidegger: Atlas of Systematic Human Anatomy. Vol. I. Basel, S. Karger AG.)

THE TEMPOROMANDIBULAR JOINT: MEDIAL ASPECT

ITEM 63

Figure 2–33 shows the medial aspect of the temporomandibular joint. The medial surface of the joint capsule is attached to the temporal bone and to the mandible. The circular arrangement of these fibers encloses the entire joint like a sleeve.

The stylomandibular ligament can be seen again from the medial surface. In addition, the *sphenomandibular ligament* is shown descending from the spine of the sphenoid bone to the lingula. In its route to the lower teeth, the inferior alveolar nerve descends between the sphenomandibular ligament and the ramus of the mandible to gain access to the mandibular foramen. This is the area, bounded medially by the sphenomandibular ligament and laterally by the ramus of the mandible, which is infiltrated in an inferior alveolar nerve block.

The sphenomandibular ligament extends from the _____ of the sphenoid bone to the _____.

QUESTION
214

---

spine . . . lingula

ANSWER

The area infiltrated with an inferior alveolar nerve block is bounded laterally by the _____ of the mandible; medially by the _____ ligament.

QUESTION
215

---

ramus . . . sphenomandibular

ANSWER

SUMMARY OF UNIT TWO

BONES OF THE SKULL

As you work through the summary of this unit on the skull, continue to use the skull for observation. Go slowly enough to palpate structures on yourself when possible. As you review structures which are not directly palpable, envision the location and relationships of these structures on yourself. In gaining expertise in head and neck anatomy, you will find it helpful to picture, for example, the precise location of your own foramen rotundum, and also to picture which structures are in front of it, which behind it, which lateral to it, and which medial.

Six bones comprise the cranium: frontal, parietal, temporal, ethmoid, sphenoid, and occipital. Eight different bones make up the bony face: nasal, lacrimal, maxilla, zygoma, palatine, vomer, inferior nasal concha, and mandible.

The typical joint between bones of the skull is a suture. A suture is formed by connective tissue fibers joining jagged edges of bone. Main sutures on the top of the skull include the sagittal, coronal, and lambdoidal. The junction of the sagittal and coronal sutures is called the bregma; the junction of the sagittal and lambdoidal sutures is called the lambda. The only freely movable joint in the skull is the temporomandibular joint.

ANTERIOR ASPECT OF THE SKULL

The principal bones of the anterior aspect of the skull are the frontal, maxillae, and mandible. Prominent markings on the frontal bone include the frontal eminence, the superciliary ridge, and the glabella. The supraorbital margin leading into the orbit usually has a single foramen, or notch, called the supraorbital foramen, which lodges nerves and arteries. When there are two notches, as sometimes occurs, the more prominent one is called the supraorbital foramen and the less common one, the frontal notch.

The orbit is made up of parts of several bones, including the frontal, zygoma, maxilla, lacrimal, ethmoid, sphenoid, and palatine. The round opening into the apex of the orbit is the optic canal, which lodges the optic nerve (second cranial) and the ophthalmic artery. The superior orbital fissure transmits the ophthalmic vein as well as nerves to the muscles which move the eyeball. The inferior orbital fissure contains the infraorbital nerve and artery, which run along a canal in the floor of the orbit and surface at the infraorbital foramen on the maxilla.

Bones which form the framework of the nose include the maxillae, nasal bones, and two bones which make up the septum: the vertical plate of the ethmoid and the vomer.

The maxilla and zygoma form the skeleton of the cheek. Foramina in the zygoma accommodate the zygomatic nerve, which is sensory to skin of the upper cheek. The part of the maxilla which holds teeth is termed the alveolar process.

Markings on the anterior surface of the mandible include the mental protuberance and mental foramen. The mental foramen provides exit for the mental nerve.

LATERAL ASPECT OF THE SKULL

In a lateral view of the skull, all the bones seen from the superior and anterior aspects are visible, as well as the temporal bone and part of the greater wing of the sphenoid bone. Three general areas of the temporal bone have been described: the squamous portion, the tympanic portion, and the petrous portion. The zygomatic process of the temporal bone extends anteriorly from the lower part of the squamous portion. On the lower surface of the zygomatic process is the mandibular fossa, the point of articulation of the temporomandibular joint. The long, slender styloid process is located anteromedial to the mastoid process.

Main areas of the mandible include the body, alveolar process, ramus, coronoid process, and condyle. The condyle articulates with the temporal bone in the temporomandibular joint. The concave mandibular notch is between the coronoid process and the condyle; the concave coronoid notch is on the anterior edge of the ramus.

The temporal and infratemporal fossae have particular importance in dental studies because of the numerous arteries and nerves contained within these spaces. In addition, these fossae are crossed by most of the muscles of mastication. These areas are, generally, deep to the zygomatic bone.

On the medial wall of the infratemporal fossa is a slitlike opening, the pterygomaxillary fissure. This fissure leads inward to the pterygopalatine fossa, an area which also carries nerves and arteries important in general functioning of the mouth.

BASE OF THE SKULL: INFERIOR ASPECT

The inferior aspect of the skull presents many foramina which are the sites of entrance and exit of cranial nerves and arteries. All the nerves gaining entry into the cranial vault, and all the arteries and veins supplying the tissue of the brain, must enter the base of the skull through various openings.

Viewing the inferior aspect of the skull with the mandible removed, we see, anteriorly, the hard palate. The bony framework of the roof of the mouth is composed of the palatine processes of the maxilla anteriorly and the horizontal plates of the palatine bones posteriorly. The suture extending down the midline between the two fused maxillae is the medial palatine suture. The suture between the palatine bone and the maxilla is the transverse palatine suture.

The incisive fossa penetrates the anterior midline region of the palatine process. The greater and lesser palatine foramina penetrate the posterolateral region of the horizontal plates. All these foramina transmit nerves and vessels to their respective areas. Pterygoid processes are important to the dental specialist because these processes provide attachment for muscles of mastication.

The groove for the auditory tube extends posterolaterally from the posterior part of the scaphoid fossa. Important foramina are positioned near this oblique groove: the foramen ovale, which transmits the mandibular division of the trigeminal (fifth cranial) nerve and the foramen spinosum, which transmits an artery to the meninges. Medial to the groove for the auditory tube is the foramen lacerum, the point of entry of the internal carotid artery into the cranial vault.

The mandibular fossa is formed by the posterior boundary of the squamous portion of the temporal bone, and the anterior boundary of the tympanic portion. These two bones join to form a tympanosquamous fissure. In some skulls the tegmen tympani projects into the suture as a wedge. Since the tegmen tympani is part of the petrous portion, the resulting fissures are named accordingly: the petrosquamous and the petrotympanic fissures.

Between the styloid process and the mastoid process is the stylomastoid foramen, which transmits the facial (seventh cranial) nerve to muscles of facial expression. Medial to the styloid process is a large opening, the jugular foramen, which transmits the internal jugular vein as well as the glossopharyngeal, vagus, and accessory (ninth, tenth, and eleventh cranial) nerves.

The extremely prominent foramen magnum is located in the posterior part of the base of the skull. This large opening contains the lower boundary of the medulla oblongata where it becomes continuous with the cervical region of the spinal cord. Occipital condyles, seen from the lower surface of the skull, are the points of articulation of the skull with the first cervical vertebra. The hypoglossal canal, an opening through the anterior part of the condyles, transmits the hypoglossal (twelfth cranial) nerve. Tubercles near the foramen magnum provide attachment for muscles of the neck and shoulder and muscles of the pharynx.

The mandible, viewed from the interior surface, presents several small projections in the anterior midline. These are the genial tubercles, or mental spine, which furnish muscle attachments.

The oblique mylohyoid line runs superiorly and posteriorly, separating two fossae for salivary glands: the sublingual fossa anteriorly and the submandibular fossa posteriorly. The clinically significant mandibular foramen is located on the medial surface of the ramus overhung by a bony projection, the lingula. Extending downward from the foramen is the mylohyoid groove.

BASE OF THE SKULL: INTERNAL ASPECT

Sutures seen on the outside of the skull are also visible on the inside: the sagittal, coronal, lambdoidal, and squamous sutures. In addition, a midline groove for the superior sagittal sinus and lateral grooves for the middle meningeal arteries can be seen.

The base of the skull, as seen from above, can be considered as having three levels: anterior, middle, and posterior cranial fossae. The boundary between the anterior and middle fossae is the posterior border of the lesser wings of the sphenoid bone. The boundary between the middle and posterior fossae is the petrous part of the temporal bone. Frontal lobes of the cerebrum are situated in the anterior cranial fossa; temporal lobes and midbrain lie in the middle cranial fossa; pons, medulla, and cerebellum occupy the posterior cranial fossa.

The orbital plates of the frontal bones make up most of the floor of the anterior cranial fossa. Prominent markings in the anterior fossa include the vertically projecting crista galli and the perforated cribriform plate, both parts of the ethmoid bone.

The base of the sphenoid bone and the hypophyseal fossa are located at the midline in the middle cranial fossa. Lateral to the base of the sphenoid bone is the cavernous sinus, part of the venous drainage of the brain. Anterior to the base of the sphenoid are the posterior projections of the lesser wings, the anterior clinoid processes. The transverse ridge posterior to the hypophyseal fossa is the dorsum sella turcica, from which the posterior clinoid processes project superolaterally.

The foramen rotundum, posterolateral to the anterior clinoid processes, is seen only from the interior. This foramen is the opening for the maxillary division of the trigeminal (fifth cranial) nerve. Foramina ovale, spinosum, and lacerum are complete openings through to the undersurface of the base of the skull. Foramen ovale transmits the mandibular (third) division of the trigeminal nerve (V).

The squamous and petrous parts of the temporal bone comprise the remainder of the middle cranial fossa. The trigeminal ganglion is located at the anteromedial end of the petrous ridge.

The posterior cranial fossa is formed by the occipital bone and by parts of the petrous and squamous portions of the temporal bone. The flattened base is the clivus. The cerebellum rests in the large posterolateral regions of the posterior cranial fossa; the pons and midbrain rest on the clivus.

The prominent foramen magnum is the opening through which the medulla is made continuous with the spinal cord. Vertebral arteries and the spinal roots of the accessory (eleventh cranial) nerve are also routed through this foramen. Extending inferiorly from the anterolateral regions of the foramen magnum are the occipital condyles, visible on the undersurface of the skull. The hypoglossal canal extends anteriorly through the occipital condyles.

Returning to the interior aspect, you will see that the posterior slope of the petrous bone presents a foramen entering this bone. This opening is the internal acoustic meatus, the path of blood vessels and of the facial (seventh cranial) nerve and the vestibulocochlear (eighth cranial) nerve in the inner ear. Posterior to the foramen magnum, the internal occipital crest extends up the midline to the internal occipital protuberance. Grooves leading from the back of the posterior cranial fossa lodge vessels which are a part of the venous drainage of the brain: the transverse sulcus and the sigmoid sulcus, both of which extend to the jugular foramen.

THE TEMPOROMANDIBULAR JOINT

The temporomandibular joint is the articulation of the condyle of the mandible with the mandibular fossa and articular tubercle of the temporal bone. Contraction of the lateral pterygoid muscle, in synchrony with other muscles opening the jaw, pulls the mandible forward and rotates it downward, providing both a hinge and gliding action at the joint. Synovial fluid within the joint capsule reduces friction at the joint.

The area around the mandibular foramen is infiltrated with anesthetic to provide an inferior alveolar nerve block. This space is bounded laterally by the medial surface of the ramus of the mandible and medially by the sphenoid ligament.

Bones of the cranium include

1. _____
2. _____
3. _____
4. _____
5. _____
6. _____

QUESTION
216

1. frontal   4. ethmoid

2. parietal   5. sphenoid

3. temporal   6. occipital

ANSWER

Bones of the face include

1. _____   5. _____
2. _____   6. _____
3. _____   7. _____
4. _____   8. _____

QUESTION
217

ANSWER

1. nasal
2. lacrimal
3. maxilla
4. zygoma

5. palatine
6. vomer
7. inferior nasal concha
8. mandible

QUESTION
218

The main sutures on the top of the skull are the _____, _____, and _____ sutures.

ANSWER

coronal . . . lambdoidal . . . sagittal (in any order)

QUESTION
219

The principal markings on the frontal bone are the

1. _____ eminence
2. _____ ridge
3. _____

ANSWER

frontal . . . superciliary . . . glabella

QUESTION
220

The optic (second cranial) nerve and the ophthalmic artery are transmitted in the _____ canal.

ANSWER

optic

QUESTION
221

The orbit is made up of (circle one)
A. a single bone
B. two bones
C. seven bones

ANSWER

Option C is the correct answer. The seven bones comprising the orbit are the following: frontal, zygoma, maxilla, lacrimal, ethmoid, sphenoid, and palatine.

QUESTION
222

The nerves to muscles which move the eyeball are transmitted in the superior _____ _____.

ANSWER

orbital fissure

QUESTION
223

The infraorbital nerve and artery are transmitted in the _____ _____ fissure.

ANSWER

inferior orbital

The framework of the nose is formed by the _____ and the _____ bones, plus the two bones which make up the septum.

QUESTION
224

maxillae . . . nasal

ANSWER

The septum is made up of the vertical plate of the _____ and the _____ .

QUESTION
225

ethmoid . . . vomer

ANSWER

The maxilla and zygoma make up the framework of the _____ .

QUESTION
226

cheek

ANSWER

Prominent bone markings on the anterior surface of the mandible include the _____ protuberance and the _____ foramen.

QUESTION
227

mental . . . mental

ANSWER

The mental nerve is *sensory/motor* (circle one).

QUESTION
228

sensory

ANSWER

The three general areas of the temporal bone are the _____ portion, the _____ portion, and the _____ portion.

QUESTION
229

squamous . . . tympanic . . . petrous (in any order)

ANSWER

The point of articulation of the temporomandibular joint is the _____ fossa, located on the inferior surface of the _____ bone.

QUESTION
230

mandibular . . . temporal

ANSWER

The main areas of the mandible are the
　　　　1. _____
　　　　2. _____
　　　　3. _____ process

QUESTION
231

4. _____
5. _____ process
6. _____

ANSWER

1. angle   4. ramus
2. body   5. coronoid
3. alveolar   6. condyle

QUESTION
232

The temporal and infratemporal fossae contain branches of _____ and _____, and some of the _____ of mastication.

ANSWER

arteries . . . nerves . . . muscles

QUESTION
233

The fossa which is medial to the pterygomaxillary fissure is the _____ _____ fossa.

ANSWER

pterygopalatine

QUESTION
234

The foramina visible from the inferior aspect of the skull are entrances and exits for arteries and nerves reaching or leaving the _____.

ANSWER

brain

QUESTION
235

Two sutures of the hard palate include the _____ and _____ palatine sutures.

ANSWER

transverse . . . medial

QUESTION
236

Openings in the hard palate include the _____ foramen and the greater and lesser _____ foramina.

ANSWER

incisive . . . palatine

QUESTION
237

Pterygoid processes provide attachment for muscles of _____.

ANSWER

mastication

The foramen ovale transmits the _____ division of the trigeminal (fifth cranial) nerve.

QUESTION 238

mandibular

ANSWER

The foramen spinosum transmits an artery to the _____.

QUESTION 239

meninges

ANSWER

The foramen lacerum is part of the route of the _____ _____ artery as it enters the cranium.

QUESTION 240

internal carotid

ANSWER

The consistently occurring fissure in the mandibular fossa is the _____ _____ fissure.

QUESTION 241

tympanosquamous

ANSWER

The point of origin of the sphenomandibular ligament is the _____ of the sphenoid bone.

QUESTION 242

spine

ANSWER

The stylomastoid foramen contains the facial nerve to muscles of _____ _____.

QUESTION 243

facial expression

ANSWER

The foramen magnum contains the lower boundary of the _____.

QUESTION 244

medulla

ANSWER

Points of articulation of the skull with the first cervical vertebra are the occipital _____.

QUESTION 245

ANSWER   condyles

QUESTION 246   The genial tubercles are small projections on the internal aspect of the anterior midline of the _____.

ANSWER   mandible

QUESTION 247   The oblique mylohyoid line separates two fossae for _____ glands.

ANSWER   salivary

QUESTION 248   The foramen located on the medial side of the ramus of the mandible is the _____ foramen, which transmits the inferior alveolar nerve.

ANSWER   mandibular

QUESTION 249   The bony projection medial to the mandibular foramen is the _____.

ANSWER   lingula

QUESTION 250   The anterior cranial fossa contains the _____ lobes of the cerebrum; the middle cranial fossa, the _____ lobes and the midbrain; the posterior cranial fossa, the _____ lobes and the cerebellum, pons, and medulla.

ANSWER   frontal . . . temporal . . . occipital

QUESTION 251   The posterior border of the lesser wing of the sphenoid bone is the boundary between the _____ and _____ cranial fossae.

ANSWER   anterior . . . middle

QUESTION 252   The ridge between the middle and posterior cranial fossae is the _____ part of the _____ bone.

ANSWER   petrous . . . temporal

The anterior cranial fossa is made up of parts of the _____, _____, and _____ bones.

QUESTION 253

frontal . . . ethmoid . . . sphenoid (in any order)

ANSWER

The crista galli and cribriform plate are parts of the _____ bone.

QUESTION 254

ethmoid

ANSWER

Bones entering into formation of the middle cranial fossa include the _____ and the _____ bones.

QUESTION 255

sphenoid . . . temporal (in either order)

ANSWER

The cavernous sinus is located in the _____ cranial fossa.

QUESTION 256

middle

ANSWER

Projections anterior and posterior to the hypophyscal fossa are the _____ processes.

QUESTION 257

clinoid

ANSWER

Anterior and posterior clinoid processes and the hypophyseal fossa are all parts of the _____ _____.

QUESTION 258

sella turcica

ANSWER

Foramina in the middle cranial fossa include the foramen _____, foramen _____, foramen _____, and foramen _____.

QUESTION 259

rotundum . . . ovale . . . spinosum . . . lacerum (in any order)

ANSWER

The foramen rotundum transmits the _____ division of the trigeminal nerve (V).

QUESTION 260

maxillary

ANSWER

QUESTION
261

Foramen _____ transmits the mandibular division of the trigeminal nerve (V).

ANSWER

ovale

QUESTION
262

The apex of the petrous bone is the location of the _____ ganglion.

ANSWER

trigeminal

QUESTION
263

The pituitary gland is lodged in the _____ fossa.

ANSWER

hypophyseal

QUESTION
264

The bones which enter into formation of the posterior cranial fossa are the _____ and _____ bones.

ANSWER

occipital . . . temporal

QUESTION
265

The base of the occipital bone anterior to foramen magnum is the _____.

ANSWER

clivus

QUESTION
266

The foramen magnum is part of the _____ bone.

ANSWER

occipital

QUESTION
267

Other foramina which open into the posterior cranial fossa include the internal _____ meatus, the _____ foramen, and the _____ canal.

ANSWER

acoustic . . . jugular . . . hypoglossal

QUESTION
268

The articulation between the temporal bone and the mandible is the _____ joint.

temporomandibular

The configuration of the articular surface of the temporal bone is to allow a
combination of _____ and _____ action as the jaw is opened.

---

hinge . . . gliding (in either order)

The action of pulling the mandible forward and rotating it downward is
accomplished by the _____ _____ muscle together with other
muscles involved in opening the jaw.

---

lateral pterygoid

Friction is reduced within the temporomandibular capsule by the presence
of _____ fluid.

---

synovial

In an inferior alveolar nerve block, anesthetic fluid enters a soft tissue space;
the ramus of the mandible provides the _____ wall of this space, and
the sphenomandibular ligament the _____ wall.

---

lateral . . . medial

PART TWO
☐
SYSTEMS

Unit Three ☐ MUSCLES OF THE HEAD AND NECK

MUSCLES OF THE HEAD ITEM 1

Most of the muscles of the head can be conveniently considered in two groups: (1) *muscles of facial expression,* and (2) *muscles of mastication.* Muscles of the face are derived embryonically from the second branchial, or hyoid, arch and are innervated by the facial nerve (cranial nerve VII). Muscles of the scalp, although not really muscles of facial expression, are also supplied by the facial nerve and will be treated with this first group. The second group of muscles of the head, the muscles of mastication, derive embryonically from the first branchial, or mandibular arch, and are innervated by the trigeminal nerve (cranial nerve V).

Other muscles of the head are those which move the eye, those which move the tongue, and muscles associated with the neck. Some of these will be dealt with in later units.

Muscles of facial expression receive their nerve supply from the _____ nerve; muscles of mastication, from the _____ nerve.

QUESTION 1

facial (cranial nerve VII) . . . trigeminal (cranial nerve V)

ANSWER

Muscles of the scalp are innervated by the same nerve as that which innervates the (circle one)
 A. muscles of facial expression
 B. muscles of mastication

QUESTION 2

ANSWER   The correct answer is A. The facial (seventh cranial) nerve, which innervates the muscles of facial expression, also innervates the muscles of the scalp.

QUESTION
3   The embryonic origin of muscles of mastication is the *first/second* (circle one) branchial arch; the origin of the muscles of facial expression is the *mandibular/hyoid* (circle one) branchial arch.

ANSWER   first . . . hyoid

ITEM 2   MUSCLES OF FACIAL EXPRESSION

Muscles of the face can be conveniently grouped as (1) muscles around and above the eye, (2) muscles around and above the mouth, and (3) muscles below the mouth. For purposes of study, it is necessary to describe each muscle as if it acted independently of the other muscles of the face. In fact, these muscles almost always act in groups. Thus, actions of paired muscles on each side of the face are usually symmetrical. A loss of this symmetry may often be an early sign of injury to the facial nerve on one side.

As you study the various muscles of the face, spend several minutes making faces at yourself in the mirror. This exercise will help you to recognize these muscles both in normal action and as they may appear in some pathological conditions.

As you work through the present unit, also refer frequently to the skull to observe the origins and insertions of various muscle groups. If you do not have a skull available, refer back to the diagrams of the frontal and lateral aspects of the skull in Unit Two, Figures 2–4 and 2–13.

QUESTION
4   In various facial expressions, muscles of the face usually function *independently/as a group* (circle one).

ANSWER   as a group

QUESTION
5   Injury of the facial (seventh cranial) nerve on one side of the face may often be detected by a lack of _____ in the functioning of the muscles on each side of the face.

ANSWER   symmetry

THE ORBICULARIS OCULI MUSCLE   ITEM 3

Facial muscles around the eye are illustrated in Figure 3–1. Note the *orbicularis oculi,* the sphincter muscle covering the rim of the orbit. This muscle has two parts: the *palpebral* part in the lids, and the *orbital* part at the rim of the orbit. The palpebral part of the orbicularis oculi originates on the medial palpebral ligament, the structure which attaches the eyelids to the medial edge of the orbital rim. Fibers of the palpebral part extend through the upper and lower lids to intermesh at the lateral edge of the eye. Contraction of the palpebral part of the orbicularis oculi muscle closes the lids gently, as in sleep.

The orbital part of the orbicularis oculi originates on the medial palpebral ligament also, as well as on the bony rim of the orbit, the nasal process of the frontal

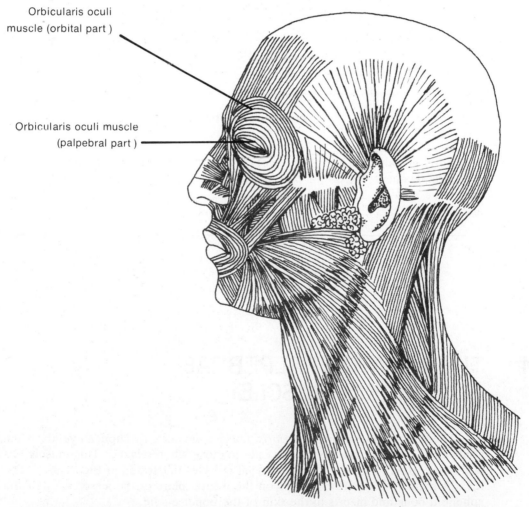

Orbicularis oculi
muscle (orbital part)

Orbicularis oculi muscle
(palpebral part)

Figure 3–1. Orbicularis oculi muscle, lateral aspect. (Redrawn from Anson [Ed.]: Morris' Human Anatomy. 12th Ed. Copyright © 1966 by McGraw-Hill, Inc. Used by permission of McGraw-Hill Book Company.)

bone, and the frontal process of the maxilla. Fibers of the orbital part extend laterally around the rim of the orbit. Contraction of the orbital part of the orbicularis oculi muscle closes the eye forcefully.

QUESTION 6

The sphincter muscle of the eye is the _____ _____ muscle.

ANSWER

orbicularis oculi

QUESTION 7

The sphincter muscle of the eye has two parts, the _____ part which closes the eyelid gently and the _____ part which closes the eyelid forcefully.

ANSWER

palpebral . . . orbital

QUESTION 8

Outer fibers of the orbicularis oculi extending around the rim of the orbit comprise the _____ part, while fibers extending through the lids comprise the _____ part of this muscle.

ANSWER

orbital . . . palpebral

QUESTION 9

Both the palpebral and orbital parts of the orbicularis oculi arise on the medial palpebral ligament; the orbital part, additionally, has points of origin on the bony rim of the _____, on the _____ process of the frontal bone, and on the _____ process of the maxilla.

ANSWER

orbit . . . nasal . . . frontal

ITEM 4   THE LEVATOR PALPEBRAE SUPERIORIS MUSCLE

The *levator palpebrae superioris* muscle elevates the upper eyelids when contracted, and permits the upper eyelid to close when relaxed. This muscle lies within the orbit, hidden by the superficial muscles illustrated in Figure 3–1. The levator palpebrae superioris arises on the orbital plate of the lesser wing of the sphenoid bone and inserts in the skin of the upper eyelid.

Actually the levator palpebrae superioris belongs to the group of ocular muscles rather than to the group of muscles of facial expression. While the muscles of facial expression are innervated by the facial nerve (VII), the levator palpebrae superioris is innervated by the oculomotor nerve (III). Injury to the oculomotor nerve, with consequent paralysis of the levator muscle, results in drooping of the upper lid, a condition known as *ptosis*.

The upper eyelid is raised by contraction of the levator _____ _____ muscle.

palpebrae superioris

The levator muscle which raises the upper eyelid originates on the orbital plate of the _____ _____ of the _____ bone and inserts into the upper lid.

lesser wing . . . sphenoid

The levator palpebrae superioris muscle is innervated by the _____ nerve.

oculomotor (third cranial)

Drooping of the upper eyelid following injury to the oculomotor nerve is termed _____.

ptosis

THE CORRUGATOR SUPERCILII AND PROCERUS MUSCLES   ITEM 5

Two small muscles near the eye, not illustrated, produce wrinkles of the forehead and nose characteristic of certain facial expressions. The first of these muscles is the *corrugator supercilii,* a slender muscular band deep to the upper part of the orbicularis oculi. The corrugator supercilii draws the skin of the forehead medially downward above the nose, producing the vertical wrinkles of the forehead characteristic of a frown. The second muscle is the *procerus,* a tiny nasal muscle which draws down the medial angle of the eyebrows to cause transverse wrinkles across the root of the nose.

QUESTION
14

Contraction of the corrugator supercilii draws the skin of the _____ medially and downward, causing vertical wrinkles in the _____, as in a frowning expression.

ANSWER

forehead . . . forehead

QUESTION
15

The procerus muscle draws down the medial edge of the eyebrows, causing transverse wrinkles across the _____ of the _____.

ANSWER

root . . . nose

ITEM 6   MUSCLES WHICH ELEVATE THE ANGLE OF THE MOUTH

Figure 3–2 shows two muscles which elevate the angle of the mouth, the *zygomaticus major* and the *zygomaticus minor*. These muscles originate on the zygomatic bone and insert into skin of the upper lip and into the orbicularis oris muscle encircling the mouth. A third muscle involved in elevating the angle of the mouth is the *levator anguli oris,* only partially visible in Figure 3–2 because it lies deep to the superficial muscles shown in this illustration. The levator anguli oris arises from the canine fossa of the maxilla and descends laterally to the angle of the mouth.

QUESTION
16

The three muscles involved in elevating the angle of the mouth are the _____ _____, the _____ _____, and the levator _____ _____.

ANSWER

zygomaticus major . . . zygomaticus minor . . . anguli oris

QUESTION
17

The muscle which arises from the canine fossa of the maxilla and inserts at the angle of the mouth is the levator _____ _____.

ANSWER

anguli oris

QUESTION
18

The zygomaticus major and zygomaticus minor originate on the _____ _____ and insert into the skin of the lip and into the _____ _____ muscle which encircles the mouth.

ANSWER

zygoma (zygomatic bone) . . . orbicularis oris

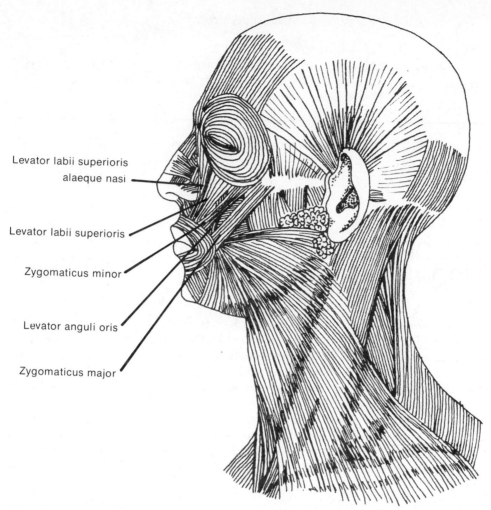

Levator labii superioris alaeque nasi

Levator labii superioris

Zygomaticus minor

Levator anguli oris

Zygomaticus major

Figure 3–2. Muscles which elevate the upper lip and angle of the mouth. (Redrawn from Anson [Ed.]: Morris' Human Anatomy. 12th Ed. Copyright © 1966 by McGraw-Hill, Inc. Used by permission of McGraw-Hill Book Company.)

MUSCLES WHICH ELEVATE THE UPPER LIP

ITEM 7

Look back to Figure 3–2 and observe the locations of the *levator labii superioris* and the *levator labii superioris alaeque nasi*. These two muscles elevate the upper lip. The levator labii superioris alaeque nasi also raises the ala of the nose.

The levator labii superioris arises from the maxilla just below the infraorbital foramen and inserts into the upper lip. The levator labii superioris alaeque nasi, lying in the sulcus between the nose and cheek, originates from the frontal process of the maxilla and inserts into the ala of the nose and into the skin of the upper lip.

The muscle which arises from the maxilla, below the infraorbital foramen, and extends to the upper lip is the levator _____ _____.

QUESTION
19

ANSWER   labii superioris

QUESTION
20

The levator labii superioris alaeque nasi originates on the frontal process of the _____ and inserts into the upper lip and into the _____ of the _____.

ANSWER   maxilla . . . ala . . . nose

ITEM 8   THE ORBICULARIS ORIS AND RISORIUS MUSCLES

The *orbicularis oris,* shown in Figure 3–3, is a sphincter muscle which closes and protrudes the mouth. It also keeps food on the occlusal surfaces of the teeth in the region of the lips. This muscle encircles the mouth and inserts obliquely into skin and mucous membranes of the upper and lower lips. Some fibers originate from the maxilla, but most arise from muscles lateral to the mouth, particularly from the buccinator muscle.

The *risorius* is a thin muscle which extends from the fascia over the parotid gland to the angle of the mouth. It is involved in the typical widening of the mouth in a smile. The fibers of insertion of the risorius, as can be seen in Figure 3–3, often fuse with the *platysma* muscle, a superficial muscle covering the neck and chin.

QUESTION
21

The orbicularis oris muscle is a _____ muscle which is comprised of fibers arising from surrounding muscles, especially fibers arising from the _____ muscle.

ANSWER   sphincter . . . buccinator

QUESTION
22

Contraction of the orbicularis oris muscle causes the mouth to _____ and to _____.

ANSWER   close . . . protrude (in either order)

QUESTION
23

The muscle which extends from the parotid fascia to the outer corner of the mouth is the _____, a muscle which helps to _____ the mouth in expressions of mirth.

ANSWER   risorius . . . widen

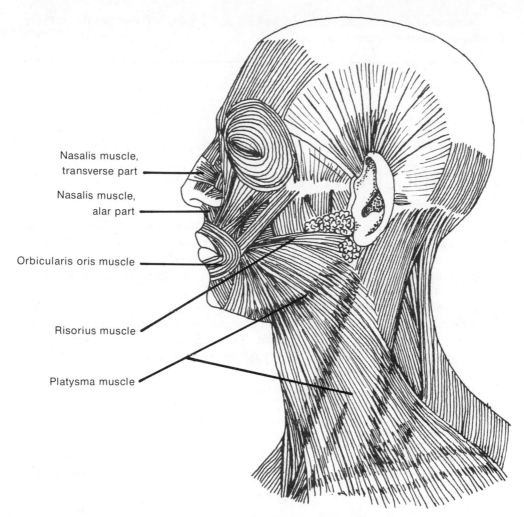

Nasalis muscle,
transverse part

Nasalis muscle,
alar part

Orbicularis oris muscle

Risorius muscle

Platysma muscle

Figure 3–3. Orbicularis oris, risorius, platysma, and nasalis muscles. (Redrawn from Anson [Ed.]: Morris' Human Anatomy. 12th Ed. Copyright © by McGraw-Hill, Inc. Used by permission of McGraw-Hill Book Company.)

THE NASALIS MUSCLE   ITEM 9

Look back to Figure 3–3 and notice the two parts of the *nasalis* muscle, the *transverse* part extending across the bridge of the nose and the *alar* part inserting into the ala of the nose. Contraction of these muscles dilates the nasal opening, widening and flattening the nose.

Fibers of the nasalis muscle which extend across the bridge of the nose comprise the _____ part; fibers inserting into the ala of the nose comprise the _____ part.

QUESTION
24

---

transverse . . . alar

ANSWER

QUESTION 25

Action of the _____ and _____ parts of the nasalis muscle causes the nasal aperture to _____.

ANSWER

transverse . . . alar . . . dilate

ITEM 10

THE BUCCINATOR MUSCLE

The *buccinator* muscle, shown in Figure 3–4, forms the anterior part of the cheek. It originates from the alveolar processes of the maxilla and mandible in the region of the molar teeth and from a ligamentous band, the pterygomandibular raphe. The pterygomandibular raphe extends from the pterygoid hamulus superiorly to the posterior edge of the mylohyoid line of the mandible inferiorly. Observe these landmarks on your skull.

Fibers of the buccinator muscle run horizontally forward to blend with the deep fibers of the orbicularis oris muscle. The buccinator pulls the angle of the mouth laterally, compresses the cheek, and keeps food on the occlusal surfaces of the teeth in the region of the cheek.

In Figure 3–4, notice the duct of the parotid gland piercing the buccinator muscle.

QUESTION 26

The buccinator muscle originates at the _____ processes of the maxilla and mandible.

ANSWER

alveolar

QUESTION 27

The ligamentous band from which some fibers of the buccinator originate is called the _____ raphe.

ANSWER

pterygomandibular

QUESTION 28

The connective tissue band from which some fibers of the buccinator arise extends from the pterygoid _____ superiorly to the _____ line of the mandible inferiorly.

ANSWER

hamulus . . . mylohyoid

QUESTION 29

The principal actions of the buccinator muscle are to
1. extend the _____ of the _____ laterally
2. compress the _____
3. keep food on the _____ _____ of the teeth

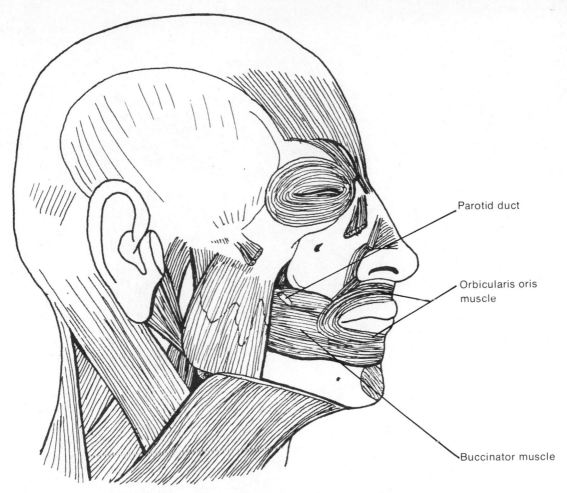

Figure 3–4. Buccinator muscle, lateral aspect. (Redrawn from Wolf-Heidegger: Atlas of Systematic Human Anatomy. Vol. I. Basel, S. Karger AG.)

1. angle . . . mouth
2. cheek
3. occlusal surfaces

ANSWER

MUSCLES WHICH ACT ON THE LOWER LIP   ITEM 11

Locate on Figure 3–5 the *depressor anguli oris* and the *depressor labii inferioris* muscles. The more superficial depressor anguli oris arises on the external oblique line of the mandible, and extends superiorly to insert at the angle of the mouth. Its function is to depress the angle of the mouth. The deeper depressor labii inferioris originates from the external oblique line medial to the mental

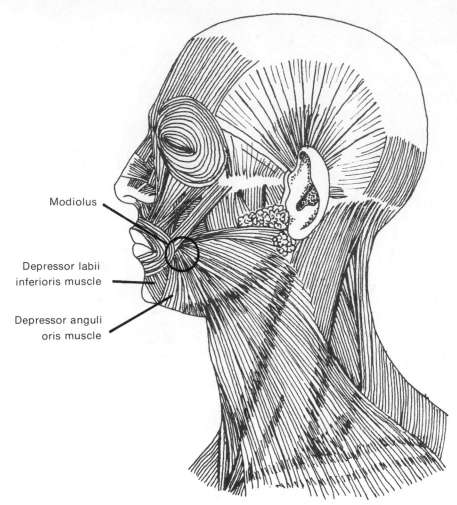

Figure 3–5. Muscles which depress the lower lip and angle of the mouth. (Redrawn from Anson [Ed.]: Morris' Human Anatomy. 12th Ed. Copyright © 1966 by McGraw-Hill, Inc. Used by permission of McGraw-Hill Book Company.)

foramen and inserts medially and superiorly into the skin of the lower lip. The depressor labii inferioris draws the lower lip downward.

The *mentalis* muscle, which does not show in Figure 3–5, arises from the anterior surface of the mandible and inserts into the lower lip. It raises the skin of the chin and protrudes the lower lip.

Notice in Figure 3–5 the region called the *modiolus*, where fibers from the depressor anguli oris, levator anguli oris, orbicularis oris, zygomaticus major, and buccinator muscles intermingle.

QUESTION
30

The function of the depressor anguli oris muscle is to depress the _____ of the _____; that of the depressor labii inferioris is to depress the _____ _____.

angle . . . mouth . . . lower lip

ANSWER

Action of the mentalis muscle draws the skin of the chin upward and causes the lower lip to _____.

QUESTION
31

protrude

ANSWER

The depressor anguli oris originates at the _____ _____ line of the mandible and inserts at the _____ of the mouth.

QUESTION
32

external oblique . . . angle

ANSWER

The depressor labii inferioris arises on the external oblique line medial to the _____ foramen and inserts into the _____ _____.

QUESTION
33

mental . . . lower lip

ANSWER

The mentalis muscle arises from the front of the _____.

QUESTION
34

mandible

ANSWER

THE EPICRANIUS AND AURICULAR MUSCLES   ITEM 12

The *epicranius* muscle of the scalp and the *auricular* muscles around the ear are shown in Figure 3–6. The epicranius muscle consists of two muscle masses, the frontal and the occipital bellies, united by a fibrous *aponeurosis* covering the superiormost part of the scalp. The epicranius draws the scalp backward, with the frontal portion raising the eyebrows in expressions of surprise. The auricular muscles, superior to and around the ear, provide very little movement.

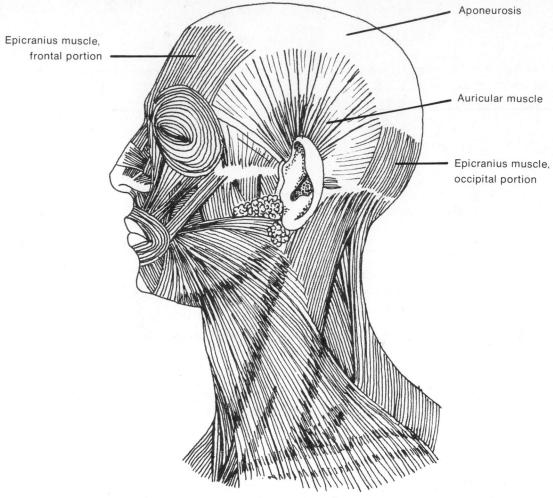

Figure 3-6. Muscles of the scalp. (Redrawn from Anson [Ed.]: Morris' Human Anatomy. 12th Ed. Copyright © 1966 by McGraw-Hill, Inc. Used by permission of McGraw-Hill Book Company.)

QUESTION
35

The two bellies of the epicranius muscle are the _____ portion and the _____ portion.

ANSWER

frontal . . . occipital (in either order)

QUESTION
36

The two portions of the epicranius muscle attach to a fibrous sheet, called the _____, which covers the superiormost part of the scalp.

ANSWER

aponeurosis

QUESTION
37

Raising the eyebrows in surprise is effected by contraction of the _____ portion of the epicranius muscle.

frontal

Muscles of the scalp above and around the ears are the _____ muscles.

auricular

REVIEW OF THE FACIAL MUSCLES

ITEM 13

As a review, the muscles of facial expression are recapitulated at this point. As you review this section, palpate these muscles on yourself as an aid to memory.

The muscles in the area around and above the eye include the orbicularis oculi which closes the eye, with its orbital and palpebral parts; the levator palpebrae superioris, which elevates the upper eyelid; the corrugator supercilii, which draws the skin of the forehead medially downward; and the procerus, which draws the medial angle of the eyebrows downward.

The angle of the mouth is elevated by three muscles: the zygomaticus major, zygomaticus minor, and levator anguli oris. The upper lip is elevated by contraction of the levator labii superioris and the levator labii superioris alaeque nasi. The orbicularis oris, which encircles the mouth, causes the mouth to close and to protrude. The risorius causes the mouth to widen in mirth. The buccinator pulls the angle of the mouth laterally.

The depressor anguli oris depresses the angle of the mouth; the depressor labii inferioris draws the lower lip down; and the mentalis protrudes the lower lip.

The transverse and alar parts of the nasalis muscle dilate the nasal aperture and widen and flatten the nose.

Muscles of the scalp include the frontal and occipital parts of the epicranius muscle, which draw the scalp backward, and the auricular muscles above and around the ear.

The principal muscles around and above the eye are the
1. _____
2. _____
3. _____
4. _____

1. orbicularis oculi
2. levator palpebrae superioris
3. corrugator supercilii
4. procerus
   (in any order)

QUESTION
40

The three muscles which elevate the angle of the mouth are the

1. _____
2. _____
3. _____

ANSWER

1. zygomaticus major
2. zygomaticus minor
3. levator anguli oris
   (in any order)

QUESTION
41

The two muscles involved in raising the upper lip are the

1. _____
2. _____

ANSWER

1. levator labii superioris
2. levator labii superioris alaeque nasi
   (in either order)

QUESTION
42

The muscle which closes and protrudes the mouth is the _____ _____; that which widens the mouth in a smile is the _____; that which pulls the angle of the mouth laterally is the _____.

ANSWER

orbicularis oris . . . risorius . . . buccinator

QUESTION
43

The transverse and alar parts of the nasalis muscle dilate the _____ _____.

ANSWER

nasal aperture (opening)

QUESTION
44

The angle of the mouth is depressed by the depressor _____ _____; the lower lip is drawn down by the depressor _____ _____; the lower lip is protruded by the _____ muscle.

ANSWER

anguli oris . . . labii inferioris . . . mentalis

QUESTION
45

One of the muscles of the scalp is the _____ muscle with frontal and occipital bellies; the muscles above and around the ear are the _____ muscles.

ANSWER

epicranius . . . auricular

QUESTION
46

Using the Word Bank, fill in the numbered blanks to correspond to the label numbers on the accompanying diagram.

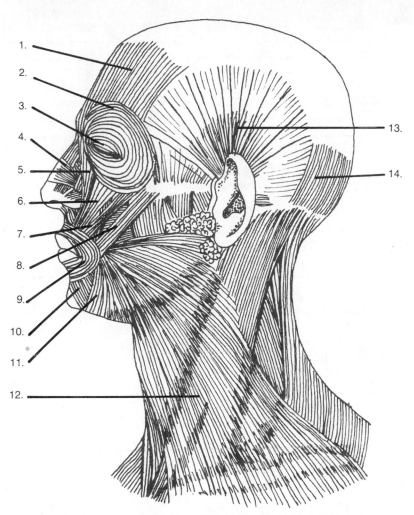

(Redrawn from Anson [Ed.] Morris' Human Anatomy. 12th Ed. Copyright © 1966 by McGraw-Hill, Inc. Used by permission of McGraw-Hill Book Company.)

Word Bank

A. auricular
B. depressor anguli oris
C. depressor labii inferioris
D. frontal part of epicranius
E. levator labii superioris
F. levator labii superioris alaeque nasi
G. nasalis
H. occipital part of epicranius
I. orbicularis oris
J. orbital part of orbicularis oculi
K. palpebral part of orbicularis oculi
L. platysma
M. zygomaticus major
N. zygomaticus minor

Labels

1. _____
2. _____
3. _____
4. _____
5. _____
6. _____
7. _____
8. _____
9. _____
10. _____
11. _____
12. _____
13. _____
14. _____

ANSWER

1.—(D) frontal part of epicranius
2.—(J) orbital part of orbicularis oculi
3.—(K) palpebral part of orbicularis oculi
4.—(G) nasalis
5.—(F) levator labii superioris alaeque nasi
6.—(E) levator labii superioris
7.—(N) zygomaticus minor
8.—(M) zygomaticus major
9.—(I) orbicularis oris
10.—(C) depressor labii inferioris
11.—(B) depressor anguli oris
12.—(L) platysma
13.—(A) auricular
14.—(H) occipital part of epicranius

ITEM 14   MUSCLES OF MASTICATION

Four muscles which act upon the mandible are traditionally grouped as the muscles of mastication. These are the *masseter, temporalis, medial pterygoid,* and *lateral pterygoid* muscles. All four of these muscles are innervated by the mandibular division of the trigeminal nerve (V_3).

Three of these muscles, masseter, temporalis, and medial pterygoid, act mainly to elevate the mandible, as in closing the jaws.

The lateral pterygoid muscle moves the condyle forward in either protrusion of the mandible (forward movement) or depression of the mandible.

Muscles of mastication include the

1. _____
2. _____
3. _____
4. _____

1. temporalis
2. masseter
3. medial pterygoid
4. lateral pterygoid
   (in any order)

Muscles of mastication are innervated by the _____ division of the trigeminal nerve (V).

mandibular

The only one of the muscles of mastication which is not involved in elevation of the mandible is the _____ _____ muscle.

lateral pterygoid

The three muscles of mastication involved in elevating the mandible are the _____ muscle, the _____ muscle, and the _____ pterygoid muscle.

masseter . . . temporalis . . . medial

THE MASSETER MUSCLE　　ITEM 15

The masseter muscle, shown in Figure 3–7, arises in the form of two heads, a superficial head and a deep head. The superficial head arises from the superficial aspect of the anterior two thirds of the lower border of the zygomatic arch. The deep head originates from the posterior third and the entire medial surface of the zygomatic arch. These two heads insert on the lateral surfaces of the ramus, the coronoid process, and the angle of the mandible. The masseter muscle elevates the mandible.

To help remember the location of the masseter muscle, clench your teeth tightly and palpate the muscle. When you have done this, relax your jaw and open your mouth very slightly and notice the softness of the relaxed masseter muscle.

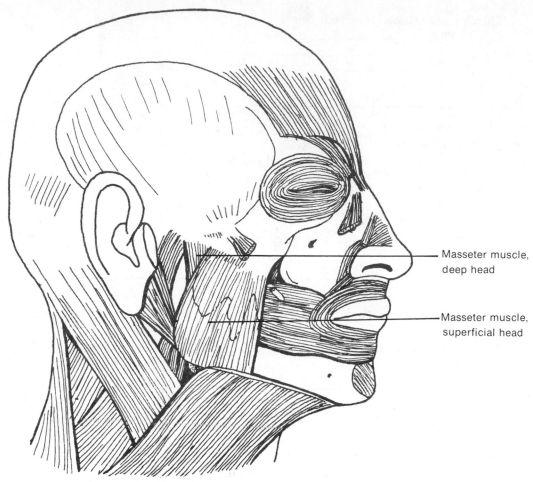

Figure 3–7. Masseter muscle, showing deep and superficial heads. (Redrawn from Wolf-Heidegger: Atlas of Systematic Human Anatomy. Vol. I. Basel, S. Karger AG.)

QUESTION
51

The superficial head of the masseter muscle originates from the anterior two thirds of the lower border of the _____ _____; the deep head, from the posterior third and the medial surface of the _____ _____.

ANSWER

zygomatic arch . . . zygomatic arch

QUESTION
52

The place of insertion of the masseter muscle is on the lateral surface of the _____ of the _____.

ANSWER

ramus . . . mandible

QUESTION
53

The action of the masseter muscle is to _____ the mandible.

ANSWER

elevate

The fanshaped temporalis muscle, shown in Figure 3–8, arises from the frontal and parietal bones below the superior temporal line and from a sheet of fascia, the temporal fascia, which extends from the superior temporal line to the zygomatic arch. Its fibers converge deep to the zygomatic arch, forming a thick tendinous band which separates the muscle into two portions as it inserts on the mandible. The superficial portion inserts on the upper lateral border of the coronoid process of the mandible. The larger, deep portion inserts as a band extending from the inner surface of the coronoid process downward along the anterior border of the ramus to the level of the mandibular third molar teeth. Innervation is by the mandibular division of the trigeminal nerve (V_3). The temporalis assists in elevation and retrusion of the mandible.

QUESTION 54

The temporalis muscle originates on the _____ and _____ bones and from the _____ fascia.

ANSWER

frontal . . . parietal . . . temporal

QUESTION 55

Fibers of the temporalis muscle lie deep to the _____ _____.

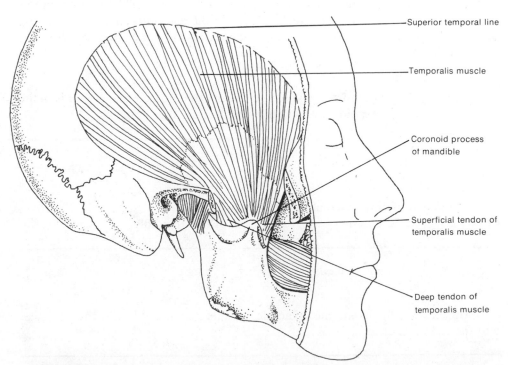

Superior temporal line

Temporalis muscle

Coronoid process of mandible

Superficial tendon of temporalis muscle

Deep tendon of temporalis muscle

Figure 3–8. Temporalis muscle, lateral aspect. (Redrawn from Wolf-Heidegger: Atlas of Systematic Human Anatomy. Vol. I. Basel, S. Karger AG.)

ANSWER   zygomatic arch

QUESTION   The superficial portion of the temporalis muscle inserts on the _____
56   process of the mandible; the deep portion inserts on the anterior border of the
_____ of the _____.

_____

ANSWER   coronoid . . . ramus . . . mandible

QUESTION   The actions of the temporalis muscle are to _____ and to
57   _____ the mandible.

_____

ANSWER   elevate . . . retrude

ITEM 17   THE MEDIAL PTERYGOID MUSCLE

Figure 3–9 shows the medial pterygoid muscle, which arises from the medial
side of the lateral pterygoid plate and from the adjacent lateral edge of the palatine
bone. The muscle descends posteriorly downward and laterally to insert on the
medial surface of the ramus and angle of the mandible. Contraction of the medial
pterygoid muscle, along with contraction of the temporalis and masseter muscles,
elevates the jaw.

QUESTION   The origins of the medial pterygoid muscle are the _____ side of the
58   _____ pterygoid plate and the _____ bone.

_____

ANSWER   medial . . . lateral . . . palatine

QUESTION   The insertion of the medial pterygoid muscle is the _____ surface
59   of the _____ and _____ of the mandible.

_____

ANSWER   medial . . . ramus . . . angle

QUESTION   Muscles which elevate the mandible are the _____, the _____,
60   and the _____ _____.

_____

ANSWER   masseter . . . temporalis . . . medial pterygoid (in any order)

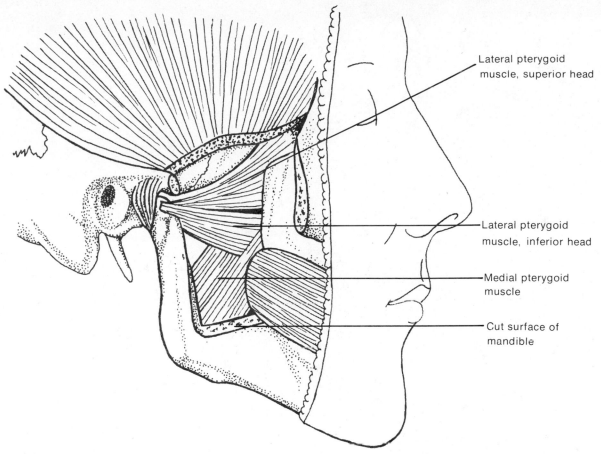

Lateral pterygoid
muscle, superior head

Lateral pterygoid
muscle, inferior head

Medial pterygoid
muscle

Cut surface of
mandible

Figure 3–9. Pterygoid muscles, lateral aspect (coronoid process and anterior half of ramus of mandible removed). (Redrawn from Wolf-Heidegger: Atlas of Systematic Human Anatomy. Vol. I. Basel, S. Karger AG.)

THE LATERAL PTERYGOID MUSCLE   ITEM 18

Look back to Figure 3–9 and observe the lateral pterygoid muscle arising by two heads. The superior head arises from the infratemporal surface of the greater wing of the sphenoid bone; the inferior head, from the lateral surface of the lateral pterygoid plate. Fibers merge as they extend horizontally backward, but insert as separate entities. The fibers of the superior part insert on the articular disk of the temporomandibular joint; the inferior fibers, in the pterygoid fovea of the mandible.

Contraction of both lateral pterygoid muscles draws the condyles forward, a movement necessary for the temporomandibular joint to open. Contraction of only one of the lateral pterygoid muscles causes a lateral shift of the mandible, or deviation to the opposite side.

Figure 3–10, a medial view, shows the medial pterygoid as it inserts on the medial aspect of the mandible and the lateral pterygoid as it inserts at the temporomandibular joint.

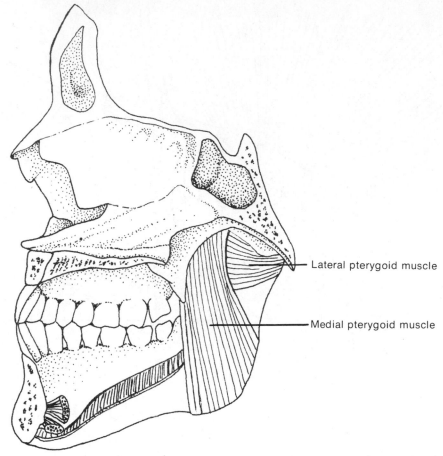

Figure 3–10. Medial and lateral pterygoid muscles, medial aspect. (Redrawn from Wolf-Heidegger: Atlas of Systematic Human Anatomy. Vol. I. Basel, S. Karger AG.)

QUESTION
61

The origin of the superior head of the lateral pterygoid muscle is the
_____ surface of the greater wing of the sphenoid bone.

ANSWER

infratemporal

QUESTION
62

The origin of the inferior head of the lateral pterygoid muscle is the
_____ surface of the lateral pterygoid plate.

ANSWER

lateral

QUESTION
63

The insertion of the upper head of the lateral pterygoid muscle is the
_____ disk of the _____ joint.

articular . . . temporomandibular

ANSWER

The insertion of the lower head of the lateral pterygoid muscle is the _____ _____ of the mandible.

QUESTION
64

pterygoid fovea

ANSWER

Bilateral contraction of the lateral pterygoid muscles draws the _____ forward to permit the _____ joint to open.

QUESTION
65

condyles . . . temporomandibular

ANSWER

Unilateral contraction of one lateral pterygoid muscle pulls the jaw toward the _____ side.

QUESTION
66

opposite

ANSWER

THE TEMPORALIS MUSCLE: LOCATION IN THE TEMPORAL FOSSA

ITEM
19

Figure 3–11, a frontal section through the muscles of mastication, illustrates the compartment in which the temporalis muscle lies. Notice how the fleshy portion of this muscle fills the temporal fossa, the depression of bone above the level of the zygomatic arch. In Figure 3–11, the temporalis muscle can be seen arising from the parietal bone, the squamous portion of the temporal bone, the lateral surface of the greater wing of the sphenoid bone, and the temporal fascia. The fascia can be seen extending from the temporal line downward to the zygomatic arch. Observe the large, extensive tendon of insertion of the temporalis muscle, which arises high in the muscle and descends to attach to the coronoid process and the anterior border of the ramus of the mandible.

Extending downward from its origin, the temporalis muscle fills the _____ fossa, a bony depression superior to the _____ arch.

QUESTION
67

temporal . . . zygomatic

ANSWER

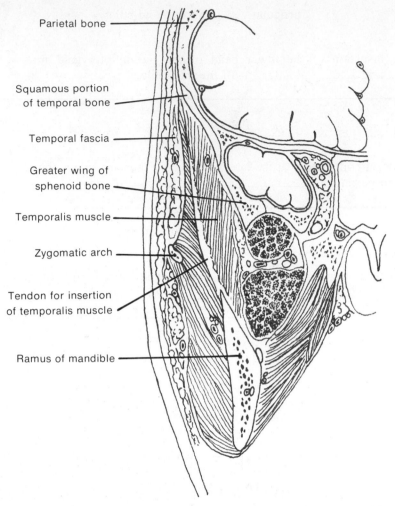

Parietal bone

Squamous portion
of temporal bone

Temporal fascia

Greater wing of
sphenoid bone

Temporalis muscle

Zygomatic arch

Tendon for insertion
of temporalis muscle

Ramus of mandible

Figure 3–11.   Frontal section through muscles of mastication, showing location of the temporalis muscle. (Redrawn from Truex and Kellner: Detailed Atlas of the Head and Neck. New York, Oxford University Press.)

QUESTION
68

The temporalis muscle takes its origin from the _____ bone, the _____ part of the temporal bone, the lateral surface of the greater wing of the _____, bone, and the temporal _____.

ANSWER

parietal . . . squamous . . . sphenoid . . . fascia

QUESTION
69

The tendon of insertion of the temporalis muscle attaches to the _____ process and the _____ border of the ramus of the mandible.

ANSWER

coronoid . . . anterior

THE MASSETER AND MEDIAL PTERYGOID MUSCLES: RELATIVE POSITIONS

ITEM 20

The frontal section shown in Figure 3–12 illustrates how the masseter and medial pterygoid muscles form a sling for the angle and ramus of the mandible. Observe that the masseter muscle occupies the same position external to the angle of the mandible as the medial pterygoid does on the inside. These two muscles act together to elevate the mandible, as in closing the mouth. In Figure 3–12, notice the superficial head of the masseter muscle arising from the inferior border of the zygomatic arch; the deep head, from the deep surface of the arch. The two heads blend and insert into the lateral surface of the coronoid process, ramus, and angle of the mandible.

The medial pterygoid muscle can be seen arising from the medial surface of the lateral plate of the pterygoid process of the sphenoid bone. Notice the insertion

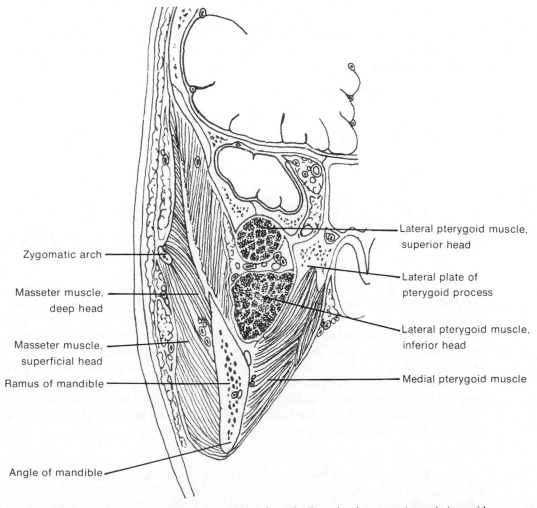

Zygomatic arch

Masseter muscle, deep head

Masseter muscle, superficial head

Ramus of mandible

Angle of mandible

Lateral pterygoid muscle, superior head

Lateral plate of pterygoid process

Lateral pterygoid muscle, inferior head

Medial pterygoid muscle

Figure 3–12. Frontal section through muscles of mastication, showing masseter and pterygoid muscles. (Redrawn from Truex and Kellner: Detailed Atlas of the Head and Neck. New York, Oxford University Press.)

of the medial pterygoid muscle on the medial aspect of the angle and ramus of the mandible.

QUESTION
70

The sling which the masseter and medial pterygoid muscles form for the angle of the mandible enables these two muscles to act in concert to _____ the mandible.

ANSWER

elevate

QUESTION
71

The two heads of the masseter muscle arise from the _____ ____ and insert into the _____ surface of the coronoid process, ramus, and angle of the mandible.

ANSWER

zygomatic arch . . . lateral

QUESTION
72

The medial pterygoid muscle originates from the lateral plate of the pterygoid process of the _____ bone and inserts on the _____ surface of the angle and ramus of the mandible.

ANSWER

sphenoid . . . medial

ITEM 21   THE LATERAL PTERYGOID MUSCLE: LOCATION IN THE INFRATEMPORAL FOSSA

The horizontal orientation of the lateral pterygoid muscle high in the infratemporal fossa, and the position of this muscle relative to the other muscles of mastication, may be seen in the frontal section shown in Figure 3–12. The smaller superior head of the lateral pterygoid and the larger inferior head have separate origins and, although they blend posteriorly, separate insertions. The separation of the two heads is apparent at the point where the frontal section shown in Figure 3–12 is made. Lying deep in the infratemporal fossa, almost the entire lateral pterygoid muscle is under cover of the temporalis muscle. Horizontally oriented, the lateral pterygoid is positioned to exert forward traction on the neck of the mandible to effect depression of the mandible.

QUESTION
73

The lateral pterygoid muscle runs *vertically/horizontally* (circle one) to draw the mandible forward.

horizontally

The location of the lateral pterygoid muscle is within the *temporal/infra-temporal* (circle one) fossa.

---

infratemporal

The superior and inferior heads of the lateral pterygoid muscle have
A. two separate origins but a single insertion
B. a single origin but two separate insertions
C. two separate origins and two separate insertions

The correct answer is C. Originating separately, the two heads blend posteriorly and then insert separately, the superior head inserting into the articular disk of the temporomandibular joint and the inferior head ending in the pterygoid fovea of the neck of the mandible.

REVIEW OF THE MUSCLES OF MASTICATION ITEM 22

This item presents a brief review of the four principal muscles of mastication. Again, palpate these muscles on yourself whenever possible. Three of these muscles, masseter, temporalis, and medial pterygoid, act mainly to elevate the mandible. The masseter has two heads, which arise from the lower border of the zygomatic arch and insert on the lateral aspect of the ramus of the mandible. The temporalis originates from the temporal line and from temporal fascia; a superficial portion inserts on the coronoid process of the mandible and a deep portion of the anterior border of the ramus of the mandible. The medial pterygoid arises from the medial aspect of the lateral pterygoid plate, and inserts on the medial surface of the ramus and angle of the mandible.

The fourth of the principal muscles of mastication, the lateral pterygoid, protrudes the mandible. Its superior head arises from the infratemporal surface of the greater wing of the sphenoid bone and inserts on the articular disk of the temporomandibular joint. The inferior head arises from the lateral aspect of the lateral pterygoid plate and inserts in the pterygoid fovea of the mandible.

In the table on page 146, fill in the names of the muscles numbered on the accompanying diagram and write in the origin and insertion of each muscle. (The masseter muscle does not appear in the accompanying illustration; however, fill in the origin and insertion of the masseter where called for in the table.)

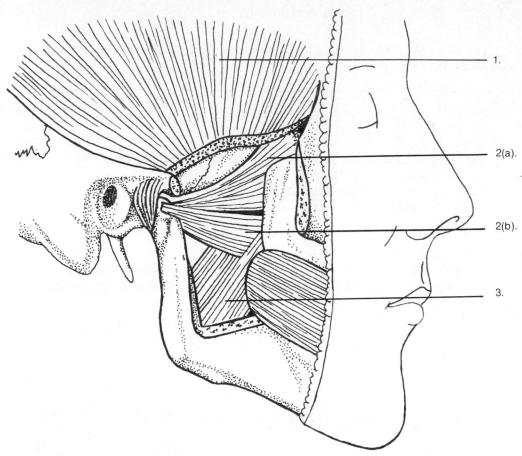

(Redrawn from Wolf-Heidegger: Atlas of Systematic Human Anatomy. Vol. I. Basel, S. Karger AG.)

Muscle	Origin	Insertion
1. _____	_____	_____
	_____	_____
2(a). _____	_____	_____
(superior head)	_____	_____
(b). _____	_____	_____
(inferior head)	_____	_____
3. _____	_____	_____
	_____	_____
4. Masseter	_____	_____

ANSWER

Muscle	Origin	Insertion
1. Temporalis	Temporal line	Coronoid process
	Temporal fascia	Anterior border of mandible
2(a). Lateral pterygoid (superior head)	Infratemporal surface of greater wing of sphenoid	Articular disk of the temporomandibular joint
(b). Lateral pterygoid (inferior head)	Lateral aspect of lateral pterygoid plate	Pterygoid fovea of mandible
3. Medial pterygoid	Medial aspect of lateral pterygoid plate	Medial surface of ramus and angle of mandible
4. Masseter	Zygomatic arch	Lateral aspect of ramus of mandible

THE SUPRAHYOID MUSCLES   ITEM 23

In addition to the four previously described muscles of mastication, several accessory muscles also act upon the mandible. These muscles, called the *suprahyoid muscles* because they are situated above the hyoid bone, appear in Figure 3–13. They include the *geniohyoid,* the *mylohyoid,* and the *digastric.* The suprahyoid muscles assist the lateral pterygoids in depressing the mandible; they assist the temporalis muscles in retracting the mandible.

The suprahyoid muscles are so named because of their position _____ to the hyoid bone.

QUESTION 77

---

superior

ANSWER

The names of the suprahyoid muscles are the _____, the _____, and the _____.

QUESTION 78

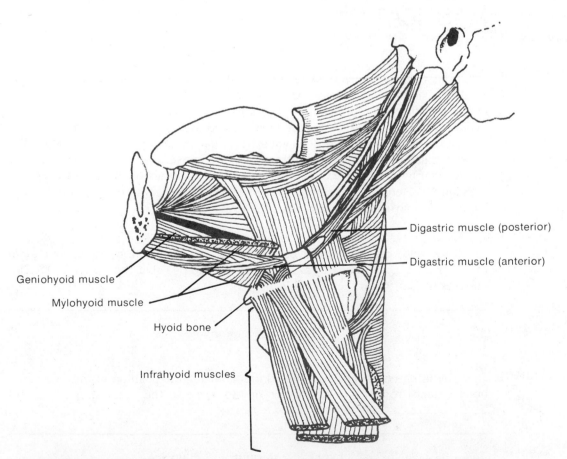

Digastric muscle (posterior)

Digastric muscle (anterior)

Geniohyoid muscle

Mylohyoid muscle

Hyoid bone

Infrahyoid muscles

Figure 3–13.   The suprahyoid and infrahyoid muscles, lateral aspect. (Redrawn from Romanes [Ed.]: Cunningham's Textbook of Anatomy. 10th Ed. New York, Oxford University Press.)

ANSWER   mylohyoid . . geniohyoid . . digastric (in any order)

QUESTION   The muscles which act in concert with the suprahyoid muscles to open the
79   jaw are the _____ _____ muscles.

ANSWER   lateral pterygoid

QUESTION   The muscles which act in concert with the suprahyoids to retract (retrude),
80   the mandible are the _____ muscles.

ANSWER   temporalis

ITEM 24   THE INFRAHYOID MUSCLES: ROLE IN MASTICATION

Look back to Figure 3–13 and observe the location of the *infrahyoid* muscles.
While the suprahyoid muscles extend from the upper border of the hyoid bone up
to the mandible, the infrahyoid muscles extend from the inferior surface of the
hyoid bone down to attach for the most part to the sternum and clavicle.

Because the hyoid bone does not articulate with other bones, its vertical level
is determined by the state of contraction of the muscles attached to its superior
and inferior borders. For example, in order for the suprahyoid muscles to depress
the mandible, tension of the infrahyoid muscles is necessary to fix the hyoid bone in
a downward position.

QUESTION   The role of the infrahyoid muscles in mastication is to maintain
81   the _____ bone in a downward position so that the _____
muscles can act upon the mandible.

ANSWER   hyoid . . . suprahyoid

QUESTION   The infrahyoid muscles involved in stabilizing the position of the _____
82   bone extend from the lower border of this bone to the _____ and
_____.

ANSWER   hyoid . . . sternum . . . clavicle

THE SUPRAHYOID MUSCLES: INNERVATION

ITEM
25

The innervation of the suprahyoid muscles is varied. The mylohoid is innervated by the mandibular division of the trigeminal nerve (V). The digastric, as you can see in Figure 3–13, is a two bellied muscle. The anterior belly, like the mylohyoid, is supplied by the mandibular division of the trigeminal nerve (V₃) while the posterior belly is supplied by the facial nerve (VII). A branch of the first cervical nerve, conducted by way of the hypoglossal nerve (XII), innervates the geniohyoid muscle.

The two suprahyoid muscles innervated by the mandibular division of the trigeminal nerve are the _____ muscle and the _____ belly of the digastric muscle.

QUESTION
83

---

mylohyoid . . . anterior

ANSWER

The first cervical nerve innervates the _____ muscle; the facial nerve, the _____ belly of the digastric muscle.

QUESTION
84

---

geniohyoid . . . posterior

ANSWER

MOVEMENTS OF THE MANDIBLE

ITEM
26

Before you study the various movements of the mandible, it is important for you to first go back to Unit Two and reread very carefully Items 59 through 63 on the temporomandibular joint. Also, if possible, you should obtain a skull and locate on it all the structures described in Unit Two, Items 59 to 63, as you review this earlier material. As you work through the present and following items, move the mandible on the skull to illustrate for yourself the various movements described. After you have reviewed thoroughly the items in Unit Two, proceed, skull in hand, with this item and the ones that follow.

There are three pairs of basic movements of the mandible: depression and elevation, protrusion and retraction, and right or left lateral shift. *Depression* lowers the mandible, thus opening the mouth; *elevation* raises the mandible, bringing the teeth into closer contact, or occlusion. *Protrusion* is a forward movement of the mandible; *retraction,* a drawing of the mandible backward. Both protrusion and retraction are possible only when the mandible is slightly, but not markedly, depressed. *Right lateral shift* is a deviation of the anterior portion of the mandible to the right; *left lateral shift,* a deviation to the left.

QUESTION
85

Movement of the mandible in a vertical plane is
A. protrusion or retraction
B. depression or elevation
C. right or left shift

ANSWER

The correct answer is B. Movement in a vertical plane is up or down, as in opening or closing the mouth.

QUESTION
86

Protrusion and retraction are movements of the mandible in
A. a vertical plane
B. a lateral plane
C. an anteroposterior plane

ANSWER

The correct answer is C. Movement in an anteroposterior plane is forward or backward, as in protruding or retracting the jaw.

QUESTION
87

Deviation of the mandible to the right or to the left is termed a _____ _____.

ANSWER

lateral shift

QUESTION
88

The term used to describe the action of the mandible which brings the teeth into closer occlusion is _____.

ANSWER

elevation

QUESTION
89

The term descriptive of the forward movement of the mandible is _____.

ANSWER

protrusion

QUESTION
90

The term used in association with opening the mouth is _____ of the mandible.

ANSWER

depression

QUESTION
91

The term which refers to the muscular action which draws the mandible backward is _____.

ANSWER

retraction

THE MUSCLES OF MASTICATION: PRINCIPLES OF ACTION

ITEM 27

Three basic generalizations apply to action of the muscles of mastication:

(1) Except in the case of occlusion, the mandible is held in position by a balance between the opposing downward pull of gravity and the depressor muscles, on the one hand, and the upward pull of the elevator muscles, on the other.

(2) Except for lateral shifts, there is symmetrical action of the muscles of mastication on the right and left sides of the head and symmetrical movement of the right and left temporomandibular joints.

(3) All movements of the mandible are brought about by groups of muscles acting in concert; no movement of the mandible can result from a single pair of muscles acting alone.

The position of the mandible is determined by a balance between the _____ pull and the _____ pull of opposing muscles.

QUESTION
92

---

downward . . . upward (in either order)

ANSWER

Corresponding muscles on the right and left act in synchrony for all movements of the mandible except _____ _____.

QUESTION
93

---

lateral shifts

ANSWER

Every movement of the mandible requires _____ action of several groups of muscles.

QUESTION
94

---

coordinated (concerted)

ANSWER

COORDINATED MUSCLE ACTIVITY IN ELEVATION OF THE MANDIBLE

ITEM 28

The combined, symmetrical action of the temporalis, masseter, and medial pterygoid muscles on both sides of the head effect the elevation of the mandible. The temporalis muscles elevate the coronoid process, while the masseters and medial pterygoids together elevate the angle of the mandible. The lateral pterygoid and suprahyoid muscles must relax as the three levator muscles exert their upward traction on the mandible.

QUESTION
95
Muscles which insert on the medial and lateral side of the ramus of the mandible, forming a sling, are the _____ and _____ _____ muscles.

ANSWER
masseter . . . medial pterygoid (in either order)

QUESTION
96
The temporalis muscle exerts an upward traction on the _____ process, the site at which this muscle attaches to the mandible.

ANSWER
coronoid

QUESTION
97
The muscles which must relax to allow the levator muscles to raise the mandible are the _____ _____ muscles and the _____ muscles.

ANSWER
lateral pterygoid . . . suprahyoid (in either order)

ITEM 29   MUSCLE ACTIONS INVOLVED IN DEPRESSION OF THE MANDIBLE

During depression of the mandible, the lateral pterygoid muscles exert a forward traction on the neck of the mandible, the superior head of the lateral pterygoid pulling the articular disk down the inclination of the articular tubercle. The suprahyoid muscles assist the lateral pterygoids in drawing down the mandible, with the infrahyoid muscles keeping the hyoid bone stabilized. The levator muscles must relax to permit the lateral pterygoid and suprahyoid muscles to depress the mandible.

QUESTION
98
Traction to draw the articular disk down the plane of the articular tubercle is exerted by the _____ head of the _____ _____ muscle.

ANSWER
superior . . . lateral pterygoid

QUESTION
99
To depress the mandible, the lateral pterygoid muscles must pull in both a _____ and a _____ direction.

forward . . . downward (in either order)   *ANSWER*

The muscles attaching to the hyoid bone which assist the lateral pterygoids to depress the mandible are called the _____ muscles; muscles which fix the hyoid bone while the mandible is being depressed are called _____ muscles.   *QUESTION* **100**

suprahyoid . . . infrahyoid   *ANSWER*

The levator muscles which must relax to allow the mandible to be depressed are the _____ muscles, the _____ muscles, and the _____ pterygoid muscles.   *QUESTION* **101**

temporalis . . . masseter . . . medial   *ANSWER*

PROTRUSION AND RETRACTION OF THE MANDIBLE   ITEM 30

In order for the mandible to protrude, it is necessary for the lateral pterygoid muscles to contract to draw the mandible forward while the suprahyoid muscles relax. The medial pterygoid muscles assist the lateral pterygoids in protrusion of the mandible. To retract the mandible, the posterior fibers of the temporalis muscles, with the assistance of the mylohyoid, digastric, and geniohyoid muscles, draw the mandible backward. Alternation of protrusion and retraction is characteristic of chewing and grinding motions.

Protrusion of the mandible is accomplished by contraction of the _____ pterygoid muscles, with assistance from the _____ pterygoid muscles; retraction, by the contraction of the posterior portion of the _____ muscles, assisted by the _____ muscles.   *QUESTION* **102**

lateral . . . medial . . . temporalis . . . suprahyoid   *ANSWER*

The mylohyoid, digastric, and geniohyoid muscles must *contract/relax* (circle one) in order for the lateral pterygoids to depress the mandible; these same muscles must *contract/relax* (circle one) for the lateral pterygoids to protrude the mandible.   *QUESTION* **103**

contract . . . relax   *ANSWER*

ITEM 31   MUSCLE ACTIONS IN LATERAL SHIFTS OF THE MANDIBLE

Simultaneous contractions of the lateral pterygoid muscles on both the right and left sides of the head will draw the condyles of the mandible forward. However, contraction of the lateral pterygoid on the right side only will cause the mandible to deviate to the left. This deviation is called a left lateral shift. Contraction of the lateral pterygoid on the left side only produces a right lateral shift. In other words, when only the lateral pterygoid on one side of the head contracts, the mandible shifts laterally to the opposite side. For a lateral shift to occur, the lateral pterygoid muscle must be relaxed on the side toward which the mandible deviates. Furthermore, the levator muscles must also relax, though not markedly.

QUESTION
104

The right lateral shift of the mandible is caused by contraction of the _____ pterygoid muscle on the _____ side of the head; a left lateral shift by contraction of the muscle on the _____ side.

ANSWER

lateral . . . left . . . right

ITEM 32   REVIEW OF THE MOVEMENTS OF MUSCLES OF MASTICATION

The table below synopsizes the actions of the muscles involved in the various movements of the mandible. As you review these movements by studying the table, perform the various movements yourself in front of a mirror, palpate the action of these muscles on yourself, and manipulate the mandible of a skull if you have one available.

Movement	Contraction	Relaxation
Elevation	Masseters Medial pterygoids Temporalis muscles	Lateral pterygoids Suprahyoids
Depression	Lateral pterygoids Suprahyoids	Masseters Medial pterygoids Temporalis muscles
Protrusion	Lateral pterygoids Medial pterygoids	Suprahyoids plus slight relaxation of levators
Retraction	Posterior portion of temporalis muscles Suprahyoids	Lateral pterygoids plus slight relaxation of levators
Right lateral shift	Left lateral pterygoid	Right lateral pterygoid plus slight relaxation of levators
Left lateral shift	Right lateral pterygoid	Left lateral pterygoid plus slight relaxation of levators

Protrusion of the mandible results from contraction of the _____ pterygoid muscles, assisted by the _____ pterygoid muscles.

QUESTION
105

---

lateral . . . medial

ANSWER

Right lateral shift requires contraction of the _____ pterygoid muscle on the _____ side; left lateral shift, contraction on the _____ side.

QUESTION
106

---

lateral . . . left . . . right

ANSWER

Retraction of the mandible is effected by contraction of the posterior fibers of the _____ muscles and contraction of the _____ muscles, while the _____ pterygoid muscles relax.

QUESTION
107

---

temporalis . . . suprahyoid . . . lateral

ANSWER

The muscles which relax to permit depression of the mandible are the _____ muscles, the _____ muscles, and the _____ pterygoid muscles.

QUESTION
108

---

temporalis . . . masseter . . . medial

ANSWER

Muscles which elevate the mandible are the _____ muscles, the _____ muscles, and the _____ pterygoid muscles.

QUESTION
109

---

temporalis . . . masseter . . . medial

ANSWER

To depress the mandible, the lateral pterygoids and suprahyoids must _____; for elevation of the mandible, the lateral pterygoids and suprahyoids must _____.

QUESTION
110

---

contract . . . relax

ANSWER

SUMMARY OF UNIT THREE

The muscles of primary concern in dentistry are those of facial expression and those of mastication. Because facial muscles attach to overlying skin, the face is highly mobile. The facial muscles, embryonically derived from the second branchial arch, can be conveniently grouped into those (1) around and above the eyes, (2) around and above the mouth, and (3) below the mouth. All are supplied by the facial (seventh cranial) nerve.

MUSCLES OF FACIAL EXPRESSION

The orbicularis oculi muscle is a sphincter muscle having two parts: the palpebral part to close the eyes gently and the orbital part to close the eyes forcefully. The levator palpebrae superioris elevates the upper eyelid. The levator, not a facial muscle in the strict sense, derives its nerve supply from the oculomotor (third cranial) nerve rather than the facial nerve (VII).

The corrugator supercilii muscle draws the skin of the forehead downward, as in frowning. The procerus muscle draws the medial angle of the eyebrows downward.

Several narrow muscles are involved in elevating the lips. The zygomaticus muscles insert into the skin of the upper lip and into the muscle encircling the mouth, the orbicularis oris. The levator labii superioris and the levator labii superioris alaeque nasi both insert into the skin of the upper lip, the latter also inserting into the ala of the nose. The nasalis muscle, too, inserts into the ala of the nose as well as extending across the bridge of the nose. The levator anguli oris elevates the angle of the mouth.

The orbicularis oris is a sphincter muscle which closes and protrudes the mouth. It surrounds the mouth, most of its fibers arising from the buccinator muscle of the cheek. The orbicularis oris keeps food on the occlusal surface of the teeth in the region of the lips. The thin risorius muscle, extending from the fascia over the parotid gland to the angle of the mouth, widens the mouth, as in an expression of mirth. The superficial platysma muscle covering the neck and chin has fibers of insertion which often fuse with those of the risorius.

The buccinator muscle, which constitutes the anterior part of the cheek, pulls the angle of the mouth laterally, compresses the cheek, and keeps food on the occlusal surface of teeth. Fibers of the buccinator intermingle with those of the orbicularis oris, levator anguli oris, depressor anguli oris, and zygomaticus major in an area called the modiolus.

Muscles which depress the lower lip are the more superficial depressor anguli oris and the deeper depressor labii inferioris. The mentalis muscle raises the skin of the chin and protrudes the lower lip.

MUSCLES OF MASTICATION

All muscles of mastication are innervated by the mandibular division of the fifth cranial nerve, the trigeminal nerve. Three muscles of mastication are involved in elevation of the mandible: the masseter, the temporalis, and the medial pterygoid. The masseter has two heads; one, the superficial head, arising from the anterior two thirds of the superficial aspect of the lower border of the zygomatic arch; the other, the deep head, from the posterior third of the deep aspect of the arch. Fibers of the fanshaped temporalis muscle converge to form a tendinous band which inserts on the coronoid process and anterior border of the mandible. The third muscle which elevates the mandible is the medial pterygoid, which arises from the medial surface of the lateral pterygoid plate of the sphenoid bone. The medial pterygoid inserts on the ramus and angle of the mandible.

The lateral pterygoid muscle extends horizontally and laterally to insert on the articular disk of the temporomandibular joint and on the pterygoid fovea of the mandible.

Accessory muscles, referred to as *suprahyoid* because of their position superior to the hyoid bone, include the mylohyoid, digastric, and geniohyoid. These muscles pull the anterior portion of the mandible downward, as well as assisting in retraction of the mandible.

ACTION OF THE MUSCLES OF MASTICATION

Movement of the mandible requires the action of groups of muscles working in concert. Except for lateral shifts, there is symmetrical action of muscles on each side of the jaw and symmetrical movement at the two temporomandibular joints. Except during occlusion, the mandible is held in position by a balance between depressor and levator muscles. The principal movements of the mandible include protrusion, retraction, depression, elevation, and lateral shift. For protrusion, the lateral pterygoid must contract, and the suprahyoids relax; for retraction, lateral pterygoids must relax while suprahyoids and the posterior portion of the temporalis contract. For depression, lateral pterygoids and suprahyoids must contract and temporalis and masseters relax; for elevation, lateral pterygoids and suprahyoids must relax while levator muscles contract. For a right lateral shift, the lateral pterygoid on the left must contract, while the lateral pterygoid on the right side relaxes.

Gentle closing of the eyes is effected by the _____ part of the orbicularis occuli muscle; forcible closing by the _____ part.

QUESTION 111

---

palpebral . . . orbital

ANSWER

Innervation of the muscles of facial expression is from branches of the _____ nerve, although the levator palpebrae superioris muscle, which raises the upper eyelid, receives its motor supply from the _____ nerve.

QUESTION 112

---

facial (seventh cranial) . . . oculomotor (third cranial)

ANSWER

The corrugator supercilii muscles draw the skin of the _____ downward, while the procerus muscle of the nose draws down the medial angle of the _____.

QUESTION 113

---

forehead . . . eyebrows

ANSWER

QUESTION
114

The zygomaticus major and zygomaticus minor muscles are involved in elevating the _____ of the mouth.

ANSWER

angle

QUESTION
115

The levator labii superioris alaeque nasi muscle attaches to both upper lip and ala of the nose; a related muscle attaching to the upper lip is the levator _____ _____ muscle, while another muscle attaching to the ala of the nose is the _____ muscle.

ANSWER

labii superioris . . . nasalis

QUESTION
116

The levator _____ _____ muscle elevates the angle of the mouth.

ANSWER

anguli oris

QUESTION
117

The sphincter muscle which surrounds the mouth and acts to protrude and close the mouth is the _____ _____.

ANSWER

orbicularis oris

QUESTION
118

The muscle which keeps food on the occlusal surface of the teeth in the region of the lips is the _____ _____ muscle; in the region of the cheek, the _____ muscle.

ANSWER

orbicularis oris . . . buccinator

QUESTION
119

The risorius muscle extends over the _____ gland to the _____ of the mouth, its fibers of insertion fusing with those of the _____ muscle.

ANSWER

parotid . . . angle . . . platysma

QUESTION
120

The muscle which compresses the cheek and pulls the angle of the mouth to the side is the _____ muscle.

ANSWER

buccinator

The modiolus is an area lateral to the _____ of the mouth where fibers of several muscles _____.

QUESTION
121

---

angle . . . intermingle (converge)

ANSWER

The angle of the mouth is depressed by the depressor _____ _____ muscle.

QUESTION
122

---

anguli oris

ANSWER

The lower lip is depressed by the depressor _____ _____ muscle; it is protruded by the _____ muscle.

QUESTION
123

---

labii inferioris . . . mentalis

ANSWER

The effect of contractions of the masseter, temporalis, and medial pterygoid muscles is _____ of the mandible.

QUESTION
124

---

elevation

ANSWER

The suprahyoid muscles include the _____, the _____, and the _____ muscles.

QUESTION
125

---

mylohyoid . . . digastric . . . geniohyoid (in any order)

ANSWER

The two movements of the mandible which require contraction of the suprahyoid muscles are _____ and _____.

QUESTION
126

---

depression . . . retraction (in either order)

ANSWER

The two movements of the mandible which require relaxation of the suprahyoid muscles are _____ and _____.

QUESTION
127

---

elevation . . . protrusion (in either order)

ANSWER

The two movements of the mandible which require contraction of the lateral pterygoids are _____ and _____.

QUESTION
128

ANSWER

depression . . . protrusion (in either order)

QUESTION
129

The two movements of the mandible which require relaxation of the lateral pterygoids are _____ and _____ .

ANSWER

elevation . . . retraction (in either order)

QUESTION
130

When the lateral pterygoid and suprahyoid muscles contract to depress the mandible, there must be relaxation of the _____, the _____, and the _____ _____ muscles.

ANSWER

temporalis . . . masseter . . . medial pterygoid

QUESTION
131

In a lateral shift, the _____ _____ muscle on the side opposite the movement contracts while the corresponding muscle on the other side relaxes.

ANSWER

lateral pterygoid

Unit Four □ GROSS STRUCTURES OF THE BRAIN

DIVISIONS OF THE BRAIN

The brain is generally divided into three regions, as shown in Figure 4–1: the *cerebral hemispheres*, the *cerebellum*, and the *brain stem*. The brain stem is subdivided into four areas: the *diencephalon, midbrain, pons*, and *medulla*. The right and left cerebral hemispheres are incompletely separated by the deep *longitudinal fissure*. Inferior to this fissure the two hemispheres are joined by a broad band of nerve fibers called the *corpus callosum*. The corpus callosum can be clearly seen in Figure 4–1.

The three main divisions of the brain are the _____ hemispheres, the _____, and the _____ stem.

QUESTION 1

---

cerebral . . . cerebellum . . . brain

ANSWER

The diencephalon, midbrain, pons, and medulla are subdivisions of the _____ _____.

QUESTION 2

---

brain stem

ANSWER

The corpus callosum is a band of _____ fibers connecting the two _____ _____.

QUESTION 3

---

nerve . . . cerebral hemispheres

ANSWER

161

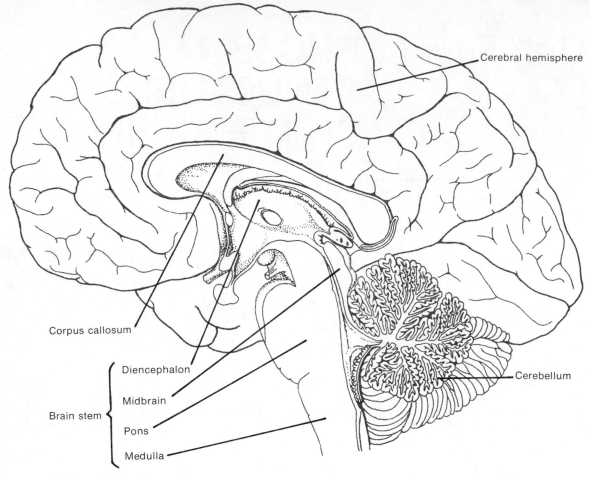

Figure 4-1.   Right half of brain, medial aspect. (Redrawn from Wolf-Heidegger: Atlas of Systematic Human Anatomy. Vol. III. Basel, S. Karger AG.)

ITEM 2   COMPOSITION OF THE BRAIN

The brain is composed of billions of nerve cells, or *neurons*. The cell bodies of neurons having related functions are aggregated into clusters called *nuclei,* which form part of the gray matter of the brain. The remaining substance of the brain is composed of nerve fibers, which make up the white matter. A bundle of nerve fibers with a common origin and destination constitutes a *tract*. The tracts provide afferent and efferent connections between different areas of the brain and between the brain and the spinal cord.

QUESTION
4

A cluster of cell bodies of neurons which have related functions is called a _____.

nucleus   *ANSWER*

A bundle of nerve fibers within the brain is referred to as a _____.   *QUESTION*
5

---

tract   *ANSWER*

The afferent and efferent tracts connect various areas within the _____   *QUESTION*
and also connect the brain itself with the _____ _____.   **6**

---

brain . . . spinal cord   *ANSWER*

THE CEREBRAL HEMISPHERES   ITEM
3

The cerebral hemispheres have an outer layer, the *cortex,* composed of an
aggregate of diffusely located nerve cell bodies, and an inner region comprising
tracts and nuclei. The outer surface of each cerebral hemisphere, shown in the
lateral view in Figure 4–2, is marked by the presence of a series of grooves, known
as *sulci,* with convolutions of brain substance, called *gyri,* protruding between
them. Deeper furrows between the gyri are called *fissures.* Although the pattern
of gyri and sulci shows considerable variation, it is sufficiently constant to permit
naming those which commonly appear.

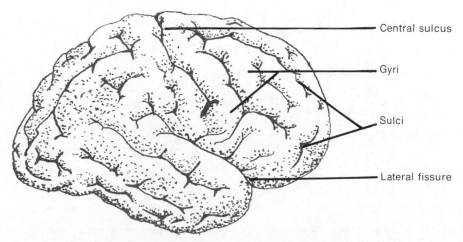

Figure 4–2.   Brain, lateral view, showing gyri and sulci.

QUESTION
7

The _____ comprises the outer layer of the cerebral hemispheres; fiber _____ and _____ comprise the inner region.

ANSWER

cortex . . . tracts . . . nuclei

QUESTION
8

The convolutions of brain substance protruding on the outer surface of the cerebral hemispheres are termed _____; the grooves between the protrusions are called _____ or _____.

ANSWER

gyri . . . sulci . . . fissures

ITEM 4   LOBES AND FISSURES OF THE CEREBRAL HEMISPHERES

Each cerebral hemisphere has five lobes: *frontal, parietal, temporal, occipital,* and *insula.* The first four of these lobes appear in Figure 4–3. The fifth lobe, the insula, does not appear, since it is deep to the upper temporal lobe and can be seen only when the temporal lobe is retracted downward.

Notice in Figure 4–3 how the *central sulcus* separates the frontal and parietal lobes. The *lateral fissure,* deeper than the central sulcus, separates the temporal lobe inferiorly from the frontal and parietal lobes superiorly. The third fissure of the brain, the *longitudinal fissure,* is the most prominent of all. Not visible from the lateral view, but shown in the superior aspect in Figure 4–4, the longitudinal fissure separates the two cerebral hemispheres.

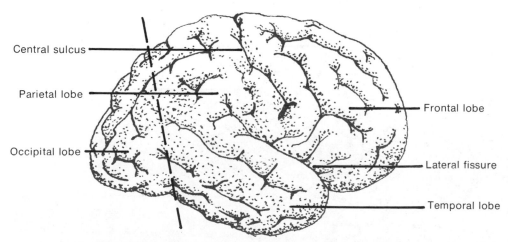

Figure 4–3. Right cerebral hemisphere, showing lobes of brain.

The frontal and parietal lobes of the cerebral hemispheres are separated by the _____ sulcus.

QUESTION
9

central

ANSWER

The longitudinal fissure separates the two _____ _____.

QUESTION
10

cerebral hemispheres

ANSWER

The groove separating the frontal and parietal lobes superiorly from the temporal lobe inferiorly is the _____ _____.

QUESTION
11

lateral fissure

ANSWER

THE LOBES WITHIN THE CRANIUM: LOCATION

ITEM 5

The frontal lobes occupy the anterior cranial fossa; the temporal lobes, the middle cranial fossa; the occipital lobes, the upper part of the posterior cranial fossa above the cerebellum. The parietal lobes are located in the upper region of the brain between the frontal and occipital lobes. The insula lies deep to the temporal lobe.

Match the lobes of the cerebral hemispheres with their proper locations by placing the appropriate letter from column B in the parentheses of column A.

QUESTION
12

Column A	Column B
( ) 1. frontal	A. above the cerebellum
( ) 2. parietal	B. middle cranial fossa
( ) 3. temporal	C. deep to the temporal lobe
( ) 4. occipital	D. anterior cranial fossa
( ) 5. insula	E. upper region between frontal and occipital lobes

1.—(D), 2.—(E), 3.—(B), 4.—(A), 5.—(C)

ANSWER

ITEM 6   LOBES OF THE CEREBRAL HEMISPHERES: FUNCTIONAL ROLES

The frontal lobe, as a whole, is involved in abstract thought, although little is known about the mechanisms operative in such thought. One area of the frontal lobe, the precentral gyrus, is the location of neuron cell bodies whose processes are responsible for voluntary muscle control.

The parietal lobe contains the center which integrates incoming stimuli and formulates appropriate speech reactions to these stimuli. A specific area of the parietal lobe, the postcentral gyrus, is the site of reception of conscious sensations of pressure, pain, touch, and temperature.

The temporal lobe receives auditory stimuli, and some evidence also links this area to the function of recent memory. The occipital lobe is largely concerned with vision. The function of the insula is virtually unknown.

QUESTION 13

The region of the brain which is involved in abstract thought is the _____ lobe.

ANSWER

frontal

QUESTION 14

Cell bodies of neurons involved in control of voluntary muscles are located in the _____ gyrus of the frontal lobe.

ANSWER

precentral

QUESTION 15

Sensations of pain, temperature, touch, and pressure are received in the _____ gyrus of the parietal lobe.

ANSWER

postcentral

QUESTION 16

Auditory sensations are received in the _____ lobe; visual sensations, in the _____ lobe.

ANSWER

temporal . . . occipital

QUESTION 17

The center in which speech is formulated and initiated is located in the _____ lobe.

ANSWER

parietal

SUPERIOR ASPECT OF THE BRAIN   ITEM 7

Figure 4–4 shows the superior aspect of the brain. The deep longitudinal fissure, referred to in Items 1 and 4, can be seen in the midline, separating the two cerebral hemispheres. Notice the three lobes of the cerebrum which are visible from the superior view: the frontal, parietal, and occipital lobes. Observe also the prominent central sulcus dividing the frontal lobe from the parietal lobe. Anterior

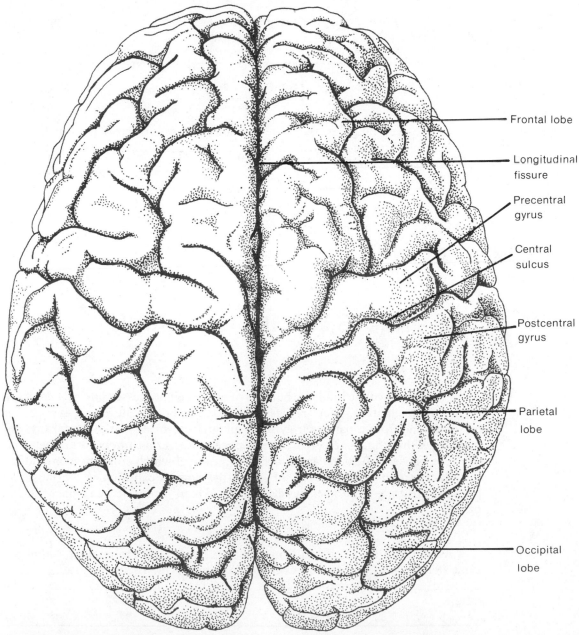

Figure 4–4. Brain, superior aspect. (Redrawn from Wolf-Heidegger: Atlas of Systematic Human Anatomy. Vol. III. Basel, S. Karger AG.)

to the central sulcus is the precentral gyrus of the frontal lobe, the brain center for voluntary muscle control. Posterior to the central sulcus is the postcentral gyrus, the center for awareness of pressure, pain, touch and thermal sensations.

QUESTION
18

The deep midline groove which separates the right and left cerebral hemispheres is termed the _____ _____.

ANSWER

longitudinal fissure

QUESTION
19

The precentral gyrus, the center for motor control, is located in the _____ lobe, anterior to the _____ sulcus.

ANSWER

frontal . . . central

QUESTION
20

The postcentral gyrus, the center for consciousness of pressure, touch, pain, and thermal sensations, is located in the _____ lobe, posterior to the _____ sulcus.

ANSWER

parietal . . . central

ITEM 8   THE TRACTS WITHIN THE BRAIN

Fiber tracts of the brain are bundles of nerve cell processes having a common origin and destination. They are classified into three broad categories. *Association tracts* extend from a particular gyrus to an adjacent or distant gyrus, always remaining within the same cerebral hemisphere. *Projection tracts* form fiber connections between the brain and spinal cord, some of which cross from one side to the other. *Commissural tracts,* of which the corpus callosum is the most important, are transverse fiber bundles which extend from one hemisphere to the other.

QUESTION
21

Association tracts extend from one _____ to another within the same hemisphere; projection tracts extend between the brain and _____ _____; commissural tracts extend from one _____ to the other.

ANSWER

gyrus . . . spinal cord . . . hemisphere

Tracts which always remain in the same hemisphere are called _____ tracts; those which always cross from one hemisphere to the other hemisphere are called _____ tracts; those which pass between the brain and the spinal cord are called _____ tracts.

---

association . . . commissural . . . projection

THE VENTRICLES OF THE BRAIN   ITEM 9

The ventricles of the brain are connecting cavities which contribute to formation, circulation, and reabsorption of the cerebrospinal fluid which surrounds the brain and spinal cord as a protective shock absorber. The ventricles are four in number: two lateral *ventricles,* the *third ventricle,* and the *fourth ventricle.* Figure 4–5 shows the location of the four ventricles as well as the narrow channels connecting them. The anterior part of each of the two lateral ventricles communicates with the third ventricle through an *interventricular foramen.* In Figure 4–5, notice the *cerebral aqueduct* joining the third and fourth ventricles. *Medial* and *lateral apertures* allow cerebrospinal fluid to flow from the fourth ventricle into the subarachnoid space surrounding the brain and spinal cord.

The openings between the two lateral ventricles and the third ventricle are called _____ foramina.

---

interventricular

The cerebral aqueduct is the narrow connecting passage between the _____ ventricle and the _____ ventricle.

---

third . . . fourth

Through the single medial and two lateral apertures of the fourth ventricle, cerebrospinal fluid flows from this ventricle into the _____ space which surrounds the brain.

---

subarachnoid

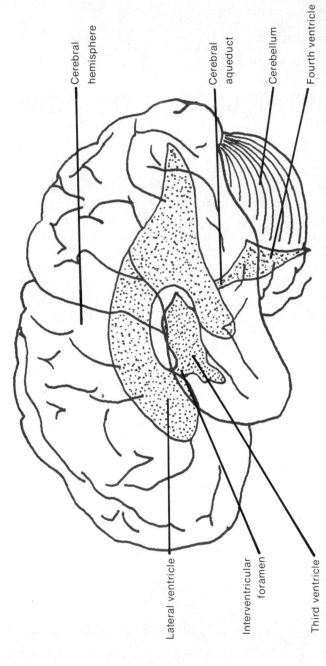

Figure 4–5. Ventricles of brain, lateral view. (Redrawn from Curtis: Introduction to the Neurosciences. Philadelphia, W. B. Saunders Co.)

Cerebral hemisphere

Cerebral aqueduct

Cerebellum

Fourth ventricle

Lateral ventricle

Interventricular foramen

Third ventricle

The cerebrospinal fluid circulating through the subarachnoid space surrounding the brain is originally elaborated in the _____ of the brain.

QUESTION
26

ventricles

ANSWER

THE COMMISSURAL TRACTS IN THE CEREBRUM: LOCATION

ITEM 10

Figure 4–6, a horizontal section through the cerebral hemispheres, shows the location of several important tracts of the brain. Notice the two segments of the corpus callosum, the prominent commissural tract which joins the two hemispheres. The *genu* of the corpus callosum appears anterior to the lateral ventricles, and the *splenium* of the corpus callosum appears posterior to the third ventricle. The anterior column of a second commissural tract, the *fornix*, can be seen posterior to the genu of the corpus callosum.

The corpus callosum is (circle one)
A. an association tract
B. a commissural tract
C. a projection tract

QUESTION
27

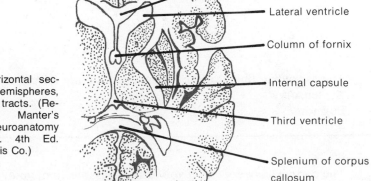

Figure 4–6. Horizontal section through cerebral hemispheres, showing commissural tracts. (Redrawn from Gatz: Manter's Essentials of Clinical Neuroanatomy and Neurophysiology. 4th Ed. Philadelphia, F. A. Davis Co.)

Genu of corpus callosum

Lateral ventricle

Column of fornix

Internal capsule

Third ventricle

Splenium of corpus callosum

ANSWER   The correct answer is B. This commissural tract extends from one hemisphere to the other. Association tracts, on the other hand, extend from gyrus to gyrus within a hemisphere and are involved in the elaborate functional correlation of diverse cortical operations within a single hemisphere. The projection tracts, you should recall, communicate between brain and spinal cord.

ITEM 11   THE INTERNAL CAPSULE

Turn back to Figure 4–6 and note the location of the *internal capsule,* an important projection tract. The internal capsule is a prominent band of ascending sensory and descending motor fibers connecting the brain and the spinal cord. The region of the internal capsule is clinically important because rupture of a small blood vessel in the area (stroke) can interfere with efferent tracts descending from the cortex, with resultant paralysis. Rupture of a small vessel in this area can also interfere with afferent tracts, resulting in sensory loss.

QUESTION 28   A cerebrovascular accident in the area of the internal capsule can cause paralysis by interfering with the (circle one)
A. ascending tracts
B. descending tracts

ANSWER   The correct answer is B. The descending tracts are efferent, or motor, fibers from the cortex to the spinal cord. Interruption of the conduction of motor impulses, occasioned by a stroke in one of the hemispheres, can affect motor control on the opposite side of the body.

QUESTION 29   The ascending fibers of the internal capsule are (circle one)
A. sensory
B. motor

ANSWER   The correct answer is A. If you missed this question, you were just not thinking. As pointed out in the answer to Question 28, the motor fibers of the internal capsule descend from brain to spinal cord. The ascending fibers are afferent, bringing sensation from the spinal cord to the cerebral cortex.

THE BASAL GANGLIA   ITEM 12

The *basal ganglia* are paired masses of gray matter, or nuclei, embedded in the white matter of the cerebral hemispheres. Figure 4–7, a horizontal section through the cerebrum, shows three of these subcortical nuclei: the *caudate nucleus,* the *putamen,* and the *globus pallidus.* Acting together, these nuclei modify muscular activity by facilitating or inhibiting motor neurons as particular muscle movements demand.

The basal ganglia are subcortical _____ which facilitate or inhibit innervation to _____.

QUESTION 30

nuclei . . . muscles

ANSWER

As a review of the major nuclei and tracts of the brain, write in the numbered spaces the names of the corresponding numbered structures on the diagram on page 174. Consult Figures 4–6 and 4–7 only if you find it necessary to do so.

QUESTION 31

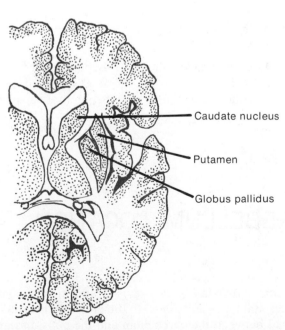

Figure 4–7. Horizontal section through cerebral hemispheres, showing basal ganglia. (Redrawn from Gatz: Manter's Essentials of Clinical Neuroanatomy and Neurophysiology. 4th Ed. Philadelphia, F. A. Davis Co.)

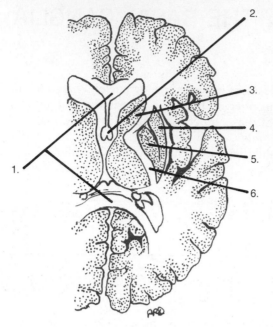

(Redrawn from Gatz: Manter's Essentials of Clinical Neuroanatomy and Neurophysiology. 4th Ed. Philadelphia, F. A. Davis Co.)

Labels

1. _____
2. _____
3. _____
4. _____
5. _____
6. _____

ANSWER

1. corpus callosum   4. putamen
2. fornix   5. globus pallidus
3. caudate nucleus   6. internal capsule

ITEM 13   THE CEREBELLUM: LOCATION

The *cerebellum,* shown in Figure 4–8, is located in the posterior cranial fossa, inferior to the occipital lobes and dorsal to the pons and medulla. The fourth ventricle is interposed between the cerebellum and the pons and medulla. Superior, middle, and inferior *cerebellar peduncles,* or nerve tracts, connect the cerebellum to the midbrain, pons, and medulla, respectively.

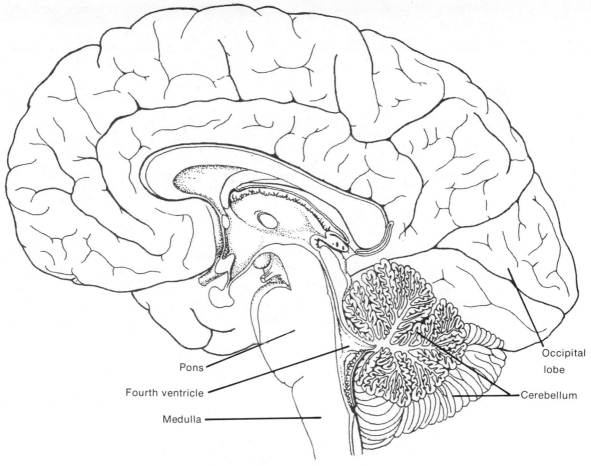

Figure 4–8. Brain, medial aspect, showing location of cerebellum. (Redrawn from Wolf-Heidegger: Atlas of Systematic Human Anatomy. Vol. III. Basel, S. Karger AG.)

The region of the cranium in which the cerebellum is situated is called the _____ _____ fossa.

QUESTION 32

---

posterior cranial

ANSWER

The ventricle of the brain between the cerebellum and the brain stem is the _____ ventricle.

QUESTION 33

---

fourth

ANSWER

The cerebellar peduncles are three separate nerve tracts connecting the cerebellum with three different regions of the brain stem as follows: the superior cerebellar peduncle connects with the _____; the middle cerebellar

QUESTION 34

peduncle connects with the _____; and the inferior cerebellar peduncle connects with the _____.

ANSWER   midbrain . . . pons . . . medulla

ITEM 14   STRUCTURES OF THE CEREBELLUM

The cerebellum is composed of two lateral *cerebellar hemispheres,* which fuse near the midline in a narrow portion called the *vermis.* The surface of the hemispheres is deeply grooved to form concentric folds called *folia.* The right side of the body is under the influence of the right cerebellar hemisphere and the left side under the influence of the left hemisphere, an arrangement in direct contrast to the contralateral influence of the cerebral hemispheres. The efferent and afferent pathways of the cerebellum are involved in coordination of the action of muscle groups throughout the body and in the maintenance of equilibrium.

QUESTION 35   The vermis is the portion near the midline where the two cerebellar _____ fuse.

ANSWER   hemispheres

QUESTION 36   The anatomical term by which the folds of the external cerebellar cortex are designated is _____.

ANSWER   folia

QUESTION 37   The functions of the cerebellum include coordination of the action of groups of _____ and maintenance of _____.

ANSWER   muscles . . . equilibrium

QUESTION 38   The right cerebellar hemisphere exerts control over the _____ side of the body; the right cerebral hemisphere, over the _____ side.

ANSWER   right (same) . . . left (opposite)

STRUCTURES OF THE DIENCEPHALON: LOCATION OF THE THALAMUS

ITEM 15

The superiormost part of the brain stem is the diencephalon. Two important structures of the diencephalon are the *thalamus* and the *hypothalamus*. The thalamus, as can be seen in Figure 4–9, comprises paired groups of nuclei located near the midline of each cerebral hemisphere, lateral to the third ventricle.

The diencephalon is part of the *brain stem/cerebrum* (circle one).

QUESTION 39

---

brain stem

ANSWER

The fluid filled cavity separating the right thalamus from the left thalamus is the slitlike _____ ventricle.

QUESTION 40

---

third

ANSWER

STRUCTURES OF THE THALAMUS

ITEM 16

The nuclei which make up the thalamus are cell bodies of neurons in the ascending sensory pathways from the spinal cord to the brain. The thalamus serves as a relay station for afferent impulses making their way to the cerebral cortex. Thus, in the thalamus, fibers carrying sensations of pain, temperature, pressure, and touch make their final synapse with other cell bodies which send processes to the postcentral gyrus. The postcentral gyrus, you will recall, is the sensory area of the cerebral cortex.

The thalamus contains call bodies of neurons which carry sensory impulses from the _____ _____ to the _____.

QUESTION 41

---

spinal cord . . . brain

ANSWER

The area of the brain to which the thalamus relays sensations of pain, temperature, and pressure is the (circle one)
A. postcentral gyrus
B. precentral gyrus

QUESTION 42

The correct answer is A. The postcentral gyrus is the sensory area of the brain, located posterior to the central sulcus in the parietal lobe. The precentral gyrus is a motor area in the frontal lobe, anterior to the central sulcus.

ITEM 17   THE HYPOTHALAMUS

The hypothalamus, shown in Figure 4–10, is the most ventral portion of the diencephalon. It forms the floor and lower lateral walls of the third ventricle. The hypothalamus is composed of a group of nuclei situated in a roughly triangular area inferior to the thalamus.

Although it is a relatively small area of the brain, the hypothalamus is involved in an amazingly large number of vital functions. Nuclei in the hypothalamus, with their afferent and efferent tracts, have a regulatory influence on the rate of the heart and its contractile strength, on gastrointestinal motility and secretory activity, and on certain metabolic functions.

QUESTION
43

Nuclei of the hypothalamus are associated with (circle one)

A. afferent nerve tracts only
B. efferent nerve tracts only
C. afferent and efferent tracts

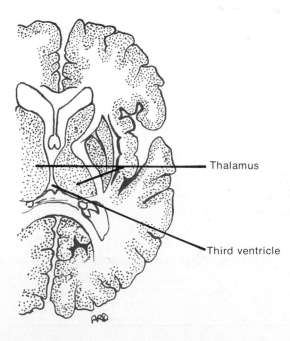

Figure 4–9. Horizontal section through cerebral hemispheres, showing location of thalamus. (Redrawn from Gatz: Manter's Essentials of Clinical Neuroanatomy and Neurophysiology. 4th Ed. Philadelphia, F. A. Davis Co.)

Thalamus

Third ventricle

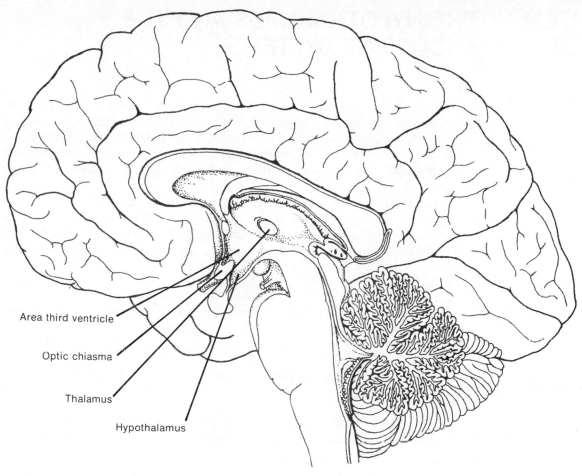

Area third ventricle

Optic chiasma

Thalamus

Hypothalamus

Figure 4–10. Right half of brain, medial aspect, showing location of the hypothalamus. (Redrawn from Wolf-Heidegger: Atlas of Systematic Human Anatomy. Vol. III. Basel, S. Karger AG.)

The correct answer is C.

ANSWER

Important visceral activities which the hypothalamus has a part in regulating include (1) the rate and contractile strength of the _____, (2) motility and secretory activity of the _____ system, and (3) a number of _____ functions.

QUESTION
44

heart . . . gastrointestinal . . . metabolic

ANSWER

The hypothalamus is located inferior to the _____ and ventro-lateral to the _____ ventricle of the brain.

QUESTION
45

thalamus . . . third

ANSWER

ITEM 18

THE HYPOTHALAMUS AND THE ENDOCRINE SYSTEMS

The hypothalamus serves as a neural "funnel" to channel input from the central nervous system into hormonal mechanisms. The hormonal mechanisms, in turn, regulate visceral activity. The hypothalamus is strategically located just above the *hypophysis,* or pituitary gland. Through its neural and vascular connections with the hypophysis, the hypothalamus exerts its control over the endocrine system.

Some nuclei of the hypothalamus, such as those which regulate such diverse conditions as body temperature, appetite, and satiety, do not directly involve endocrine function. The hypothalamus is also implicated in behavioral and visceral expressions of many emotional states, such as flushing, and gastrointestinal disturbance.

QUESTION 46

The hypothalamus exercises its influence over endocrine systems via its communication with the _____.

ANSWER

hypophysis (pituitary gland)

QUESTION 47

Nonendocrine regulatory functions of the hypothalamus include control of the _____ of the body and of _____ for food.

ANSWER

temperature . . . appetite

QUESTION 48

The hypothalamus controls visceral activities indirectly in that efferent impulses from the central nervous system are funneled through the hypothalamus into _____ mechanisms.

ANSWER

hormonal (endocrine)

QUESTION 49

The hypothalamus is implicated in the visceral disturbances accompanying many states of _____.

ANSWER

emotion

STRUCTURES OF THE DIENCEPHALON AND MIDBRAIN

ITEM 19

On the ventral aspect of the brain stem, shown in Figure 4–11, a number of important structures in the region of the diencephalon and midbrain can be seen. Notice the *cerebral peduncle,* or crus cerebri, on each side of the midbrain and in the area where the midbrain merges with the diencephalon. These peduncles comprise ascending and descending projection tracts which extend upward to become continuous with fibers of the internal capsule.

The part of the brain stem immediately inferior to the diencephalon and cerebral hemispheres and immediately superior to the pons is called the _____.

QUESTION
50

---

midbrain

ANSWER

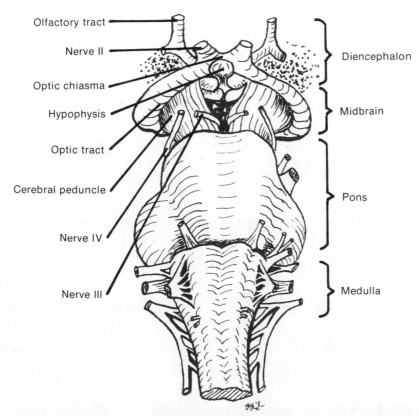

Figure 4–11. Brain stem, ventral aspect, showing structures of diencephalon and midbrain. (Redrawn and modified from Truex and Carpenter: Strong and Elwyn's Human Neuroanatomy. 5th Ed. Baltimore, The Williams and Wilkins Co.)

QUESTION
51

The cerebral peduncles are (circle one)

A. association tracts   B. commissural tracts   C. projection tracts

ANSWER

The correct answer is C. Projection tracts connect the spinal cord and brain stem with cerebral centers. Association tracts, on the other hand, are confined within a single hemisphere, while commissural tracts connect the two hemispheres.

QUESTION
52

The cerebral peduncles are continuous with fibers of the _____ capsule.

ANSWER

internal

QUESTION
53

The cerebral peduncles carry (circle one)

A. ascending fibers only
B. descending fibers only
C. ascending and descending fibers

ANSWER

The correct answer is C. The cerebral peduncles are continuous with the internal capsule, and contain ascending sensory fibers as well as descending motor fibers.

ITEM 20   THE INTERPEDUNCULAR FOSSA

Look back to Figure 4–11 and notice the region between the cerebral peduncles. This area is called the *interpeduncular fossa*. This fossa contains the *hypophysis* (pituitary gland) and the point of emergence of the *oculomotor* (third cranial) *nerve*. Also notice in Figure 4–11, anterior to the cerebral peduncles, the location of the *optic* (second cranial) *nerves;* their prominent crossing, the *optic chiasma;* and the *optic tract*. Anterior to the optic nerves, the *olfactory tract* is seen. Also observe in Figure 4–11 how the *trochlear* (fourth cranial) *nerve,* after emerging from the dorsal aspect of the brain stem, appears on the ventral surface at the upper level of the pons.

QUESTION
54

The hypophysis is located in the area between the cerebral peduncles called the _____ fossa.

ANSWER

interpeduncular

QUESTION
55

The optic nerves (II), optic chiasma, and optic tract lie (circle one)

A. within the interpeduncular fossa
B. anterior to the cerebral peduncles

The correct answer is B, as a quick glance at Figure 4–11 will show.   *ANSWER*

The trochlear nerve (IV) emerges from the   QUESTION
A. dorsal surface of the brain stem   56
B. ventral surface of the brain stem

The correct answer is A. Although the fourth cranial nerve curves around   *ANSWER*
the brain stem to appear on the ventral surface where the upper level of the pons
joins the midbrain, its point of emergence is on the dorsal surface.

In the numbered spaces below write the names of the corresponding numbered   QUESTION
structures on the accompanying diagram.   57

Labels

1. _____
2. _____
3. _____
4. _____
5. _____
6. _____

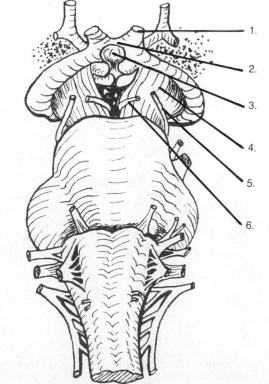

(Redrawn and modified from Truex and
Carpenter: Strong and Elwyn's Human Neuro-
anatomy. 5th Ed. Baltimore, The Williams and
Wilkins Co.)

1. optic nerve (II)
2. optic chiasma
3. hypophysis (pituitary gland)

4. cerebral peduncle
5. trochlear nerve (IV)
6. oculomotor nerve (III)

ITEM 21   THE PONS

The pons, seen from the ventral aspect in Figure 4–12, presents a distinct band of transverse fibers which appear to extend from the cerebellar hemispheres, dorsal to the pons, around the brain stem. The ventral surface of the pons, which occupies the basilar part of the occipital bone, is grooved longitudinally for the *basilar artery,* one of the arteries to the brain. A prominent feature of the pons is the emergence of the fifth cranial nerve, the *trigeminal nerve.* On a horizontal line between the pons and the medulla, three more cranial nerves can be seen emerging: the *abducens* (VI), *facial* (VII), and *vestibulocochlear* (VIII) nerves.

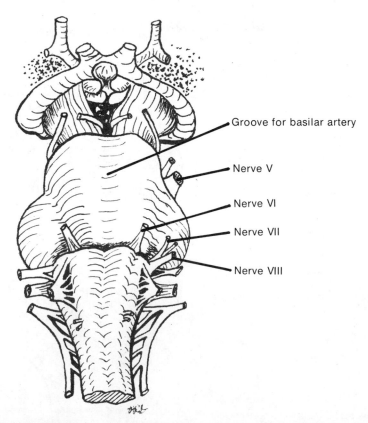

Groove for basilar artery

Nerve V

Nerve VI

Nerve VII

Nerve VIII

Figure 4–12.   Brain stem, ventral aspect, showing structures of pons. (Redrawn and modified from Truex and Carpenter: Strong and Elwyn's Human Neuroanatomy. 5th Ed. Baltimore, The Williams and Wilkins Co.)

The prominent longitudinal groove on the ventral surface of the pons is the groove for the _____ artery.

---

basilar

The most prominent cranial nerve seen emerging from the ventral surface of the pons is the _____ nerve.

---

trigeminal (V)

The cranial nerves emerging between the pons and medulla are the _____ nerve, the _____ nerve, and the _____ nerve.

---

abducens (VI) . . . facial (VII) . . . vestibulocochlear (VIII)

In the numbered spaces on page 186 write in the names of the corresponding numbered structures on the diagram below.

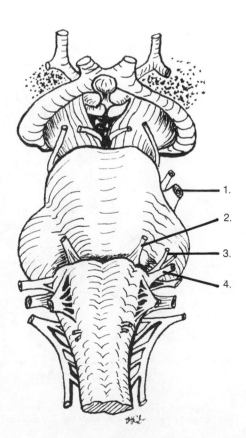

(Redrawn and modified from Truex and Carpenter: Strong and Elwyn's Human Neuro-anatomy. 5th Ed. Baltimore, The Williams and Wilkins Co.)

Labels

1. _____ nerve
2. _____ nerve
3. _____ nerve
4. _____ nerve

ANSWER

1. trigeminal (V)
2. abducens (VI)

3. facial (VII)
4. vestibulocochlear (VIII)

ITEM 22   THE MEDULLA

The medulla, seen from the ventral aspect in Figure 4–13, is the lower region of the brain stem. Notice the longitudinal groove at the midline of the medulla, the *anterior median fissure*. Two additional grooves, the *anterolateral sulcus* and the *posterolateral sulcus,* run parallel and lateral to this median fissure. The anterolateral sulcus is the site of emergence of the hypoglossal (twelfth cranial) nerve.

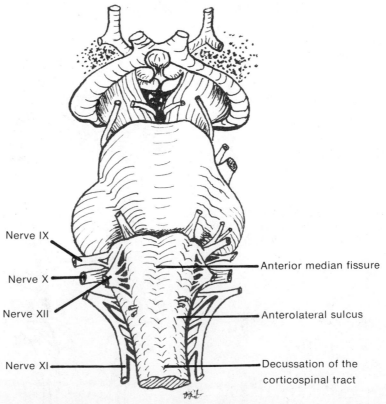

Nerve IX

Nerve X

Nerve XII

Nerve XI

Anterior median fissure

Anterolateral sulcus

Decussation of the corticospinal tract

Figure 4–13.   Medulla, ventral aspect. (Redrawn and modified from Truex and Carpenter: Strong and Elwyn's Human Neuroanatomy. 5th Ed. Baltimore, The Williams and Wilkins Co.)

The posterolateral sulcus, which is hidden in Figure 4–13, carries the glosso-pharyngeal (ninth cranial) nerve, the vagus (tenth cranial) nerve, and the accessory (eleventh cranial) nerve.

The glossopharyngeal (IX), vagus (X), and accessory (XI) nerves emerge from the _____ sulcus; the hypoglossal nerve (XII) emerges from the _____ sulcus.

QUESTION
62

---

posterolateral . . . anterolateral

ANSWER

The longitudinal groove along the midline of the medulla is called the _____ _____ fissure.

QUESTION
63

---

anterior median

ANSWER

THE CORTICOSPINAL TRACT   ITEM 23

Look back to Figure 4–13 and observe the prominent *decussation of the corticospinal tract*. Fibers of this projection tract extend from the motor cortex in the precentral gyrus of the cerebrum through the internal capsule, midbrain, and pons. In the medulla, most of the fibers of the corticospinal tract cross in the decussation to reach anterior horn cells in the spinal cord below.

Motor fibers of the corticospinal tract originate in the _____ gyrus of the cerebrum.

QUESTION
64

---

precentral

ANSWER

Structures through which fibers of the corticospinal tract pass en route to the medulla where they decussate are the _____ capsule, the _____, and the _____.

QUESTION
65

---

internal . . . midbrain . . . pons

ANSWER

In the decussation, most of the fibers of the corticospinal tract _____ before extending to the anterior horn cells in the _____ _____.

ANSWER

cross . . . spinal cord

ITEM 24 THE NUCLEI OF CRANIAL NERVES IN THE BRAIN STEM

Located in the diencephalon, midbrain, pons, and medulla are various aggregates of nerve cell bodies. These nuclei are associated with the cranial nerves. The cranial nerves are treated in some detail in Unit Five, where their central connections are discussed. This item serves as a transition from Unit Four to Unit Five by pointing out the localization of the various cranial nerve nuclei in the brain stem.

With the single exception of the olfactory nerve (I), all cranial nerves have nuclei in the brain stem; their sites of emergence have been illustrated in various items of this unit. The nucleus of the optic nerve (II) is in the diencephalon; nuclei of the oculomotor (III) and trochlear (IV) nerves are in the midbrain. Nuclei of the trigeminal nerve (V) are located throughout the midbrain, pons, medulla, and the upper cervical spinal cord. Nuclei of the abducens (VI), facial (VII), and vestibulocochlear (VIII) nerves are in the pons; nuclei of the glossopharyngeal, vagus, accessory, and hypoglossal nerves (IX, X, XI, and XII) are in the medulla.

QUESTION
67
As a review of the sites of emergence of the cranial nerves, write in the numbered spaces below the names of the corresponding nerves in the accompanying diagram.

Labels

1. _____ nerve
2. _____ nerve
3. _____ nerve
4. _____ nerve
5. _____ nerve
6. _____ nerve
7. _____ nerve
8. _____ nerve
9. _____ nerve
10. _____ nerve
11. _____ nerve
12. _____ nerve

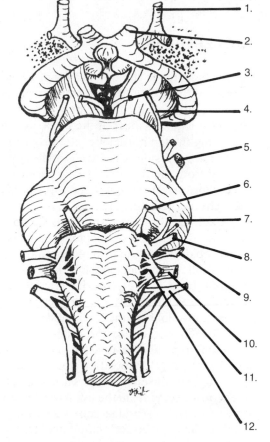

1.
2.
3.
4.
5.
6.
7.
8.
9.
10.
11.
12.

(Redrawn and modified from Truex and Carpenter: Strong and Elwyn's Human Neuro-anatomy. 5th Ed. Baltimore, The Williams and Wilkins Co.)

1. olfactory (I)	7. facial (VII)
2. optic (II)	8. vestibulocochlear (VII)
3. oculomotor (III)	9. glossopharyngeal (IX)
4. trochlear (IV)	10. vagus (X)
5. trigeminal (V)	11. accessory (XI)
6. abducens (VI)	12. hypoglossal (XII)

ANSWER

SUMMARY OF UNIT FOUR

The brain includes two cerebral hemispheres, the cerebellum and the brain stem. The brain stem is subdivided into diencephalon, midbrain, pons, and medulla. The substance of the brain is made up of nuclei and tracts. Nuclei are groups of cell bodies of neurons which have related functions within the brain. Tracts are bundles of nerve cell processes which provide afferent and efferent connections between the different areas of the brain and between the brain and the spinal cord.

THE CEREBRUM

The cortex is the outer layer of brain cells. Fiber tracts and nuclei form the interior of the cerebrum. The outer surface of the cerebrum is composed of a series of convolutions called gyri, between which run furrows or grooves called sulci. From the lateral aspect of the brain a deep groove, the lateral fissure, is seen demarcating the temporal lobe inferiorly from the frontal and parietal lobes superiorly. The central sulcus is a transverse groove which separates the frontal lobe anteriorly from the parietal lobe posteriorly. The most prominent of the grooves in the cerebrum is the longitudinal fissure which extends down the midline, separating the right and left hemispheres.

Each cerebral hemisphere is composed of five lobes: (1) the frontal lobe occupies the anterior cranial fossa and lies deep to the frontal bone; (2) the parietal lobe is posterior to the frontal lobe and occupies a region deep to the parietal bone of the skull; (3) the occipital lobe is posterior to the parietal lobe and lies deep to the occipital bone in the posterior cranial fossa; (4) the temporal lobe occupies the middle cranial fossa in a region deep to the temporal bone; (5) the insula is deep to the temporal lobe at the lateral fissure.

The fiber tracts of the brain are bundles of nerve cell processes having a common origin and destination. The three general types of fiber tracts are: (1) projection tracts, (2) association tracts, and (3) commissural tracts. Projection tracts are composed of sensory fibers ascending from the spinal cord to the brain or motor fibers descending from the brain to the spinal cord. Association tracts extend from gyrus to gyrus or bridge across several gyri, always remaining within the same cerebral hemisphere. Commissural tracts extend from one cerebral hemisphere to the other. The most prominent commissural tract is the corpus callosum.

The ventricles are cavities within brain substance which contain cerebrospinal fluid. This fluid, which circulates through ventricles and subarachnoid space, serves as a protective shock-absorber. There are two lateral ventricles, the slitlike third ventricle, and the fourth ventricle. The ventricles interconnect and are continuous with subarachnoid space. The lateral ventricles connect with the third ventricle through interventricular foramina. The connecting passage between the third and fourth ventricles is the cerebral aqueduct. The fourth ventricle communicates with subarachnoid space through a single medial and two lateral apertures.

In a horizontal section through the cerebral hemispheres, one can observe the vital internal capsule, which is composed of ascending and descending projection tracts connecting the cerebrum with the spinal cord. Also visible in a horizontal section are paired nuclei called basal ganglia, which are embedded in the cerebral hemispheres. Three of the more important basal ganglia are the caudate nucleus, the putamen, and the globus pallidus. This group of nuclei modify motor control of the skeletal muscles.

THE CEREBELLUM

The cerebellum is located in the posteriormost part of the posterior cranial fossa, deep to the occipital bone. The surface of the cerebellum shows narrow convolutions, or folia. The two cerebellar hemispheres join in an area called the vermis. Cerebellar peduncles connect the cerebellum with various regions of the brain stem. The cerebellum functions in connection with coordination of muscle actions and maintenance of equilibrium.

THE DIENCEPHALON AND MIDBRAIN

The superiormost region of the brain stem is the diencephalon, in which the thalamus and hypothalamus are located. The thalamus is situated between the internal capsule laterally and the third ventricle medially. This bilateral aggregation of nuclei is an important site of synapses of ascending fiber tracts. In the thalamus, neurons carrying pain, temperature, touch, and pressure sensations make their final synaptic connections before reaching the postcentral gyrus, the sensory area of the cerebral cortex. The hypothalamus is a group of nuclei and tracts inferior to the thalamus; it forms the floor and part of the lower lateral walls of the third ventricle. The hypothalamus is involved with neural input into the hypophysis and is an extremely important area for regulation of visceral activity.

The ventral surface of the midbrain forms the cerebral peduncles, two prominent projection tracts between the cerebrum and the spinal cord. The area between the cerebral peduncles, called the interpeduncular fossa, contains the hypophysis. The optic nerves (II) and their crossing, the optic chiasma, are anterior to the cerebral peduncles. The oculomotor nerve (III) makes its superficial exit from the brain near the midline between the midbrain and the pons. The trochlear (IV) nerve emerges dorsally and extends around the midbrain ventrally in the same region.

THE PONS AND MEDULLA

The pons resembles a wide band of fibers continuous with the cerebellum. The groove for the basilar artery extends longitudinally on the ventral surface of the pons. The prominent fibers of the trigeminal nerve (V) make their superficial exit from the ventrolateral region of the pons. At the juncture between the pons and medulla, the abducens (VI), facial (VII), and vestibulocochlear (VIII) nerves exit. Four cranial nerves emerge from the ventral surface of the medulla: the glossopharyngeal (IX), vagus (X), and accessory (XI) nerves, from the posterolateral sulcus; the hypoglossal (XII) nerve, from the anterolateral sulcus.

Fibers of the corticospinal tract, extending from the precentral gyrus of the cerebral cortex through the midbrain and pons, decussate, or cross, in the medulla before descending to the spinal cord.

Located in the medulla and pons, as well as in the midbrain and diencephalon, are various aggregates of nerve cell bodies, or nuclei, associated with the cranial nerves.

The main divisions of the brain include the two _____ hemispheres, the _____, and the brain _____.

QUESTION
68

ANSWER   cerebral . . . cerebellum . . . stem

QUESTION   The four subdivisions of the brain stem are the _____, the
69   _____, the _____, and the _____.

ANSWER   diencephalon . . . midbrain . . . pons . . . medulla (in any order)

QUESTION   Nuclei of the brain are aggregates of nerve cell _____; tracts are
70   bundles of nerve cell _____.

ANSWER   bodies . . . processes (fibers)

QUESTION   A group of cell bodies of neurons having related functions is called a_____
71   _____; a group of nerve cell processes having a common origin and destination
             is called a _____.

ANSWER   nucleus . . . tract

QUESTION   The surface layer of the cerebral hemispheres is called the cerebral _____
72   _____.

ANSWER   cortex

QUESTION   The interior of the cerebrum is made up of _____ and _____.
73

ANSWER   nuclei . . . tracts

QUESTION   Convolutions on the surface of the cerebrum are called _____; furrows be-
74   tween the convolutions are called _____.

ANSWER   gyri . . . sulci

QUESTION   The prominent horizontal groove on the lateral surface of each cerebral hemi-
75   sphere is called the _____ fissure; the vertical groove visible on the
             lateral surface is the _____ sulcus; the midline groove separating the
             two hemispheres is called the _____ fissure.

ANSWER   lateral . . . central . . . longitudinal

Anterior to the parietal lobe of the brain is the _____ lobe; posterior to the parietal lobe is the _____ lobe; inferior to the parietal lobe is the _____ lobe.

---

frontal . . . occipital . . . temporal

Ascending and descending tracts between brain and spinal cord are _____ _____ tracts; tracts from gyrus to gyrus within a hemisphere are _____ tracts; tracts between the two hemispheres are _____ tracts.

---

projection . . . association . . . commissural

The ventricles of the brain are cavities which are involved in the elaboration, circulation, and reabsorption of _____ fluid.

---

cerebrospinal

The lateral ventricles communicate with the third ventricle through _____ foramina; the third ventricle with the fourth ventricle through the cerebral _____; the fourth ventricle with subarachnoid space through lateral and medial _____.

---

interventricular . . . aqueduct . . . apertures

The tightly packed band of ascending and descending projection tracts within the substance of the brain is called the internal _____.

---

capsule

The globus pallidus, putamen, and caudate nucleus are referred to collectively as the _____ ganglia.

---

basal

The nucleus in the diencephalon where most ascending sensory fiber tracts synapse is the _____.

---

thalamus

QUESTION
83

The structure of the diencephalon responsible for neural input into the endocrine system is the _____.

ANSWER

hypothalamus

QUESTION
84

The two ascending and descending projection tracts which primarily constitute the ventral surface of the midbrain are called cerebral _____.

ANSWER

peduncles

QUESTION
85

Viewed from the ventral aspect of the brain stem, the optic nerve (II) and the olfactory tract are anterior to the _____ _____.

ANSWER

cerebral peduncles

QUESTION
86

The oculomotor nerve (III) makes its superficial exit near the midline between the _____ and the _____.

ANSWER

midbrain . . . pons

QUESTION
87

The cranial nerve which exits on the dorsal surface of the midbrain and extends around the brain stem to appear on the ventral surface is the _____ _____ nerve.

ANSWER

trochlear (IV)

QUESTION
88

The abducens (VI), facial (VII), and vestibulocochlear (VIII) nerves make their superficial exit on a horizontal line between the _____ and the _____.

ANSWER

pons . . . medulla

QUESTION
89

The trigeminal nerve (V) exits from the ventrolateral surface of the _____.

ANSWER

pons

The glossopharyngeal (IX), vagus (X), and accessory (XI) nerves emerge from the posterolateral sulcus of the _____; the hypoglossal (XII) nerve emerges from the anterolateral sulcus of the _____.

---

medulla . . . medulla

Fibers of the _____ tract decussate, or cross, in the medulla before extending down to the spinal cord.

---

corticospinal

Unit Five □ THE CRANIAL NERVES

| ITEM 1 | THE CRANIAL NERVES: INTRODUCTION |

The twelve pairs of cranial nerves provide afferent (sensory) and efferent (motor) connections between the brain stem and innervated structures. Most of the cranial nerves extend to structures of the head and neck. The vagus nerve, however, has processes which extend to viscera in the thorax and abdomen.

This unit will present an overview of the cranial nerves. The four cranial nerves particularly relevant to the practice of dentistry will receive more detailed treatment in subsequent units. These nerves are the trigeminal, or fifth cranial, nerve; the facial, or seventh cranial, nerve; the glossopharyngeal, or ninth cranial, nerve; and the vagus nerve, also known as the tenth cranial.

The discussion in this unit will emphasize the locations of the cranial nerves, their pathways from origin to destination, and the major structures which they innervate. Classification of fiber types in terms of functional components will also be introduced in this unit.

QUESTION 1

While the cranial nerves mainly innervate the head and neck, one of the cranial nerves also innervates viscera of the thorax and abdomen, namely the _____ nerve.

ANSWER

vagus

QUESTION 2

The four cranial nerves of special significance for dental anatomy are the _____ nerve, the _____ nerve, the _____ _____ nerve, and the _____ nerve.

ANSWER   trigeminal . . . facial . . . glossopharyngeal . . . vagus (in any order)

TERMINOLOGY: NUCLEUS

ITEM 2

Several specific terms are used in describing aggregates of nerve cell bodies found in the central nervous system, and their processes. The term *nucleus* applies to an aggregate of nerve cell bodies located within the central nervous system (brain and spinal cord). Nuclei containing nerve cell bodies of motor neurons of the cranial nerves are located in the midbrain, pons, and medulla. Other nuclei in the central nervous system are associated with sensory neurons. The latter nuclei form regions of synaptic connection along the sensory pathway from the periphery to the thalamus and cerebrum.

A group of nerve cell bodies within the central nervous system is called a _____ .

QUESTION 3

nucleus

ANSWER

Nuclei are associated with both _____ and _____ neurons.

QUESTION 4

motor . . . sensory (in either order)

ANSWER

Motor nuclei of cranial nerves are located in the _____ , in the _____ , and in the _____ .

QUESTION 5

midbrain . . . pons . . . medulla (in any order)

ANSWER

TERMINOLOGY: GANGLION

ITEM 3

A *ganglion* is a group of nerve cell bodies situated outside the brain and spinal cord. Some of these ganglia contain cell bodies of sensory neurons carrying special and general sensations from periphery to brain. Other ganglia associated with the cranial nerves belong to the parasympathetic division of the autonomic nervous system. These parasympathetic ganglia contain cell bodies of postganglionic motor neurons, whose peripheral processes distribute to smooth muscle, cardiac muscle, and glands.

QUESTION
6

A group of nerve cell bodies within the central nervous system is called a _____, while such an aggregate outside the central nervous system is called a _____.

ANSWER

nucleus . . . ganglion

QUESTION
7

The types of cell bodies which may be found in ganglia are those of (circle one)
A. sensory neurons only
B. motor neurons only
C. either sensory or motor neurons

ANSWER

The correct answer is C. Some ganglia contain bodies of sensory neurons; other ganglia, cell bodies of motor neurons.

QUESTION
8

Ganglia of the parasympathetic division of the autonomic nervous system contain cell bodies of *sensory/motor* (circle one) neurons.

ANSWER

motor

QUESTION
9

Motor neurons of the parasympathetic division distribute to _____ muscle, _____ muscle, or to _____.

ANSWER

smooth . . . cardiac . . . glands

ITEM 4   TERMINOLOGY: TRACT, NERVE, AND PLEXUS

A *tract* is defined as a group of nerve cell processes within the central nervous system. Tracts have a common origin and destination and occupy a definite position, but do not always constitute a compact bundle, since fibers from various tracts may be mingled.

A *nerve* is defined as a bundle of neuronal processes outside the central nervous system. Some nerves are totally sensory; some, totally motor; some mixed.

A *plexus,* also located outside the central nervous system, is a site of intermingling and regrouping of peripheral nerve fibers deriving from diverse origins.

Place a checkmark before structures which are situated outside the central nervous system

(   ) A. nerve
(   ) B. tract
(   ) C. plexus

QUESTION
10

You should have marked A and C.

ANSWER

A *tract/nerve* (circle one) usually forms a more compact bundle.

QUESTION
11

---

nerve

ANSWER

A network which regroups converging nerve fibers outside the central nervous system is called a *ganglion/plexus* (circle one).

QUESTION
12

---

plexus

ANSWER

FUNCTIONAL COMPONENTS OF THE CRANIAL NERVES

ITEM 5

Some cranial nerves are composed of a single type of fiber, referred to as a single *functional component*. Other cranial nerves contain several functional components. The terms used to identify functional components refer to the functions performed by each type of fiber contained within a given nerve.

As a class, the several specialized fiber types are referred to by the generic term, _____ _____.

QUESTION
13

---

functional components

ANSWER

ITEM 6

THE TYPES OF FUNCTIONAL COMPONENTS

The following descriptive terms are used within functional component terminology.

(1) *General, special.* The term *general* refers to stimuli conducted throughout the entire body, whereas *special* refers to stimuli conducted to or from structures associated with localized senses, e.g., sight, hearing, taste, and smell. General components are common to both cranial and spinal nerves, while special components are found in cranial nerves only.

(2) *Somatic, visceral. Somatic* refers to the skin and the muscles of the body wall, whereas *visceral* refers to organs within the body cavities.

(3) *Afferent, efferent. Afferent,* or sensory, means that the direction of conduction is toward the central nervous system; *efferent,* or motor, means that conduction is away from the central nervous system.

QUESTION 14

Functional components common to both cranial and spinal nerves are called _____, while those proper to cranial nerves only are called _____.

ANSWER

general . . . special

QUESTION 15

The adjective used to refer to functional components related to the skin and the muscles of body wall is _____; those components relating to organs within the body cavity are described as _____.

ANSWER

somatic . . . visceral

QUESTION 16

The direction of conduction of efferent neurons is *toward/away from* (circle one) the central nervous system; the direction of conduction of afferent neurons is *toward/away from* (circle one) the brain or spinal cord.

ANSWER

away from . . . toward

ITEM 7

GENERAL FUNCTIONAL COMPONENTS OF THE CRANIAL NERVES

When afferent fibers are termed *general afferent,* this means that these fibers carry sensations of pain, temperature, touch, and pressure from widely distributed receptors to the brain. The term *general,* as applied to efferent fibers, includes all motor fibers to skeletal muscles, smooth muscle, cardiac muscle, or glands.

Various combinations of the terms are used to describe the four general component types: *somatic, visceral, afferent,* and *efferent*: (1) general somatic afferent, abbreviated GSA; (2) general somatic efferent, abbreviated GSE; (3) general visceral afferent, abbreviated GVA; and (4) general visceral efferent, abbreviated GVE.

Fibers which carry impulses from receptors distributed generally over the body are called *general somatic* _____ or *general visceral* _____.

QUESTION
17

afferent . . . afferent

ANSWER

Motor impulses to skeletal muscles are carried by fibers which have a general somatic _____ component.

QUESTION
18

efferent

ANSWER

In the spaces provided, write the meanings of the following abbreviations.
1. GSA: _____
2. GSE: _____
3. GVA: _____
4. GVE: _____

QUESTION
19

1. GSA: general somatic afferent
2. GSE: general somatic efferent
3. GVA: general visceral afferent
4. GVE: general visceral efferent

ANSWER

GENERAL SOMATIC COMPONENTS   ITEM 8

General somatic afferent fibers transmit incoming sensations of pain, temperature, touch, and pressure from the body wall to the spinal cord and brain. GSA fibers also transmit proprioceptive impulses from skeletal muscles, tendons, and joint capsules to produce subconscious awareness of muscle tension and joint position.

General somatic efferent fibers convey motor impulses to skeletal muscles.

QUESTION
20
In addition to sensations of pain, temperature, pressure, and touch, proprioceptive impulses are also conveyed by GSA fibers from _____ muscles, from _____, and from _____ capsules.

ANSWER

skeletal . . . tendons . . . joint

QUESTION
21
Impulses carried outward to skeletal muscles travel over (circle one)
A. GSA fibers
B. GSE fibers

ANSWER

The correct answer is B. General somatic efferent, or GSE, fibers carry the motor impulses to skeletal muscles.

ITEM 9   GENERAL VISCERAL COMPONENTS

General visceral afferent fibers transmit pain from the viscera. GVA fibers also conduct specialized afferent impulses such as those concerned with blood pressure and regulation of other visceral activities.

General visceral efferent fibers transmit outgoing impulses to smooth muscle, cardiac muscle, or glands.

QUESTION
22
GVA fibers convey sensations of pain from _____, as well as incoming impulses associated with _____ pressure and other _____ activity.

ANSWER

viscera . . . blood . . . visceral

QUESTION
23
GVE fibers carry motor impulses to _____ muscle, to _____ muscle, or to _____.

ANSWER

smooth . . . cardiac . . . glands

SPECIAL FUNCTIONAL COMPONENTS OF THE CRANIAL NERVES

In addition to the four *general* functional components, which are common to both cranial and spinal nerves, there are also three *special* functional components which are found only in cranial nerves: special somatic afferent (SSA), special visceral afferent (SVA), and special visceral efferent (SVE). There are no special somatic efferent fibers.

SSA fibers are related to sight and hearing; SVA fibers, to taste and smell.

Place a checkmark before the type of fiber which has no *special* functional component

   (   ) A. somatic afferent
   (   ) B. somatic efferent
   (   ) C. visceral afferent
   (   ) D. visceral efferent

QUESTION
24

The checkmark should be placed before B. There are no special somatic efferent fibers.

ANSWER

Sight and hearing involve special _____ afferent fibers, while taste and touch involve special _____ afferent fibers.

QUESTION
25

---

somatic . . . visceral

ANSWER

SPECIAL VISCERAL EFFERENT COMPONENTS

Special visceral efferent fibers convey outgoing impulses to muscles embryologically derived from the mesoderm of branchial arches. These muscles include the muscles of mastication, the muscles of facial expression, and the muscles of the pharynx and larynx. The importance to dentistry of muscles supplied by SVE fibers is obvious.

SVE fibers are of special concern to dental practitioners because of the particular muscles which these fibers innervate, namely, the muscles of _____, the muscles of _____ expression, and muscles of the _____ and the _____.

QUESTION
26

ANSWER   mastication . . . facial . . . pharynx . . . larynx

QUESTION   Muscles embryologically derived from the mesoderm of branchial arches are
27   innervated by _____ _____ efferent fibers.

ANSWER   special visceral

ITEM 12   THE OLFACTORY NERVE

The *olfactory nerve* (cranial nerve I) transmits the sense of smell. It contains
only one functional component, special visceral afferent. Figure 5–1 illustrates
the route of the olfactory, or first cranial, nerve. The receptors for smell are
located in membranes which line the upper region of the nasal cavity. Fibers
ascend through the *cribriform plate* of the ethmoid bone and synapse in the
olfactory bulb on the undersurface of the frontal lobe. Processes of secondary
neurons then extend through the *olfactory tract* and brain substance to terminate

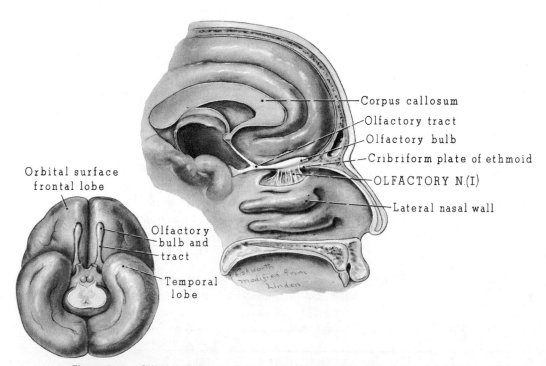

Figure 5–1. Olfactory nerve (I). (From Jacob and Francone: Structure and Function in Man. 3rd
Ed. Philadelphia, W. B. Saunders Co.)

in the uncus of the parahippocampal gyrus on the undersurface of the temporal lobe.

The single functional component of cranial nerve I is (circle one)
A. GSA: general somatic afferent
B. GVA: general somatic afferent
C. SSA: special somatic afferent
D. SVA: special visceral afferent

QUESTION
28

The correct answer is D, special visceral afferent. The sense of smell, like the sense of taste, is conveyed by SVA fibers.

ANSWER

The receptors for smell are located in the membranous lining of the upper _____ cavity.

QUESTION
29

---

nasal

ANSWER

Fibers of the olfactory nerve (I) synapse in the olfactory _____.

QUESTION
30

---

bulb

ANSWER

Secondary fibers whose cell bodies are located in the olfactory bulb are termed the olfactory _____.

QUESTION
31

---

tract

ANSWER

Central processes of olfactory fibers terminate in gyri located in the _____ lobe.

QUESTION
32

---

temporal

ANSWER

The olfactory nerve enters the skull through the _____ plate of the ethmoid bone.

QUESTION
33

---

cribriform

ANSWER

ITEM 13   THE OPTIC NERVE

Cranial nerve II, the *optic nerve,* transmits sight from the retina of the eye to the brain. The optic nerve contains a single functional component, which is special somatic afferent. Figure 5–2 shows the route of the optic nerve. Receptors for sight are located in the retina. After synapsing in the retina, the optic nerve extends posteriorly through the optic canal to enter the anterior cranial fossa. Once inside the cranial cavity, fibers of the nerve converge toward the *optic chiasma,* located just anterior and superior to the sella turcica. In the optic chiasma, medial fibers cross to join lateral fibers of the nerve from the opposite side. Fibers proximal to the optic chiasma are termed the *optic tract.*

QUESTION
34

Like the olfactory nerve (I), the optic nerve (II) conveys a single functional component; the single component of the optic nerve is special _____ afferent, whereas the single component of the olfactory nerve is special _____ afferent.

ANSWER

somatic . . . visceral

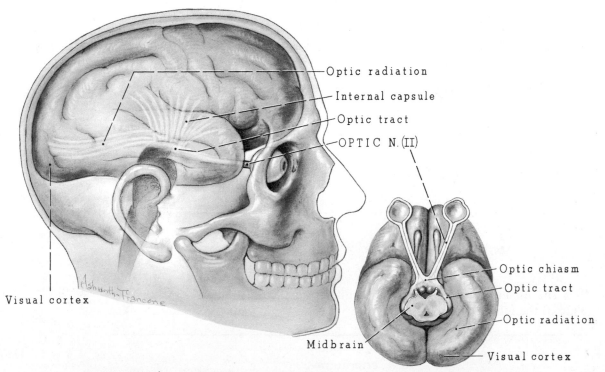

Figure 5–2.   Optic nerve (II). (From Jacob and Francone: Structure and Function in Man. 3rd Ed. Philadelphia, W. B. Saunders Co.)

The optic nerve synapses in the _____ of the eye.

---

retina

The optic nerve (II) enters the cranium through the _____ canal and converges posteromedially toward the optic _____.

---

optic . . . chiasma

In the optic chiasma, _____ fibers of each optic nerve cross to join _____ fibers of the opposite optic nerve.

---

medial . . . lateral

Fibers extending posteriorly from the optic chiasma toward the brain are termed the optic _____.

---

tract

THE OPTIC TRACT ITEM 14

The optic tract extends from the optic chiasma to the lateral geniculate body of the thalamus. Axons of neurons originating in the lateral geniculate body form *optic radiations,* indicated in Figure 5–2, which extend posteriorly to the *visual cortex* of the occipital lobe. When impulses reach the occipital cortex, visual awareness occurs.

Within the brain, the optic tract proper extends from the optic _____ to the lateral geniculate body of the _____.

---

chiasma . . . thalamus

QUESTION
40   Fibers of the optic tract which originate in the thalamus and extend to the visual cortex in the _____ lobe of the brain constitute the optic _____.

ANSWER

occipital . . . radiations

ITEM   NERVES TO THE EYE MUSCLES:
15   THE OCULOMOTOR NERVE

The *oculomotor nerve* (III) carries general somatic efferent fibers to four of the six extrinsic eye muscles which move the eyeball: the *superior, inferior,* and *medial rectus muscles,* and the *inferior oblique muscle.* The oculomotor nerve also supplies the *levator palpebrae superioris muscle,* which raises the eyelid. In addition to GSE fibers, the oculomotor nerve also carries general visceral efferent fibers which are parasympathetic to the sphincter muscle of the pupil and to ciliary muscles which accommodate the lens for near vision.

Examine Figure 5–3 and notice where the oculomotor nerve exits from the brain near the midline junction of the midbrain and pons. Figure 5–3 also shows two of the extrinsic muscles of the eye innervated by the oculomotor nerve, the superior and inferior recti.

QUESTION
41   GSE fibers of the oculomotor nerve innervate _____ muscles of the eye; GVE fibers of the oculomotor nerve innervate the _____ muscle of the pupil and the _____ muscles of the lens.

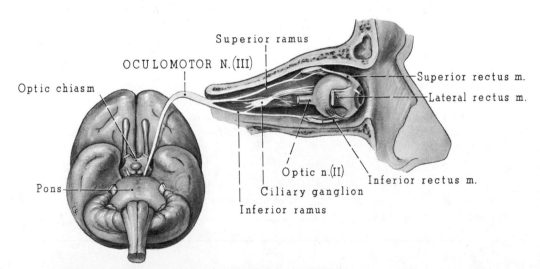

Figure 5–3. Pathway of the oculomotor nerve (III). (From Jacob and Francone: Structure and Function in Man. 3rd Ed. Philadelphia, W. B. Saunders Co.)

extrinsic . . . sphincter . . . ciliary   *ANSWER*

The point of exit from the brain of the oculomotor nerve (III) is the junction   *QUESTION*
of the _____ and the _____.   **42**

---

midbrain . . . pons (in either order)   *ANSWER*

NERVES TO THE EYE MUSCLES: ITEM
THE TROCHLEAR NERVE   16

The *trochlear nerve* (IV) can be seen in Figure 5–4 as it appears on the ventral surface of the upper pons. The single muscle innervated by the trochlear nerve, the *superior oblique muscle,* is shown from the superior view of the eyeball.

The trochlear nerve innervates the *superior rectus/superior oblique* (circle   *QUESTION*
one) muscle.   **43**

---

superior oblique   *ANSWER*

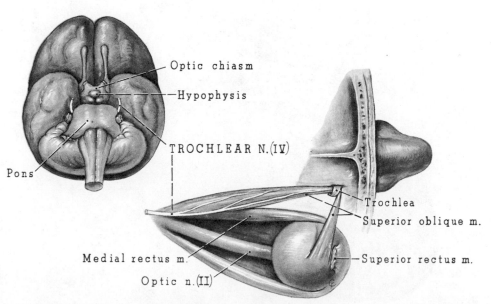

Figure 5–4. Pathway of the trochlear nerve (IV). (From Jacob and Francone: Structure and Function in Man. 3rd Ed. Philadelphia, W. B. Saunders Co.)

ITEM 17   NERVES TO THE EYE MUSCLES: THE ABDUCENS NERVE

The *abducens nerve* (VI) carries general somatic efferent fibers which supply the *lateral rectus* muscle of the eye. In Figure 5–5, notice the superficial exit of the abducens nerve at the ventral midline junction of the pons and the medulla.

QUESTION 44

The lateral rectus muscle is innervated by the _____ nerve.

ANSWER

abducens

QUESTION 45

The inferior oblique muscle is innervated by the _____ nerve.

ANSWER

oculomotor

QUESTION 46

The superior oblique muscle is innervated by the _____ nerve.

ANSWER

trochlear

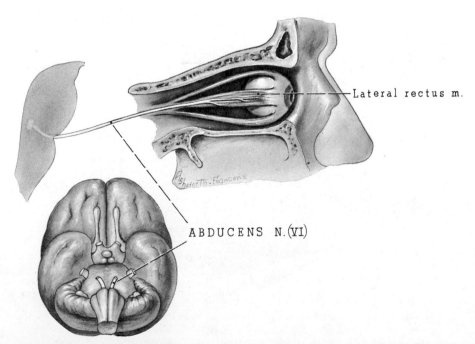

Figure 5–5. Pathway of the abducens nerve (VI). (From Jacob and Francone: Structure and Function in Man. 3rd Ed. Philadelphia, W. B. Saunders Co.)

The abducens nerve exits from the brain at the junction of the _____ and the _____.

QUESTION
47

---

pons . . . medulla (in either order)

ANSWER

The medial rectus, superior rectus, inferior rectus, and inferior oblique muscles are innervated by the _____ nerve.

QUESTION
48

---

oculomotor

ANSWER

Before each of the extrinsic eye muscles listed in Column A place the letter from Column B which corresponds to the nerve which innervates that muscle.

QUESTION
49

Column A	*Column B*
( ) 1. superior oblique muscle	A. abducens nerve (VI)
( ) 2. inferior oblique muscle	B. trochlear nerve (IV)
( ) 3. superior rectus muscle	C. oculomotor nerve (III)
( ) 4. inferior rectus muscle	
( ) 5. lateral rectus muscle	
( ) 6. medial rectus muscle	

1.—(B); 2.—(C); 3.—(C); 4.—(C); 5.—(A); 6.—(C)

ANSWER

THE TRIGEMINAL NERVE: FUNCTIONAL COMPONENTS   ITEM 18

The trigeminal nerve (cranial nerve V) is composed of both afferent and efferent fibers, with afferent fibers predominating.

The sensory component of the trigeminal nerve is general somatic afferent. It conveys sensations of pain, temperature, touch, and pressure from most of the skin and mucous membranes of the head.

The motor component of nerve V is special visceral efferent, providing motor innervation to the muscles of mastication. Proprioceptive fibers of the muscles of mastication, their tendons, and the temporomandibular joint are considered general somatic afferent. Proprioceptive impulses convey the state of muscle contraction, the degree of joint angulation, and the tension of tendons to the central nervous system, which responds with efferent impulses to effect the appropriate modification of muscle activity.

QUESTION
50

Two types of fibers comprise the trigeminal nerve (V), afferent and efferent. The more predominant type is the _____.

ANSWER

afferent

QUESTION
51

Before each item in Column A, place the letter from Column B which corresponds to the type of functional component of the fibers listed.

Column A	Column B
( ) 1. sensory fibers of the trigeminal nerve (V)	A. SVA
	B. SSA
( ) 2. motor fibers of the trigeminal nerve (V)	C. SVE
	D. GSA
	E. GSE
	F. GVA
	G. GVE

ANSWER

1. —(D); 2. —(C)

QUESTION
52

General somatic afferent fibers of the fifth cranial (trigeminal) nerve convey sensations of _____, _____, _____, and _____.

ANSWER

pain . . . temperature . . . touch . . . pressure (in any order)

QUESTION
53

The proprioceptive impulses carried by GSA fibers are unconscious sensations from muscles of _____, from _____, and from the _____ joint.

ANSWER

mastication . . . tendons . . . temporomandibular

QUESTION
54

The motor component of the trigeminal nerve (V) is termed _____ _____ efferent.

ANSWER

special visceral

THE TRIGEMINAL NERVE: DIVISIONS

The trigeminal nerve (V) is composed of three divisions: the ophthalmic division (V_1), the maxillary division (V_2), and the mandibular division (V_3). The ophthalmic and maxillary divisions are entirely sensory; the mandibular division, both sensory and motor.

The three divisions of the trigeminal nerve are the

1. _____
2. _____
3. _____

ophthalmic . . . maxillary . . . mandibular

The two divisions of the trigeminal nerve (V) which are composed entirely of general somatic afferent fibers are the _____ division and the _____ division.

ophthalmic . . . maxillary

The division of the trigeminal nerve (V) which contains both general somatic afferent and general visceral efferent fibers is the _____ division.

mandibular

THE TRIGEMINAL NERVE: THE OPHTHALMIC DIVISION

Figure 5–6 shows the cutaneous distribution of the trigeminal nerve (V). The ophthalmic division (V_1), entirely sensory, carries general somatic afferent fibers from structures related to the eye, and from the skin of the forehead, eyelids, and nose. It also conveys sensory input from mucous membranes and some of the paranasal sinuses.

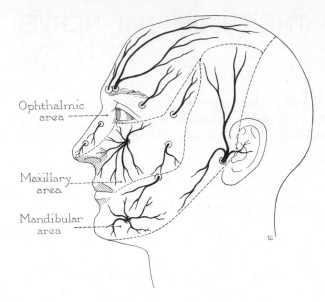

Ophthalmic
  area

Maxillary
  area

Mandibular
  area

Figure 5–6. Cutaneous distribution of the trigeminal nerve (V); redrawn from Gray. (From King and Showers: Human Anatomy and Physiology. 6th Ed. Philadelphia, W. B. Saunders Co.)

QUESTION
58

The ophthalmic division is sensory to structures related to the _____, skin of the _____ and nose, and to some of the paranasal _____. _____.

ANSWER

eye . . . forehead . . . sinuses

THE TRIGEMINAL NERVE: THE MAXILLARY DIVISION

The maxillary division of the trigeminal nerve (V) carries general somatic afferent fibers from skin of the cheek, lower eyelid, nose, and upper lip. In addition, the maxillary division (V_2) supplies the mucous membranes of the maxillary sinus, nasopharynx, roof of the mouth, tonsils, and gingivae, as well as innervating the maxillary teeth.

QUESTION
59

The maxillary division of the trigeminal nerve is
A. entirely afferent
B. entirely efferent
C. both afferent and efferent

ANSWER

The correct answer is A. Like the ophthalmic division, the maxillary division of the trigeminal nerve is entirely sensory; specifically, it is general somatic afferent.

The maxillary division is sensory to _____ of the cheek, _____ membranes of the maxillary region, and maxillary _____.

skin . . . mucous . . . teeth

THE TRIGEMINAL NERVE: ITEM
THE MANDIBULAR DIVISION 22

The mandibular division of the trigeminal nerve (V) contains both sensory and motor fibers. General somatic afferent fibers convey pain, temperature, touch, and pressure from the region of the lower jaw. Special visceral efferent fibers supply the muscles of mastication. The specific muscles innervated by the mandibular division will be discussed in Unit Six, where the trigeminal nerve, because of its central importance in dentistry, will be given detailed consideration.

Place a checkmark before the functional components proper to the mandibular division of the trigeminal nerve (V).
( ) A. GSA
( ) B. GVA
( ) C. GSE
( ) D. GVE
( ) E. SVA
( ) F. SSA
( ) G. SVE

You should have marked A, general somatic afferent, and G, special visceral efferent.

The sensory fibers of the mandibular division of cranial nerve V convey sensations of _____, _____, _____, and _____.

pain . . . temperature . . . touch . . . pressure (in any order)

The efferent fibers of the mandibular division of the trigeminal nerve convey motor impulses to muscles of _____.

mastication

ITEM 23   THE TRIGEMINAL NERVE: PATHWAY

Figure 5–7 shows branches of the trigeminal nerve (V) as they approach the trigeminal ganglion, where the cell bodies of the afferent components are located. The ophthalmic division enters the skull through the superior orbital fissure which is not shown. Note the maxillary division (V_2) entering the skull at the foramen rotundum, and the mandibular division (V_3), entering at the foramen ovale. Cell bodies of the motor fibers of the trigeminal nerve are located in the pons. Note the superficial exit of the trigeminal nerve from the ventral surface of the pons.

QUESTION
64

Match each division of the trigeminal nerve with its site of entrance into the cranial vault.

Column A	Column B
( ) 1. ophthalmic division	A. foramen ovale
( ) 2. maxillary division	B. superior orbital fissure
( ) 3. mandibular division	C. foramen rotundum

ANSWER

1.—(B) 2.—(C); 3.—(A)

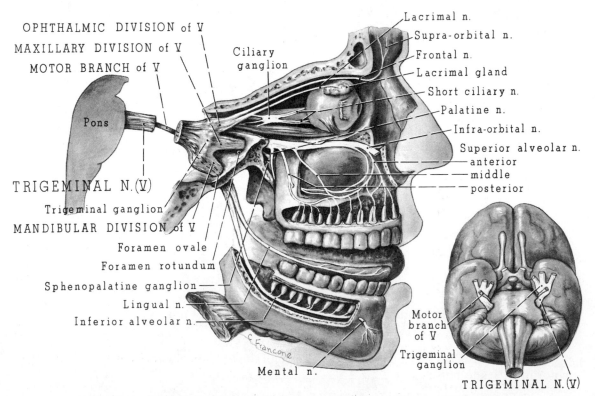

Figure 5–7.   Trigeminal nerve (V). (From Jacob and Francone: Structure and Function in Man. 3rd Ed. Philadelphia, W. B. Saunders Co.)

Cell bodies of the sensory fibers of all three divisions of the trigeminal nerve are located in the _____ ganglion.

QUESTION 65

---

trigeminal

ANSWER

Cell bodies of the motor component of the trigeminal nerve are located in the _____.

QUESTION 66

---

pons

ANSWER

THE FACIAL NERVE: FUNCTIONAL COMPONENTS   ITEM 24

The facial nerve, cranial nerve VII, carries motor fibers, sensory fibers, and a parasympathetic component which is also considered motor in function. The several components of the facial nerve include general somatic afferent, general visceral afferent, general visceral efferent, special visceral afferent, and special visceral efferent.

In the list below, check the five functional components carried by the facial nerve.

   (   ) A. GSA
   (   ) B. GSE
   (   ) C. GVA
   (   ) D. GVE
   (   ) E. SSA
   (   ) F. SVA
   (   ) G. SVE

QUESTION 67

You should have placed check marks before A, C, D, F, and G.

ANSWER

THE FACIAL NERVE: PATHWAY   ITEM 25

Both motor and sensory components of the facial nerve (VIII) leave the brain at the junction of the pons and medulla, as shown in the insert of Figure 5–8. All components go through the internal acoustic meatus to enter the petrous part of the temporal bone. Within bone, various fibers are given off to go their divergent routes. These fibers will be discussed in a later unit.

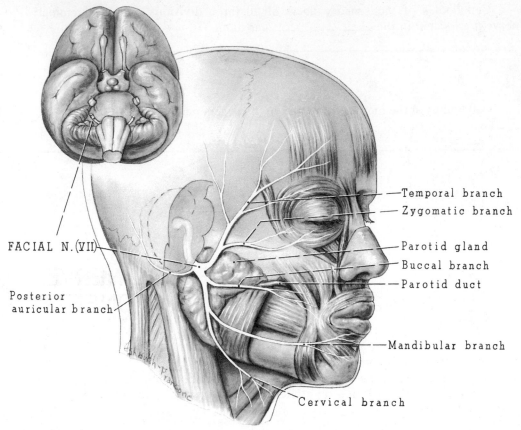

FACIAL N. (VII)

Posterior
auricular branch

Temporal branch
Zygomatic branch
Parotid gland
Buccal branch
Parotid duct
Mandibular branch
Cervical branch

Figure 5–8.   Facial nerve (VII). (From Jacob and Francone: Structure and Function in Man. 3rd Ed. Philadelphia, W. B. Saunders Co.)

Special visceral efferent fibers exit through the stylomastoid foramen to supply muscles of facial expression, as shown in Figure 5–8.

QUESTION
68

The facial nerve (VII) enters the petrous part of the temporal bone at the _____ _____ meatus.

ANSWER

internal acoustic

QUESTION
69

SVE fibers of the facial nerve (VII) leave the skull at the _____ foramen to supply the muscles of _____ _____.

ANSWER

stylomastoid . . . facial expression

The vestibulocochlear nerve, cranial nerve VIII, is concerned with equilibrium and hearing. All its fibers, like those of the optic nerve (II), are special somatic afferent. When you study Figure 5–9, you will notice that the receptors for sensory data pertaining to equilibrium and hearing are located in the inner ear. From this point, central processes exit from the posterior surface of the petrous bone through the internal auditory meatus, and enter the brain at the inferolateral border of the pons.

Sensations relating to equilibrium and hearing are carried by the _____ nerve.

QUESTION 70

---

vestibulocochlear

ANSWER

The fibers of the vestibulocochlear nerve are *special visceral afferent/special somatic afferent* (circle one).

QUESTION 71

The correct answer is special somatic afferent.

ANSWER

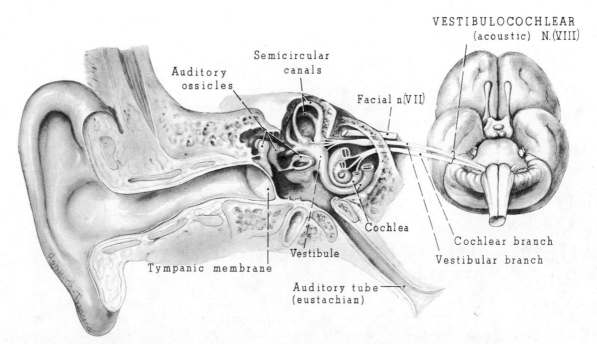

Figure 5–9. Vestibulocochlear nerve (VIII). (From Jacob and Francone: Structure and Function in Man. 3rd Ed. Philadelphia, W. B. Saunders Co.)

QUESTION
72

The sensations with which the vestibulocochlear nerve is involved are those relating to _____ and _____ .

ANSWER

equilibrium . . . hearing (in either order)

ITEM 27

THE GLOSSOPHARYNGEAL NERVE: FUNCTIONAL COMPONENTS

The glossopharyngeal nerve, cranial nerve IX, distributes principally to the tongue and pharynx, as its name implies. The ninth cranial nerve carries the same five functional components as does the facial nerve (VII): general somatic afferent, general visceral afferent, general visceral efferent, special visceral afferent, and special visceral efferent.

QUESTION
73

Place a checkmark before each functional component in the list below which is proper to the glossopharyngeal nerve (IX).

(   ) A. GSA
(   ) B. GSE
(   ) C. GVA
(   ) D. GVE
(   ) E. SSA
(   ) F. SVA
(   ) G. SVE

ANSWER

You should have placed checks before A, C, D, F, and G.

QUESTION
74

The glossopharyngeal nerve carries the same five functional components as are carried by the _____ nerve.

ANSWER

facial

ITEM 28

THE GLOSSOPHARYNGEAL NERVE: PATHWAY

Figure 5–10 shows the superficial exit of the glossopharyngeal nerve (IX) as it leaves the brain at the superolateral border of the ventral medulla. Emerging from the skull at the jugular foramen, the glossopharyngeal nerve provides taste and general sensory fibers to the posterior third of the tongue and to the pharyngeal mucosa. Motor fibers supply a single muscle of the pharynx, the

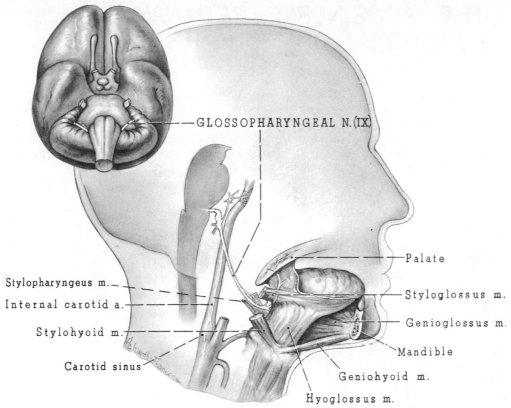

GLOSSOPHARYNGEAL N. (IX)

Stylopharyngeus m.
Internal carotid a.
Stylohyoid m.
Carotid sinus

Palate
Styloglossus m.
Genioglossus m.
Mandible
Geniohyoid m.
Hyoglossus m.

Figure 5–10. Glossopharyngeal nerve (IX). (From Jacob and Francone: Structure and Function in Man. 3rd Ed. Philadelphia, W. B. Saunders Co.)

stylopharyngeus muscle, and also provide parasympathetic innervation to the parotid gland.

The glossopharyngeal nerve (IX) leaves the brain at the superolateral surface of the ventral _____.

QUESTION 75

medulla

ANSWER

The glossopharyngeal nerve supplies the pharynx, the _____ third of the tongue, and the _____ gland.

QUESTION 76

posterior . . . parotid

ANSWER

ITEM 29   THE VAGUS NERVE: PATHWAY AND FUNCTIONAL COMPONENTS

Figure 5–11 shows the exit and distribution of the vagus nerve (X). Its fibers leave the ventral surface of the medulla just inferior to the glossopharyngeal nerve (IX), exit from the skull through the jugular foramen, and descend through the neck in the carotid sheath.

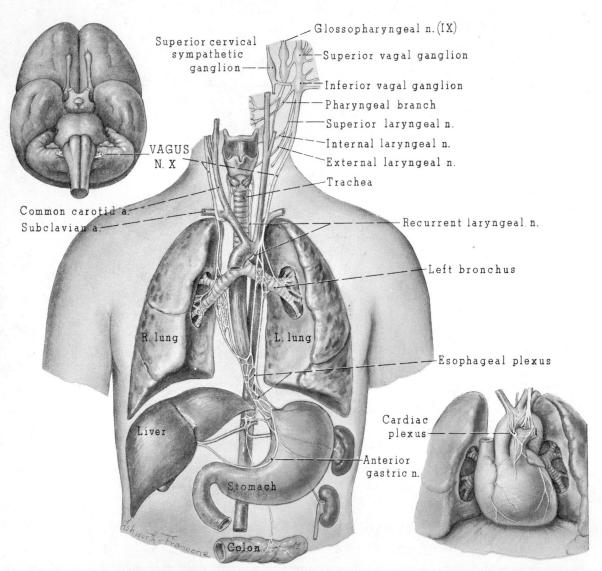

Figure 5–11. Vagus nerve (X). (From Jacob and Francone: Structure and Function in Man. 3rd Ed. Philadelphia, W. B. Saunders Co.)

The vagus nerve has both efferent and afferent components, precisely the same functional components as the facial and glossopharyngeal nerves. These components include general somatic afferent, general visceral afferent, general visceral efferent, special visceral afferent, and special visceral efferent. Most of the fibers of the vagus nerve are general visceral efferent, supplying parasympathetic innervation to thoracic and abdominal viscera.

The superficial exit of the vagus nerve (X) from the brain is the ventral surface of the _____.

QUESTION
77

---

medulla

ANSWER

The vagus nerve exits from the skull at the _____ foramen, along with the _____ nerve.

QUESTION
78

---

jugular . . . glossopharyngeal

ANSWER

Functional components of the vagus nerve are of the same types as components represented in the _____ and _____ nerves.

QUESTION
79

---

facial . . . glossopharyngeal (in either order)

ANSWER

General visceral efferent fibers of the vagus nerve are parasympathetic to _____ and _____ viscera.

QUESTION
80

---

thoracic . . . abdominal (in either order)

ANSWER

ITEM 30   THE SPINAL ACCESSORY NERVE: PATHWAY AND FUNCTIONAL COMPONENTS

The spinal accessory nerve, also known as the eleventh cranial nerve, contains both cranial and spinal parts. The pathways of both portions can be seen in Figure 5–12.

The spinal part of cranial nerve XI supplies special visceral efferent innervation to the sternocleidomastoid and trapezius muscles in the neck.

The cranial part of the spinal accessory nerve is composed of four or five rootlets below those of the vagus nerve on the lateral part of the medulla. Passing through the jugular foramen, the cranial fibers join the vagus nerve near the foramen and, in effect, constitute the inferior laryngeal branch of the vagus, providing special visceral efferent innervation to muscles of the larynx.

QUESTION 81

The functional component of both the cranial and spinal portions of the accessory nerve is _____ _____ efferent.

ANSWER

special visceral

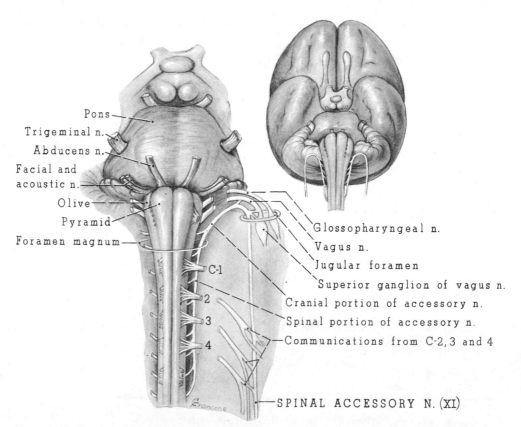

Figure 5–12. Spinal accessory nerve (XI). (From Jacob and Francone: Structure and Function in Man. 3rd Ed. Philadelphia, W. B. Saunders Co.)

Fibers of the cranial portion of the accessory nerve (XI) travel with the _____ nerve to innervate muscles of the _____.

---

vagus . . . larynx

The spinal portion of the accessory nerve provides motor innervation to two muscles in the neck, the _____ muscle and the _____ muscle.

---

sternocleidomastoid . . . trapezius (in either order)

THE HYPOGLOSSAL NERVE: PATHWAY AND FUNCTIONAL COMPONENTS

In Figure 5–13, observe the origin and pathway of the hypoglossal nerve, cranial nerve XII. A series of rootlets on the ventral surface of the medulla unites near the hypoglossal canal. After passing through the canal, the hypoglossal nerve becomes closely associated with the vagus and accessory nerves, (X) and (XI).

Extending to the floor of the mouth and tongue, the general somatic efferent fibers of the hypoglossal nerve supply the hyoglossus, styloglossus, geniohyoid, and genioglossus muscles as well as all the intrinsic muscles of the tongue.

Proprioceptive fibers associated with the hypoglossal nerve, like those of all cranial nerves, are termed general somatic afferent. These afferent connections from all skeletal muscles of the head are carried to each respective muscle in the same sheath as the general somatic efferent fibers.

The motor component of the hypoglossal nerve (XII) is general _____ _____.

---

somatic efferent

The hypoglossal nerve, after it has passed through the hypoglossal canal, is closely associated with the _____ nerve and the _____ nerve.

---

vagus . . . spinal accessory (in either order)

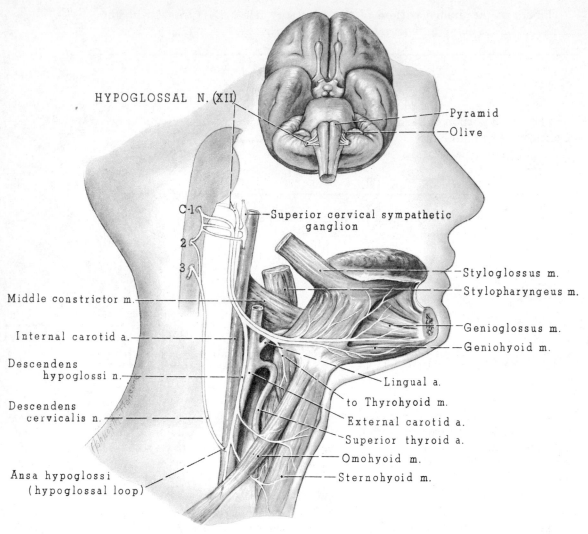

HYPOGLOSSAL N. (XII)

Pyramid
Olive

Superior cervical sympathetic ganglion

C-1
2
3

Middle constrictor m.

Internal carotid a.

Descendens hypoglossi n.

Descendens cervicalis n.

Ansa hypoglossi (hypoglossal loop)

Styloglossus m.
Stylopharyngeus m.

Genioglossus m.
Geniohyoid m.

Lingual a.
to Thyrohyoid m.
External carotid a.
Superior thyroid a.
Omohyoid m.
Sternohyoid m.

Figure 5–13.   Hypoglossal nerve (XII). (From Jacob and Francone: Structure and Function in Man. 3rd Ed. Philadelphia, W. B. Saunders Co.)

QUESTION
86

The hypoglossal nerve XII supplies, in addition to the hypoglossus, stylo-glossus, geniohyoid, and genioglossus muscles, all the intrinsic muscles of the _____.

ANSWER

tongue

QUESTION
87

Afferent fibers for proprioception are termed _____ _____ afferent.

ANSWER

general somatic

Each cranial nerve which contains general somatic efferent fibers supplying the skeletal muscles also contains general somatic afferent fibers concerned with

QUESTION
88

_____ .

proprioception

ANSWER

THE CRANIAL NERVES: SITES OF EXIT

ITEM 32

Figure 5–14, the internal aspect of the skull, shows the foramina through which the various cranial nerves exit from the brain. As you locate each foramen, associate with it the cranial nerve or nerves which it transmits. The *cribriform plate* transmits the olfactory nerve (I); the *optic canal,* the optic nerve (II); the *superior orbital fissure,* the oculomotor (III), trochlear (IV), and abducens (VI) nerves, as well as the ophthalmic division (V_1) of the trigeminal nerve (V). The maxillary division (V_2) of the trigeminal nerve exits through the *foramen rotundum;* the mandibular division (V_3), through the *foramen ovale.* The *internal acoustic meatus* transmits the facial and vestibulocochlear nerves (VII and VIII); the *jugular foramen,* the glossopharyngeal, vagus, and accessory nerves (IX, X, and XI); the *hypoglossal canal,* the hypoglossal nerve (XII).

As a review of the foramina which transmit the various cranial nerves, match each number in Column A with an appropriate letter from Column B.

QUESTION
89

Column A	*Column B*
( ) 1. olfactory nerve (I)	A. cribriform plate
( ) 2. optic nerve (II)	B. foramen ovale
( ) 3. oculomotor nerve (III)	C. foramen rotundum
( ) 4. trochlear nerve (IV)	D. hypoglossal canal
( ) 5. trigeminal nerve (V), opthalmic division	E. internal acoustic meatus
	F. jugular foramen
( ) 6. trigeminal nerve (V), maxillary division	G. optic canal
	H. superior orbital fissure
( ) 7. trigeminal nerve (V), mandibular division	
( ) 8. abducens nerve (VI)	
( ) 9. facial nerve (VII)	
( ) 10. vestibulocochlear nerve (VIII)	
( ) 11. glossopharyngeal nerve (IX)	
( ) 12. vagus nerve (X)	
( ) 13. spinal accessory nerve (XI)	
( ) 14. hypoglossal nerve (XII)	

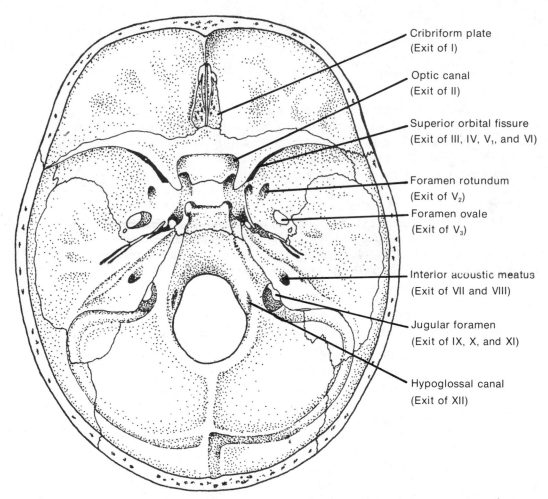

Figure 5-14.   The skull, internal aspect, showing sites of exit of cranial nerves. (Redrawn from Wolf-Heidegger: Atlas of Systematic Human Anatomy. Vol. I. Basel, S. Karger AG.)

ANSWER

1.—(A)	8.—(H)
2.—(G)	9.—(E)
3.—(H)	10.—(E)
4.—(H)	11.—(F)
5.—(H)	12.—(F)
6.'—(C)	13.—(F)
7.—(B)	14.—(D)

FUNCTIONAL COMPONENTS AND CELL COLUMNS

ITEM 33

Functional components associated with the various cranial nerves have nuclei spatially arranged into cell columns located throughout the brain stem. Figures 5–15, 5–16, and 5–17 show the arrangement of cell columns in the brain stem, viewed from the median sagittal surface. General somatic efferent and special visceral efferent fibers to skeletal muscles are shown as stippled areas. General visceral efferent cell columns, representing parasympathetic preganglionic fibers, are shown as crosshatched areas. General somatic afferent and special visceral afferent columns are shown as clear areas. General visceral afferent and special somatic afferent fibers are not identified in the illustrations.

Nuclei containing cell bodies of efferent neurons are the origins of particular nerves. Nuclei associated with sensory neurons are sites of synapse, since cell bodies of primary sensory neurons are found in peripheral ganglia.

Cell columns in the brain stem represent _____ associated with motor and sensory components of the cranial nerves.

QUESTION 90

nuclei

ANSWER

The specific sites in the brain in which cell columns are found are localized throughout the (circle one)
A. medulla
B. midbrain
C. brain stem

QUESTION 91

The correct answer is C. Cell columns are situated throughout the brain stem, some nuclei of a given column being in the medulla, some in the pons, and still others in the midbrain.

ANSWER

ITEM
·34

THE GSE AND SVE CELL COLUMN
AT MIDBRAIN LEVELS

In Figure 5–15, locate the combined general somatic efferent and special visceral efferent column (stippled areas). Notice that the cell bodies of these motor neurons innervating skeletal muscles are represented throughout the brain stem. At midbrain levels, this cell column represents the nucleus of the trochlear nerve (IV) and that portion of the nucleus of the oculomotor nerve (III) from which fibers emanate to supply extrinsic eye muscles. Note the superficial exits of fibers of each of these two cranial nerves; fiber exits of the oculomotor nerve, on the ventral surface of the brain; of the trochlear nerve, on the dorsal surface.

QUESTION
92

Nuclei, by definition, are aggregates of _____ _____ of neurons located in the central nervous system.

ANSWER

cell bodies

QUESTION
93

Motor nuclei of the oculomotor (III) and trochlear (IV) nerves are located in the _____.

ANSWER

midbrain

ITEM
35

THE GSE AND SVE CELL COLUMN
AT PONTILE LEVELS

At pontile levels, the general somatic efferent and special visceral efferent cell column (stippled areas of illustrations) includes the motor nuclei of the trigeminal (V), abducens (VI), and facial (VII) nerves. Note in Figure 5–15 the superficial exits of these cranial nerves from the ventral surface of the pons. Note also the *genu,* or bend, of the facial nerve as it loops dorsally, then ventrally around the abducent nucleus.

QUESTION
94

Motor nuclei to skeletal muscle of cranial nerves which originate in the pons include nuclei of the _____, the _____, and the _____ nerves.

ANSWER

trigeminal . . . abducens . . . facial (in any order)

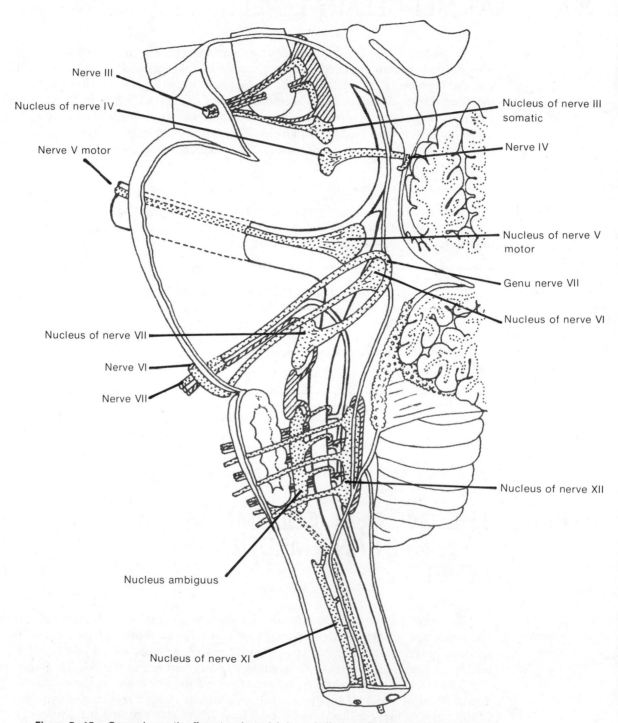

Figure 5–15. General somatic efferent and special visceral efferent cell columns in the brain stem viewed from the median sagittal surface. (Redrawn from Truex and Carpenter: Human Neuroanatomy. 6th Ed. Baltimore, Williams & Wilkins Co.)

ITEM 36
THE GSE AND SVE CELL COLUMN AT MEDULLARY LEVELS

In Figure 5–15, observe the general somatic efferent and special visceral efferent cell column (stippled area) in the medulla. At medullary levels, this cell column represents the nucleus of the hypoglossal nerve (XII), which innervates the tongue; the nucleus of the accessory nerve (XI), which descends into the cervical cord; and the *nucleus ambiguus*. The accessory nerve innervates the sternocleidomastoid and trapezius muscles. The nucleus ambiguus represents cell bodies of the vagus nerve (X), processes of which innervate muscles of the pharynx and larynx.

QUESTION
95

Motor cell columns in the medulla include the nucleus of the _____ _____ nerve to the tongue, and the nucleus of the _____ nerve to the sternocleidomastoid and trapezius muscles.

ANSWER

hypoglossal . . . accessory

QUESTION
96

The motor nucleus of the vagus nerve is called the nucleus _____. It contains cell bodies whose fibers supply muscles of the _____ and _____.

ANSWER

ambiguus . . . pharynx . . . larynx

ITEM 37
THE GVE CELL COLUMN AT MIDBRAIN AND MEDULLARY LEVELS

Examine Figure 5–16 and locate the general visceral efferent cell column (crosshatched areas). The components of this column represent the parasympathetic preganglionic fibers to smooth muscle, cardiac muscle, and glands. GVE nuclei are found at midbrain and medullary levels, but not at the pontine level.

The *visceral nucleus of the oculomotor nerve* may be found in the midbrain. These fibers of nerve III supply intrinsic eye muscles which regulate adjustments of the pupil to varying light intensities. These fibers also regulate the tension on the lens to accommodate for near and distant vision.

At the medullary level in the GVE column there are two nuclei: (1) the *dorsal motor nucleus of the vagus nerve (X)*, supplying thoracic and abdominal viscera; and (2) the *salivatory nucleus*, providing parasympathetic innervation to the salivary glands.

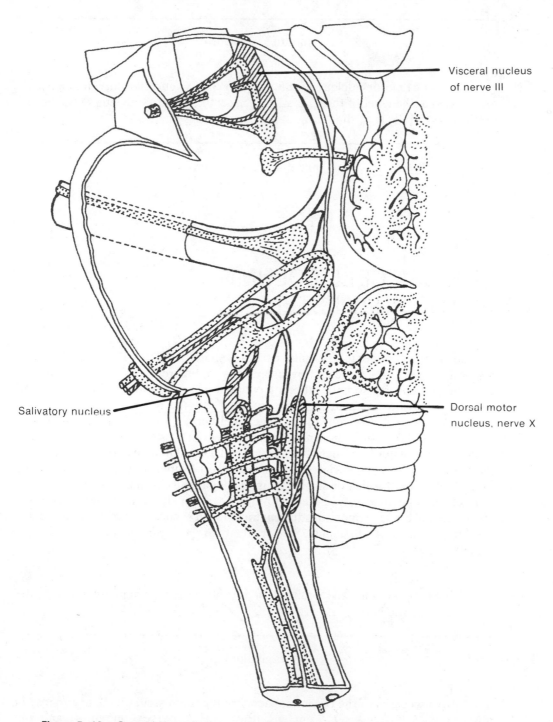

Figure 5–16. General visceral efferent cell column in the brain stem, viewed from the median sagittal surface. (Redrawn from Truex and Carpenter: Human Neuroanatomy. 6th Ed. Baltimore, The Williams and Wilkins Co.)

QUESTION
97

Nuclei in the GVE column supply motor innervation to glands, and to _____ muscle and _____ muscle.

ANSWER

smooth . . . cardiac

QUESTION
98

The dorsal motor nucleus of the vagus nerve (X) and the salivatory nucleus are located at the level of the _____; the visceral nucleus of the oculo-motor nerve (III), is at the _____ level.

ANSWER

medulla . . . midbrain

ITEM 38

THE GSA CELL COLUMN IN THE BRAIN STEM

Sensory components of cranial nerves, general somatic afferent and special visceral afferent, are indicated by clear lines in Figure 5–17. General visceral afferent and special somatic afferent columns are not shown. The trigeminal nerve (V) provides the principal sensory input into the brain stem.

Follow the sensory root of the trigeminal nerve (V) as it enters the ventral pons. Fibers of the fifth cranial nerve extend superiorly as the *mesencephalic tract* of the trigeminal nerve. Other fibers synapse in a small nucleus in the dorsal pons, the sensory nucleus of the trigeminal nerve. Still other fibers of the trigeminal nerve extend inferiorly through midbrain, pons, medulla, and cervical cord as the *spinal tract of the trigeminal nerve*. Central processes from all three areas representing the trigeminal nerve synapse in adjacent nuclei with secondary neurons, processes of which ascend to the thalamus. Sensory fibers of the trigeminal nerve are general somatic afferent.

QUESTION
99

Sensory input into the brain stem is transmitted principally through the _____ nerve.

ANSWER

trigeminal

QUESTION
100

GSA processes of the trigeminal nerve in the brain stem divide to synapse in the _____ nucleus, the _____ nucleus, and the _____ nucleus of the trigeminal nerve.

ANSWER

mesencephalic . . . sensory . . . spinal

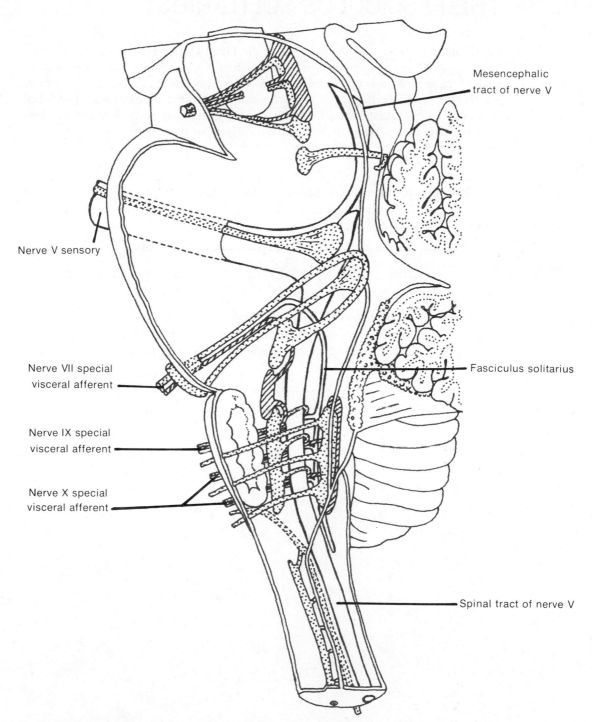

Figure 5–17.   General somatic afferent and special visceral afferent cell columns in brain stem viewed from median sagittal surface. (Redrawn from Truex and Carpenter: Human Neuroanatomy. 6th Ed. Baltimore, Williams & Wilkins Co.)

ITEM 39   THE SVA CELL COLUMN OR THE FASCICULUS SOLITARIUS

Note in Figure 5–17 the location of the facial (VII), glossopharyngeal (IX), and vagus (X) nerves on the ventral brain stem. Observe how some fibers from each of these three nerves extend dorsally to converge as the *fasciculus solitarius*. These nerves and the fasciculus solitarius convey the sensation of taste. The facial nerve carries SVA taste fibers from the anterior two thirds of the tongue; the glossopharyngeal nerve, fibers from the posterior third of the tongue; the vagus nerve, fibers from the base of the tongue.

QUESTION
101

Special visceral afferent fibers for the sensation of taste, carried in the _____ nerve, the _____ nerve, and the _____ nerve, converge as the fasciculus _____.

ANSWER

facial . . . glossopharyngeal . . . vagus . . . solitarius

QUESTION
102

Taste sensations from the anterior two thirds of the tongue are carried by the _____ nerve; sensations from the posterior third of the tongue, by the _____ nerve; sensations from the base of the tongue, by the _____ nerve.

ANSWER

facial . . . glossopharyngeal . . . vagus

SUMMARY OF UNIT FIVE

The twelve pairs of cranial nerves provide sensory and motor connections between the brain stem and the structures of the head and neck. The vagus nerve also extends to viscera of the thorax and abdomen.

The term *nucleus* designates an aggregate of nerve cell bodies contained within the brain and spinal cord; the term ganglion, an aggregate outside the brain and spinal cord. Sensory ganglia contain cell bodies of fibers conveying sensation to the brain; motor ganglia contain cell bodies whose peripheral processes innervate muscles of the head. Motor ganglia are associated with parasympathetic postganglionic cell bodies whose fibers innervate smooth muscle, cardiac muscle, and glands. A bundle of nerve cell processes located outside the central nervous system constitutes a nerve; a group contained within the brain or spinal cord, a tract. Some nerves are composed of sensory fibers only; some, of motor fibers only; some are composed of both sensory and motor fibers.

FUNCTIONAL COMPONENTS

The term *functional components* is the generic term for descriptive designations of the particular types of fibers contained in various nerves. Afferent, or sensory, fibers bring sensation *to* the central nervous system; efferent, or motor, fibers conduct impulses *away from* the central nervous system. Somatic fibers transmit sensory data from the skin or the skeletal muscles of the body wall; visceral fibers conduct data pertaining to viscera within the body cavities, to smooth muscles, or to glands. Somatic afferent fibers are called *general* if they convey sensations from widely distributed receptors. They are called *special* if they convey specific sensations of sight, hearing, taste, or smell. Efferent fibers, both somatic and visceral, are all designated as general except for one type: motor fibers to muscles embryonically derived from the mesoderm of the branchial arches are called special visceral efferent.

Altogether, there are seven different types of functional components, four general and three special. The general components are: (1) general somatic afferent, abbreviated GSA; (2) general somatic efferent, or GSE; (3) general visceral afferent, or GVA; and (4) general visceral efferent, or GVE. The special components are: (1) special somatic afferent, abbreviated SSA; (2) special visceral afferent, or SVA; and (3) special visceral efferent, or SVE. There are no special somatic efferent components.

The four designations of general components apply to both cranial and spinal nerves; the three designations of special components, to cranial nerves only.

GSA fibers convey sensations of pain, temperature, touch, and pressure, as well as proprioceptive sensations of muscular tension and joint position. GSE fibers convey motor impulses to muscles of the tongue and to extrinsic eye muscles. GVA fibers are concerned with visceral pain, blood pressure levels, and other sensory inputs necessary for regulation of visceral activity. GVE fibers carry motor impulses to smooth muscles, cardiac muscles, or glands. SSA fibers relate to sight and hearing; SVA fibers, to taste and smell. SVE fibers convey motor impulses to branchiomeric muscles such as those of mastication and facial expression, and to muscles of the pharynx and larynx.

CRANIAL NERVES

The olfactory nerve, cranial nerve I, is special visceral afferent only, and transmits the sensations of smell. The olfactory nerve makes its way from epithelial cells in the upper membrane lining of the nose through the cribriform plate of the ethmoid bone to synapse in the olfactory bulb. Its terminal processes extend to the temporal lobe.

The optic nerve, cranial nerve II, employs SSA fibers to convey sensations affecting the sense of sight. Receptors of the optic nerve are located in the retina of the eye. Fibers enter the middle cranial fossa through the optic canal, cross in the optic chiasma, and, as the optic tract, extend to the lateral geniculate body of the thalamus. From the thalamus, optic radiations extend to the visual cortex of the occipital lobe.

The oculomotor, trochlear, and abducens nerves (cranial nerves III, IV, and VI) innervate extrinsic muscles of the eye. All three carry GSE fibers to the skeletal muscles and, in addition, the oculomotor nerve (III) carries GVE fibers to the sphincter muscle of the pupil of the eye. Originating in nuclei situated in the midbrain and pons, cranial nerves III, IV, and VI enter the orbit by way of the superior orbital fissure. The trochlear nerve (IV) innervates the superior oblique muscle; the abducens nerve, the lateral rectus muscle; the oculomotor nerve (VI), all the remaining extrinsic eye muscles.

The trigeminal nerve, cranial nerve V, carries both motor and sensory fibers, with sensory fibers predominating. Its motor nucleus, located in the pons, sends SVE fibers to the muscles of mastication. At the point of the large trigeminal ganglion, the trigeminal nerve separates into its three major divisions: the ophthalmic, the maxillary, and the mandibular divisions. The ophthalmic and maxillary divisions are entirely sensory; the mandibular division has both sensory and motor components.

GSA fibers of the ophthalmic division convey sensation from structures related to the eyes, forehead, and nose. GSA fibers of the maxillary division convey sensations originating in the cheeks, lower eyelids, upper lip, maxillary sinus, roof of the mouth, tonsils, upper teeth, and related structures. GSA fibers of the mandibular division convey such sensations as pain and touch from the region of the lower jaw. The branchiomeric SVE fibers of the mandibular division carry motor impulses to the muscles of mastication.

The facial nerve, cranial nerve VII, contains five functional components: GSA, GVA, GVE, SVA, and SVE. The GVE fibers of the facial nerve subdivide within the parotid gland and spread to all the muscles of facial expression.

The vestibulocochlear nerve, cranial nerve VIII, is entirely sensory, carrying SSA components which convey sensations relating to hearing and equilibrium from receptors in the inner ear to the central nervous system.

The glossopharyngeal nerve, cranial nerve IX, is both afferent and efferent. Like the facial nerve, the glossopharyngeal nerve has five functional components: GSA, GVA, GVE, SVA, and SVE. In company with the vagus and accessory nerves, the glossopharyngeal nerve emerges from the cranium through the jugular foramen.

The vagus nerve, cranial nerve X, carries the same five types of functional components as are found in nerves VII and IX: GSA, GVA, GVE, SVA, and SVE. The majority of the fibers of the vagus nerve supply GVE innervation to thoracic and abdominal viscera.

The spinal accessory nerve, cranial nerve XI, contains fibers which originate from both the medulla and the cervical spinal cord. These fibers leave the cranium through the jugular foramen, as do fibers of the glossopharyngeal and vagus nerves. The functional component of the spinal accessory nerve is special visceral efferent. Along with the fibers of nerves IX and X, the SVE fibers of cranial nerve XI supply motor innervation to muscles of the pharynx and larynx.

The hypoglossal nerve, cranial nerve XII, innervates the tongue. It carries only GSE fibers which provide motor innervation of the styloglossus, hypoglossus, and genioglossus muscles as well as of all the intrinsic muscles of the tongue.

CELL COLUMNS

Cell columns located in the midbrain represent nuclei containing cell bodies of motor nerves which innervate skeletal muscles, nuclei which are associated with the parasympathetic division of the nervous system, and nuclei in which sensory neurons synapse with secondary neurons. Nuclei of neurons which send motor impulses to skeletal muscles include part of the oculomotor complex in addition to the trochlear and abducens nuclei in the upper brain stem. Peripheral processes supply extrinsic muscles of the eye.

Motor nuclei of the trigeminal (V) and facial (VII) nerves are located in the pons. These nerves supply the muscles of mastication and the muscles of facial expression respectively. In the medulla are located motor nuclei of the accessory (XI) and hypoglossal (XII) nerves, together with the nucleus ambiguus. The latter represents cell bodies of motor neurons which supply muscles of the pharynx and larynx. The general visceral efferent cell column in the midbrain contains the parasympathetic nucleus of the oculomotor nerve (III), whose fibers innervate smooth muscles of the pupil of the eye. The GVE cell column in the medulla contains the salivatory nucleus, comprising cell bodies of the facial and glossopharyngeal nerves (VII and IX), whose fibers are parasympathetic to the salivary glands. Also located in the medulla is the dorsal motor nucleus of the vagus nerve, which is parasympathetic to thoracic and abdominal viscera.

General somatic afferent fibers of the trigeminal nerve (V) form three tracts: the mesencephalic, the sensory, and the spinal. Nuclei associated with sensory neurons are those at which synapse with secondary neurons takes place.

Sensory input from the facial, glossopharyngeal, and vagus nerves (VII, IX, and X) converges in the structure known as the fasciculus solitarius. Fibers of nerves VII, IX, and X convey sensations of taste from the anterior two thirds, the posterior third, and the base of the tongue respectively.

Nuclei are groups of nerve cell bodies located *within/outside* (circle one) the central nervous system; ganglia are nerve cell bodies found *within/outside* the central nervous system.

QUESTION
103

---

within . . . outside

ANSWER

A nerve is located *within/outside* (circle one) the central nervous system; a tract, *within/outside* (circle one) the central nervous system.

QUESTION
104

---

outside . . . within

ANSWER

QUESTION
105

The various specific designations of nerve cell fiber types are referred to by the generic term, _____ _____.

ANSWER

functional components

QUESTION
106

Fiber types which are used for both cranial and spinal nerves are designated as *general/special* (circle one) components.

ANSWER

general

QUESTION
107

Abbreviations for the four general functional components are _____, _____, _____, and _____.

ANSWER

GSA . . . GSE . . . GVA . . . GVE (in any order)

QUESTION
108

Abbreviations for the three special functional components are _____, _____, and _____.

ANSWER

SSA . . . SVA . . . SVE (in any order)

QUESTION
109

GSA fibers convey sensations of _____, _____, _____, and _____, as well as proprioceptive sensations.

ANSWER

pain . . . temperature . . . touch . . . pressure (in any order)

QUESTION
110

Proprioceptive sensations are concerned with the state of contraction of _____ and the angulation of _____.

ANSWER

muscles . . . joints

QUESTION
111

General somatic efferent fibers innervate _____ muscles.

ANSWER

skeletal

QUESTION
112

Sensations of visceral pain are conveyed by _____ _____ afferent fibers; motor impulses to smooth muscles, cardiac muscles, and glands are carried by _____ _____ efferent fibers.

general visceral . . . general visceral   *ANSWER*

The special sensations of sight and hearing are mediated by *SSA/SVA* (circle one) nerves; the sensations of taste and smell, by *SSA/SVA* (circle one) nerves.

QUESTION
113

SSA . . . SVA   *ANSWER*

Branchiomeric fibers supply muscles of _____, muscles of _____ expression, and muscles of the _____ and _____.

QUESTION
114

---

mastication . . . facial . . . pharynx . . . larynx   *ANSWER*

The optic nerve, which conveys the sensations relating to sight, contains only _____ _____ afferent fibers.

QUESTION
115

---

special somatic   *ANSWER*

After crossing at the optic chiasma, fibers of the optic nerve reach the _____ _____ body of the thalamus.

QUESTION
116

---

lateral geniculate   *ANSWER*

The extrinsic muscles of the eye are innervated by the _____ nerve, the _____ nerve, and the _____ nerve.

QUESTION
117

---

oculomotor . . . trochlear . . . abducens (in any order)   *ANSWER*

The lateral rectus muscle is innervated by the _____ nerve; the superior oblique muscle, by the _____ nerve; the remainder of the extrinsic eye muscles, by the _____ nerve.

QUESTION
118

---

abducens . . . trochlear . . . oculomotor   *ANSWER*

The three divisions of the trigeminal nerve are the _____ division, the _____ division, and the _____ division.

QUESTION
119

---

ophthalmic . . . maxillary . . . mandibular (in any order)   *ANSWER*

QUESTION
120

The division of the trigeminal nerve containing both afferent and efferent fibers is the _____ division; the other two divisions contain _____ fibers only.

ANSWER

mandibular . . . afferent (sensory)

QUESTION
121

The structure at which cranial nerve V branches into its three divisions is called the _____ ganglion.

ANSWER

trigeminal

QUESTION
122

The functional component of the sensory fibers of all three divisions of the trigeminal nerve is _____ _____ afferent.

ANSWER

general somatic

QUESTION
123

Special visceral efferent fibers of the trigeminal nerve are carried in the _____ division.

ANSWER

mandibular

QUESTION
124

Sensory fibers of the ophthalmic division of nerve V convey sensations from the region of the _____; fibers of the maxillary division convey sensations from the region of the upper _____; fibers of the mandibular division convey sensations from the region of the lower _____.

ANSWER

eye . . . jaw . . . jaw

QUESTION
125

Motor impulses to the muscles of mastication are supplied by fibers of the _____ division of the trigeminal nerve.

ANSWER

mandibular

QUESTION
126

The functional component of the facial nerve fibers which innervate the muscles of facial expression is _____ _____ efferent.

ANSWER

special visceral

The vestibulocochlear nerve carries a _____ _____ afferent component and transmits sensations from structures concerned with _____ and equilibrium.

---

special somatic . . . hearing

In abbreviated form, the three sensory components of the glossopharyngeal nerve are termed _____, _____, and _____; the two motor components of this nerve are termed _____ and _____.

GSA . . . GVA . . . SVA . . . GVE . . . SVE

The sensations of taste are conveyed by special visceral afferent fibers of three different nerves: the _____ nerve conveys sensations from the anterior two thirds of the tongue; the _____ nerve, from the posterior third of the tongue; and the _____ nerve, from the base of the tongue and the epiglottic region.

---

facial . . . glossopharyngeal . . . vagus

Together with the vagus and accessory nerves, the glossopharyngeal nerve exits from the cranium through the _____ foramen.

---

jugular

In addition to supplying motor and sensory fibers to structures related to the head and neck, the vagus nerve also provides parasympathetic innervation to the region of the _____ and _____.

---

thorax . . . abdomen (in either order)

The hypoglossal nerve carries a general _____ _____ component and supplies muscles of the _____.

---

somatic efferent . . . tongue

QUESTION
133

List the cranial nerves which supply skeletal muscles of the head.

1. _____   6. _____
2. _____   7. _____
3. _____   8. _____
4. _____   9. _____
5. _____

ANSWER

1. oculomotor (III)   6. glossopharyngeal (IX)
2. trochlear (IV)   7. vagus (X)
3. trigeminal (V)   8. accessory (XI)
4. abducens (VI)   9. hypoglossal (XII)
5. facial (VII)

QUESTION
134

The functional component of motor fibers to muscles of the eye and tongue is _____ _____ efferent.

ANSWER

general somatic

QUESTION
135

The functional component of motor fibers to muscles of mastication, facial expression, the pharynx and the larynx is _____ _____ efferent.

ANSWER

special visceral

QUESTION
136

Cranial nerves with general visceral efferent fibers include the _____, _____, _____, and _____ nerves.

ANSWER

oculomotor . . . facial . . . glossopharyngeal . . . vagus (in any order)

QUESTION
137

General somatic afferent fibers supplying most of the head are carried in the _____ nerve.

ANSWER

trigeminal

QUESTION
138

Taste is conveyed by SVA fibers of the _____, _____, and _____ nerves.

ANSWER

facial . . . glossopharyngeal . . . vagus (in any order)

Unit Six □ The Trigeminal Nerve

THE SIGNIFICANCE OF THE TRIGEMINAL NERVE IN DENTISTRY

ITEM 1

Mastery of injection techniques presupposes a detailed knowledge of cranial nerve V, the trigeminal nerve. Branches of the trigeminal nerve which may be blocked in local anesthesia must be learned in terms of their various landmarks, their relationships to other structures, and their distribution.

Sensory branches of the trigeminal nerve innervate the teeth, the mucous membranes of oral and nasal cavities, and the skin of the face. Motor branches of nerve V distribute to the muscles of mastication. Knowledge of the nerves supplying the muscles of mastication is important for the recognition of myopathies of these muscles.

Careful study of the trigeminal nerve is prerequisite to learning _____ techniques, as well as to recognizing myopathies associated with the muscles of _____.

QUESTION 1

---

injection . . . mastication

ANSWER

The trigeminal nerve supplies *sensory/motor* (circle one) branches to the teeth, the oral and nasal mucosa, and the skin of the face; it supplies *sensory/ motor* (circle one) branches to muscles of mastication.

QUESTION 2

---

sensory . . . motor

ANSWER

ORIGIN OF THE TRIGEMINAL NERVE

ITEM 2

Cell bodies of general somatic afferent fibers concerned with pain, temperature, touch, and pressure are found in the *trigeminal ganglion,* which is located at the apex of the petrous bone. Functionally as well as structurally, the trigeminal ganglion is comparable to the dorsal root ganglion of a spinal nerve. Its central processes enter the ventrolateral surface of the pons where it lies on the clivus in the posterior cranial fossa. The fibers divide within the pons, then synapse in three nuclei: (1) the *chief sensory nucleus,* (2) the *nucleus of the spinal tract,* and (3) the *mesencephalic nucleus.* The chief sensory nucleus is located in the pons; the mesencephalic nucleus is in the midbrain; the nucleus of the spinal tract runs from the pons caudally through the medulla and cervical spinal cord. From these nuclei are made various central connections which bring sensation to conscious levels, result in reflex activity, and effect various other responses.

QUESTION
3

The trigeminal nerve has both _____ fibers and _____ fibers.

ANSWER

sensory . . . motor

QUESTION
4

The sensory ganglion associated with the trigeminal nerve is the _____ _____ ganglion.

ANSWER

trigeminal

QUESTION
5

Central processes of the trigeminal nerve enter brain at the _____.

ANSWER

pons

QUESTION
6

The three sensory nuclei of the trigeminal nerve located in the midbrain are: (1) the chief _____ nucleus, (2) the nucleus of the _____ tract, and (3) the _____ nucleus.

ANSWER

sensory . . . spinal . . . mesencephalic

ITEM 3   THE MOTOR ROOT OF THE TRIGEMINAL NERVE

The motor nucleus of the trigeminal nerve, wherein lie cell bodies of efferent nerves to the muscles of mastication, is located in the dorsal pons. Along with sensory fibers, peripheral processes of motor neurons exit from the brain on the ventrolateral surface of the pons. Motor fibers exit from the skull at the foramen ovale.

In addition to efferent fibers supplying the muscles of mastication, the motor root of the trigeminal nerve also contains afferent fibers concerned with proprioception. These proprioceptive fibers have cell bodies located in the mesencephalic nucleus of the trigeminal nerve, which is found in the midbrain.

Cell bodies of motor neurons of the trigeminal nerve are located in the dorsal _____.

QUESTION 7

pons

ANSWER

This aggregate of cell bodies is termed the _____ _____ of the trigeminal nerve.

QUESTION 8

motor nucleus

ANSWER

Processes of motor neurons of the trigeminal nerve exit from the skull at the foramen _____.

QUESTION 9

ovale

ANSWER

The motor root also contains afferent fibers associated with _____ _____.

QUESTION 10

proprioception

ANSWER

DIVISIONS OF THE TRIGEMINAL NERVE   ITEM 4

At the lower border of the trigeminal ganglion, three major nerve bundles arise. These are the three major divisions of the trigeminal nerve: the *ophthalmic, maxillary,* and *mandibular* divisions. The ophthalmic and maxillary nerves are entirely sensory. The mandibular nerve contains both sensory and motor fibers.

Study Figure 6–1 closely and observe the points where each division exits from the cranium. Remember the area to which each division distributes.

The ophthalmic division, abbreviated V_1, leaves the cranial cavity through the *superior orbital fissure* to distribute to the eye and forehead.

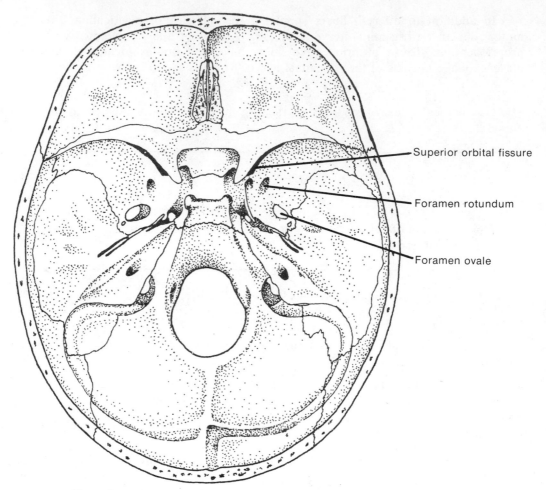

Figure 6–1. Base of the skull, superior aspect, showing points of exit of the three divisions of the trigeminal nerve (V). (Redrawn from Wolf-Heidegger: Atlas of Systematic Human Anatomy. Vol. I. Basel, S. Karger AG.)

The maxillary division, V_2, goes through the *foramen rotundum* to the upper jaw and cheek.

The mandibular division, or V_3, exits through the *foramen ovale* to the lower jaw and chin.

QUESTION
11

Match the cranial exits in Column B with the divisions of the trigeminal nerve in Column A.

Column A	*Column B*
( ) 1. ophthalmic division	A. foramen ovale
( ) 2. maxillary division	B. superior orbital fissure
( ) 3. mandibular division	C. foramen rotundum

Trigeminal division V_1 distributes to the _____ and _____; V_2, to the upper jaw and _____; V_3, to the lower jaw and _____.

---

eye . . . forehead . . . cheek . . . chin

THE OPHTHALMIC NERVE: BRANCHES   ITEM 5

The ophthalmic division of nerve V is entirely sensory. It leaves the trigeminal ganglion, passing anteriorly in a fold of dura in the lateral wall of the cavernous sinus. Just before entering the superior orbital fissure, the ophthalmic nerve divides into three branches, all of which pass through the superior orbital fissure into the orbit. The three branches, seen in Figure 6–2 on page 250 are, reading from lateral to medial, the *lacrimal,* the *frontal,* and the *nasociliary.*

Referring to Figure 6–2 if necessary, write in the numbered spaces below the names of the corresponding numbered structures on the diagram, page 251.

Labels
1. _____ nerve
2. _____ nerve
3. _____ nerve

---

1. lacrimal   2. frontal   3. nasociliary

The ophthalmic nerve is *entirely sensory/entirely motor/both sensory and motor* (circle one).

---

entirely sensory

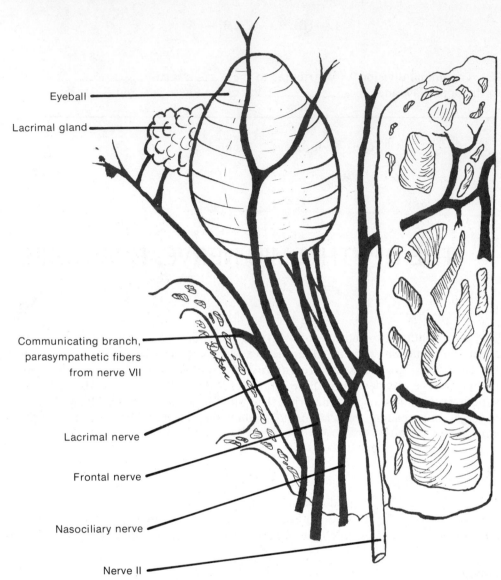

Eyeball

Lacrimal gland

Communicating branch,
parasympathetic fibers
from nerve VII

Lacrimal nerve

Frontal nerve

Nasociliary nerve

Nerve II

Figure 6–2. Branches of the ophthalmic division of the trigeminal nerve (V). (Redrawn from Woodburne: Essentials of Human Anatomy. 4th Ed. New York, Oxford University Press.)

QUESTION
15

After leaving the trigeminal ganglion, the ophthalmic nerve travels anteriorly along the lateral wall of the _____ sinus.

ANSWER

cavernous

QUESTION
16

The ophthalmic nerve divides into the lacrimal, frontal, and nasociliary branches just before intering the _____ _____ fissure.

ANSWER

superior orbital

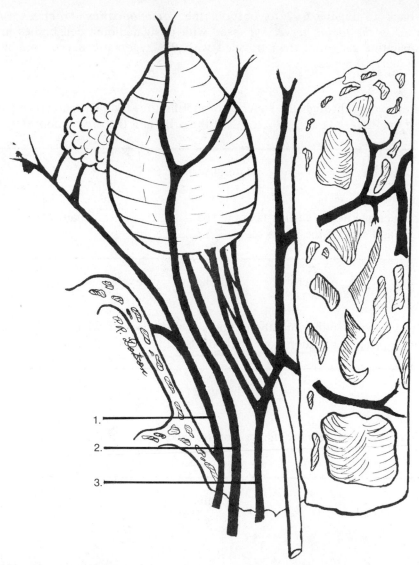

1.

2.

3.

(Redrawn from Woodburne: Essentials of Human Anatomy. 4th Ed. New York, Oxford University Press.)

THE LACRIMAL NERVE ITEM 6

Figure 6–2 depicts the route of the lacrimal branch of the ophthalmic nerve. The lacrimal nerve passes through the lateral portion of the superior orbital fissure. It then runs anteriorly through the orbit between the superior part of the lateral orbital wall and the orbital contents to reach the lacrimal gland, the conjunctiva, and the skin of the lateral portion of the upper eyelid.

In the orbit, the lacrimal nerve gains some fibers which originated as fibers controlling lacrimal gland secretion. These fibers are usually carried to the orbit in the zygomatic nerve, which is a branch of the maxillary nerve.

Refer back to Figure 6–2 to observe the *communicating branches which originated in the facial nerve,* synapsed with postganglionic cell bodies in the pterygopalatine ganglion, then traveled with the zygomatic nerve, and finally with the lacrimal nerve.

QUESTION 17

After exiting through the superior orbital fissure, the lacrimal nerve passes between the _____ _____ of the orbit and the orbital contents.

ANSWER

lateral wall

QUESTION 18

The lacrimal nerve carries fibers to the _____ gland, the _____ _____, and skin of the upper _____.

ANSWER

lacrimal . . . conjunctiva . . . eyelid

QUESTION 19

Postganglionic parasympathetic fibers, cell bodies of which are located in the pterygopalatine ganglion, join fibers of the _____ nerve.

ANSWER

lacrimal

QUESTION 20

These parasympathetic fibers control secretion of the _____ gland.

ANSWER

lacrimal

ITEM 7   THE FRONTAL NERVE

In Figure 6–3, follow the path of the frontal branch of the ophthalmic nerve. The frontal nerve passes forward above the ocular muscles and divides into two branches, a large supraorbital nerve and a smaller supratrochlear nerve.

QUESTION 21

Referring to Figure 6–3 if necessary, write in the numbered spaces below the names of the corresponding numbered structures on the diagram, page 254.

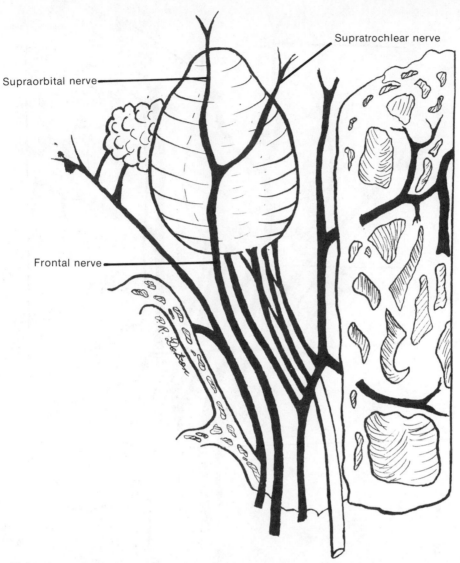

Supratrochlear nerve

Supraorbital nerve

Frontal nerve

Figure 6–3. Ophthalmic division of the trigeminal nerve (V), showing branches of the frontal nerve. (Redrawn from Woodburne: Essentials of Human Anatomy. 4th Ed. New York, Oxford University Press.)

Labels

1. _____ nerve
2. _____ nerve
3. _____ nerve

---

1. supraorbital   2. frontal   3. supratrochlear   *ANSWER*

The two main branches of the frontal nerve are the _____ nerve and the _____ nerve.   QUESTION
22

---

supraorbital . . . supratrochlear (in either order)   *ANSWER*

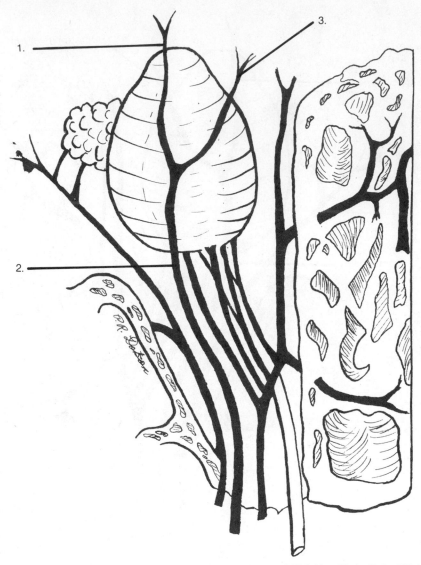

(Redrawn from Woodburne: Essentials of Human Anatomy. 4th Ed. New York, Oxford University Press.)

ITEM 8   BRANCHES OF THE OPHTHALMIC DIVISION: CUTANEOUS DISTRIBUTION

The cutaneous distribution of branches of the ophthalmic division of the trigeminal nerve may be seen in Figure 6–4. As the supraorbital nerve continues forward, it passes through the supraorbital notch, or foramen, then swings upward to supply skin of the forehead and anterior scalp, with smaller branches going to the upper eyelid and the frontal sinus.

The supratrochlear nerve runs forward and medially to reach the skin of the medial part of the forehead and the upper eyelid. Refer to Figure 6–4 to see where the supratrochlear nerve emerges from the skull.

Also in Figure 6–4, note the cutaneous distribution of the *infratrochlear nerve*, a branch of the nasociliary portion of the ophthalmic division.

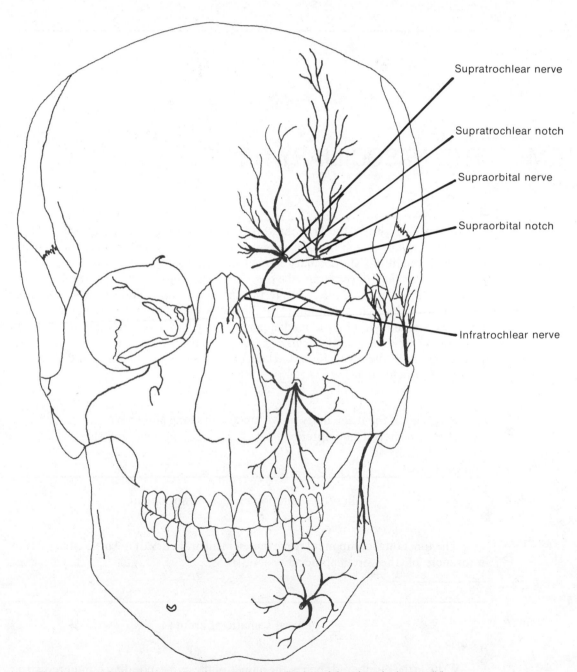

Figure 6–4. Cutaneous nerves of the ophthalmic division of the trigeminal nerve (V).

QUESTION
23

The supraorbital nerve supplies skin of the _____ and of the anterior _____.

ANSWER

forehead . . . scalp

QUESTION
24

The supratrochlear nerve is located *lateral/medial* (circle one) to the supra-orbital nerve.

ANSWER

medial

ITEM 9   THE NASOCILIARY NERVE

Figure 6–5 shows the branches of the nasociliary nerve which are given off in the orbit. *Short* and *long ciliary nerves* carry fibers for general sensation to the eyeball. In addition, short ciliary nerves carry autonomic fibers to the eye. The *posterior ethmoidal nerve* enters the posterior ethmoidal foramen to supply mucosa of the posterior ethmoid air cells and the sphenoid sinus. The *anterior ethmoidal nerve* passes through the anterior ethmoidal foramen, then branches to supply nasal mucosa and skin on the medial part of the nose. The terminal branch of the nasociliary nerve, the *infratrochlear nerve*, supplies skin of the lower lid and adjacent portion of the nose. Refer back to Figure 6–4 to see the area of distribution of the infratrochlear nerve.

QUESTION
25

Branches of the nasociliary nerve include the long and short _____ nerves, the posterior and anterior _____ nerves, and the _____ _____ nerve.

ANSWER

ciliary . . . ethmoidal . . . infratrochlear

QUESTION
26

The functional component represented in all branches of the nasociliary nerve, a branch of the ophthalmic division, is _____ _____ _____.

ANSWER

general somatic afferent

QUESTION
27

Write in the numbered spaces the names of the corresponding numbered structures on the diagram, page 258. Refer to Figure 6–5 only when necessary.

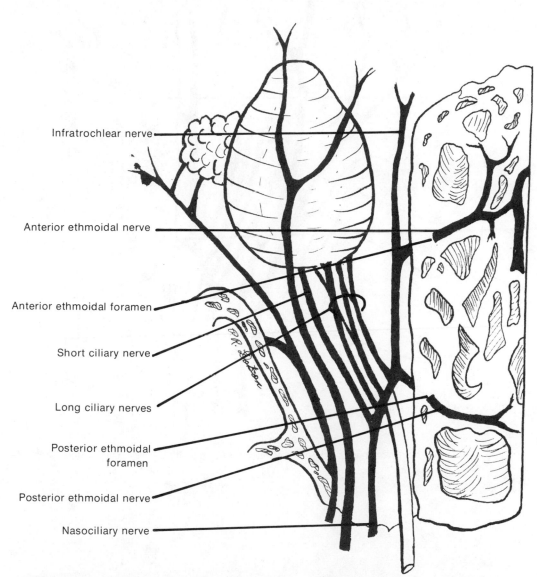

Infratrochlear nerve

Anterior ethmoidal nerve

Anterior ethmoidal foramen

Short ciliary nerve

Long ciliary nerves

Posterior ethmoidal foramen

Posterior ethmoidal nerve

Nasociliary nerve

Figure 6–5. Nasociliary branches of ophthalmic division of the trigeminal nerve (V). (Redrawn from Woodburne: Essentials of Human Anatomy. 4th Ed. New York, Oxford University Press.)

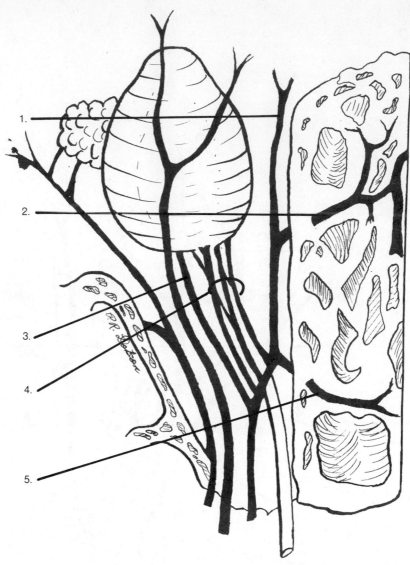

(Redrawn from Woodburne: Essentials of Human Anatomy. 4th Ed. New York, Oxford University Press.)

Labels

1. _____ nerve
2. _____ nerve
3. _____ nerve
4. _____ nerves
5. _____ nerve

ANSWER

1. infratrochlear
2. anterior ethmoidal
3. short ciliary

4. long ciliary
5. posterior ethmoidal

The maxillary division of trigeminal nerve V, like the ophthalmic division, is entirely sensory. Figure 6–6 illustrates this nerve as it courses forward from the trigeminal ganglion. Anteriorly, it extends through the dura mater on the infero-lateral surface of the cavernous sinus. A meningeal branch is given off to the dura mater of the middle cranial fossa. The maxillary nerve passes through the foramen rotundum to the pterygopalatine fossa, where several important branches are given off. The direct anterior continuation of the maxillary nerve is the infraorbital nerve, which exits from the orbit through the infraorbital foramen.

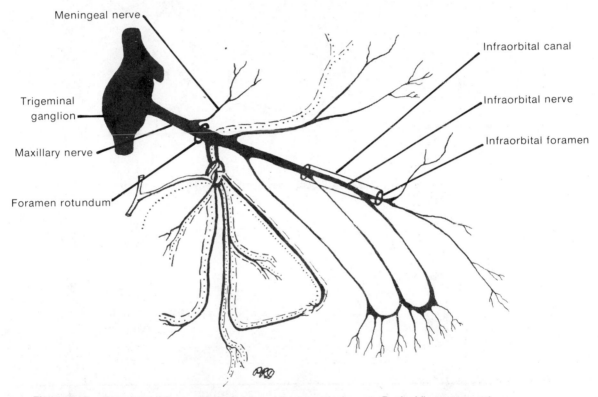

Figure 6–6. Branches of the maxillary division of the trigeminal nerve. Dashed lines represent parasympathetic fibers, and dotted lines sympathetic fibers. Both types of fibers travel with the maxillary division. (Redrawn and modified from Woodburne: Essentials of Human Anatomy. 4th Ed. New York, Oxford University Press.)

The meningeal branch of the maxillary nerve supplies the dura mater of the _____ cranial fossa.

QUESTION 28

---

middle

ANSWER

In the numbered spaces on page 260 write the names of the corresponding numbered structures on the accompanying diagram. Consult Figure 6–6 if you find it necessary.

QUESTION 29

259

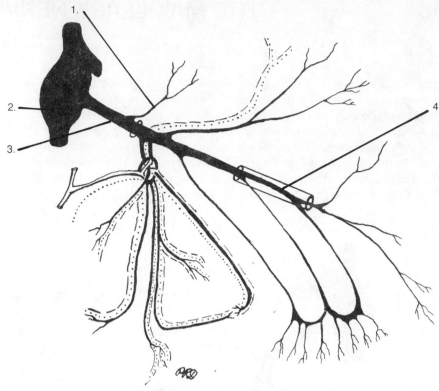

(Redrawn and modified from Woodburne: Essentials of Human Anatomy. 4th Ed. New York, Oxford University Press.)

Labels

1. _____ branch
2. _____ ganglion
3. _____ nerve
4. _____ nerve

ANSWER   1. meningeal   2. trigeminal   3. maxillary   4. infraorbital

QUESTION 30   The maxillary nerve enters the pterygopalatine fossa through the foramen _____.

ANSWER   rotundum

QUESTION 31   The infraorbital nerve, which exits from the orbit through the _____ foramen, is a direct continuation of the _____ nerve.

ANSWER   infraorbital . . . maxillary

While passing through the pterygopalatine fossa, the maxillary nerve gives off several branches, which appear in Figure 6–7. Two short *pterygopalatine branches* pass downward and enter the pterygopalatine ganglion. The *posterior superior alveolar nerve* is then given off, and superiorly a small *zygomatic nerve* enters the orbit.

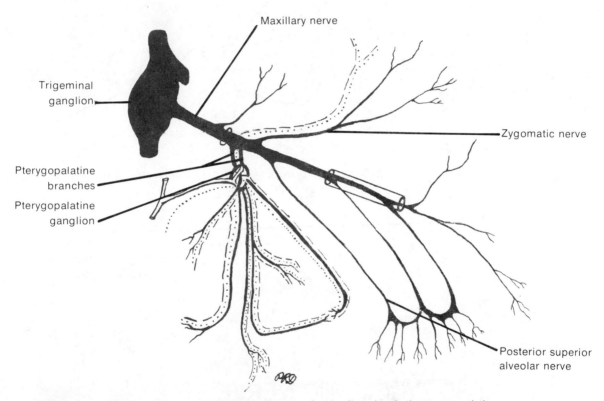

Figure 6–7. Maxillary division of the trigeminal nerve, showing branches in the pterygopalatine fossa. (Redrawn and modified from Woodburne: Essentials of Human Anatomy. 4th Ed. New York, Oxford University Press.)

In the numbered spaces below write the names of the corresponding numbered structures on the diagram, page 262. Consult Figure 6–7, if necessary.

QUESTION
32

Labels

1. _____ nerve
2. _____ nerve
3. _____ _____ _____ nerve
4. _____ ganglion
5. _____ branches

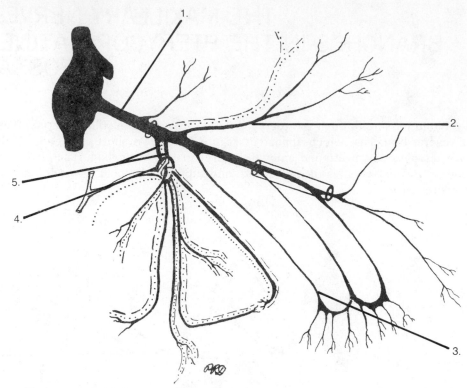

(Redrawn and modified from Woodburne: Essentials of Human Anatomy. 4th Ed. New York, Oxford University Press.)

ANSWER

1. maxillary
2. zygomatic
3. posterior superior alveolar

4. pterygopalatine
5. pterygopalatine

ITEM 12

THE ZYGOMATIC NERVE

Examine the course of the *zygomatic nerve* as shown in Figure 6–8. The zygomatic nerve arises from the superior surface of the maxillary nerve where it passes through the pterygopalatine fossa. Entering the orbit through the inferior orbital fissure, the zygomatic nerve courses on the lateral wall of the orbit, passes into the zygomatic bone through the zygomatico-orbital foramen.

QUESTION
33

The aperture through which the zygomatic nerve enters the orbit is the _____ _____ fissure.

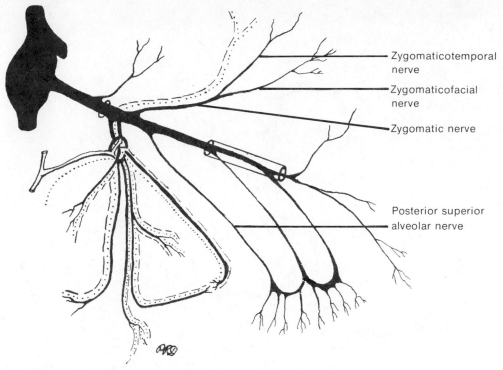

Figure 6-8. Maxillary division of the trigeminal nerve (V), showing branches of zygomatic nerve and posterior superior alveolar nerve. (Redrawn and modified from Woodburne: Essentials of Human Anatomy. 4th Ed. New York, Oxford University Press.)

inferior orbital   *ANSWER*

The zygomatic nerve enters the zygomatic bone through the _____   *QUESTION*
_____ foramen.   **34**

zygomatico-orbital   *ANSWER*

THE ZYGOMATICOFACIAL AND ZYGOMATICOTEMPORAL NERVES   ITEM 13

While coursing through the zygomatic bone, the zygomatic nerve divides into two branches, the *zygomaticofacial* and the *zygomaticotemporal nerves*. Refer to Figure 6–9 to see the distribution of these two nerves. The zygomaticofacial nerve leaves bone via the zygomaticofacial foramen on the lateral surface of the zygoma. Fibers of this nerve distribute to skin overlying the lateral surface of the zygoma.

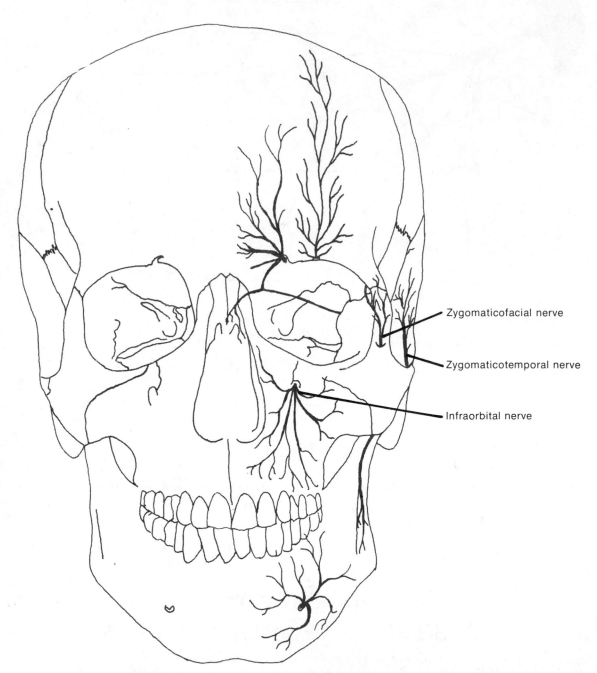

Figure 6-9. Cutaneous nerves of the maxillary division of the trigeminal nerve (V).

The zygomaticotemporal nerve leaves bone through the zygomaticotemporal foramen, which may be found in the sphenozygomatic suture. The nerve then passes upward between the temporalis muscle and the frontal bone to supply skin over the anterior fourth of the temporalis muscle.

In Figure 6–9, notice the cutaneous distribution of the terminal branches of the *infraorbital nerve:*

Within the zygomatic bone, the zygomatic nerve bifurcates into the zygomatico-_____ nerve and the zygomatico-_____ nerve.

QUESTION
35

facial . . . temporal

ANSWER

Skin over the anterior part of the temporalis muscle receives sensory innervation from the _____ nerve, while sensory supply to the skin of the lateral surface of the zygoma comes from the _____ nerve.

QUESTION
36

zygomaticotemporal . . . zygomaticofacial

ANSWER

THE POSTERIOR SUPERIOR ALVEOLAR NERVE

ITEM
14

Look back to Figure 6–8 and locate the posterior superior alveolar nerve, which supplies molar teeth and adjacent structures. This nerve, after branching off the maxillary nerve in the pterygopalatine fossa, descends through the pterygomaxillary fissure, eventually resting on the posterior surface of the maxilla.

The site at which the posterior superior alveolar nerve leaves the maxillary nerve is the _____ fossa.

QUESTION
37

pterygopalatine

ANSWER

After emerging through the pterygomaxillary fissure, the posterior superior alveolar nerve lies on the posterior surface of the _____.

QUESTION
38

maxilla

ANSWER

ITEM 15

THE POSTERIOR SUPERIOR ALVEOLAR NERVE: BRANCHES

The posterior superior alveolar nerve, which supplies sensory innervation to the molar region, branches terminally. One terminal branch descends to reach buccal gingiva of the three maxillary molar teeth and the adjacent buccal mucosa. The remaining two branches enter small foramina in the maxilla and extend through small canals in the lateral wall of the maxillary sinus forward toward the molar and premolar teeth. Branches of these nerves supply the mucous membrane of the maxillary sinus.

QUESTION
39

The posterior superior alveolar nerve carries fibers which provide *afferent/efferent* (circle one) innervation to structures supplied.

ANSWER

The posterior superior alveolar nerve is an afferent nerve. If you missed this one, reread Item 4 to regain your conception of the overall view of the three divisions of the trigeminal nerve. Only the mandibular division contains both motor and sensory fibers; the maxillary and ophthalmic divisions are entirely sensory.

QUESTION
40

The first terminal branch of the posterior superior alveolar nerve supplies afferent innervation to the ＿＿＿＿＿＿ gingiva of the maxillary molar teeth and the adjacent ＿＿＿＿＿＿ mucosa.

ANSWER

buccal . . . buccal

QUESTION
41

The second and third terminal branches of the posterior superior alveolar nerve carry GSA fibers to the ＿＿＿＿＿＿ and ＿＿＿＿＿＿ teeth and to the mucous membrane of the ＿＿＿＿＿＿ sinus.

ANSWER

molar . . . premolar . . . maxillary

ITEM 16

THE PTERYGOPALATINE BRANCHES

The *pterygopalatine branches* of the maxillary nerve, shown in Figure 6–10, are two short, thick trunks which descend from the maxillary nerve to the pterygopalatine ganglion by way of the pterygopalatine fossa. These trunks carry incoming general somatic afferent fibers which convey general sensation from the nasal and palatine mucosa. Also contained in the pterygopalatine branches are

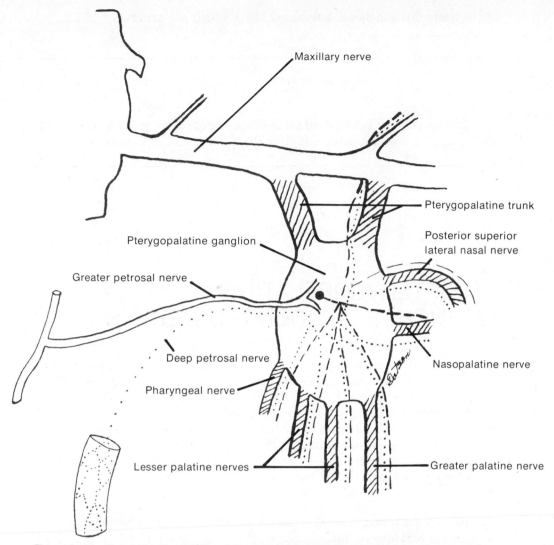

Figure 6-10. Detail showing maxillary branches which appear to arise from the pterygopalatine ganglion. (Redrawn and modified from Woodburne: Essentials of Human Anatomy. 4th Ed. New York, Oxford University Press.)

general visceral efferent fibers carrying sympathetic and parasympathetic post-ganglionic fibers.

The pterygopalatine trunks from the maxillary nerve extend from the _____ nerve to the _____ ganglion.

QUESTION
42

---

maxillary . . . pterygopalatine

ANSWER

The functional components of the pterygopalatine branches of the maxillary nerve are mainly general _____ _____, but associated with

QUESTION
43

these fibers postganglionic autonomic fibers which are general _____
_____.

---

somatic afferent . . . visceral efferent

Pterygopalatine branches of the maxillary nerve carry general sensation from
the _____ mucosa and from the _____ mucosa.

---

nasal . . . palatine

ITEM 17   THE PTERYGOPALATINE BRANCHES: ASSOCIATED NERVES

The various terminal branches of the pterygopalatine nerves appear to be
originating from the pterygopalatine ganglion, where preganglionic and postganglionic parasympathetic fibers synapse. Actually, the nerves emerging from
the pterygopalatine ganglion are mostly composed of GSA fibers from the maxillary nerve which simply pass through the ptergopalatine ganglion without chang-
ing and without synapsing. However, these pterygopalatine nerves also do contain
parasympathetic postganglionic fibers. The pterygopalatine ganglion and associated branches are shown in Figure 6–10.

Nerves emerging from the pterygopalatine ganglion contain both general
somatic afferent fibers of the _____ nerve and _____
postganglionic fibers.

---

maxillary . . . parasympathetic

ITEM 18   THE PTERYGOPALATINE GANGLION: SENSORY BRANCHES

Notice in Figure 6–10 the five sensory branches which appear to arise from the
pterygopalatine ganglion; the (1) pharyngeal, (2) lesser palatine, (3) greater palatine, (4) nasopalatine, and (5) posterior superior lateral nasal branches. Each of
these branches supplies sensory fibers to mucosa. The fibers do not synapse in
the pterygopalatine ganglion, nor are their cell bodies located there. Sensory

branches merely pass through this ganglion on their way to their cell bodies in the trigeminal ganglion.

Cell bodies of the sensory fibers passing through the pterygopalatine ganglion are actually located in the _____ ganglion.

QUESTION
46

---

trigeminal

ANSWER

Using the Word Bank, write in the numbered spaces on page 270 the names of the corresponding numbered structures on the accompanying diagram. Try to fill in all the blanks without referring to Figure 6–10.

QUESTION
47

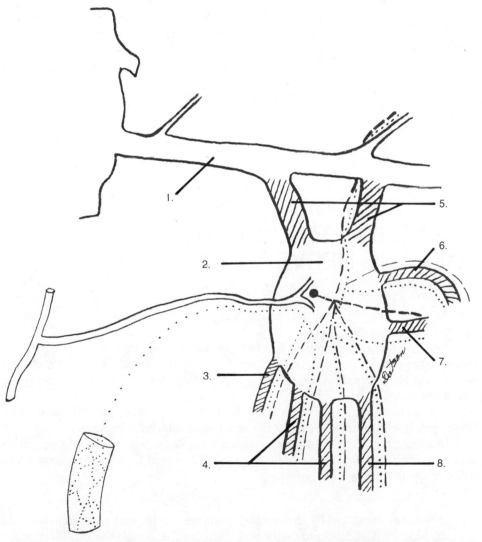

(Redrawn and modified from Woodburne: Essentials of Human Anatomy. 4th Ed. New York, Oxford University Press.)

Word Bank
greater palatine nerve
lesser palatine nerves
maxillary nerve
nasopalatine nerve
pharyngeal nerve
posterior superior lateral nasal nerve
pterygopalatine ganglion
pterygopalatine trunk

Labels

1. _____
2. _____
3. _____
4. _____
5. _____
6. _____
7. _____
8. _____

ANSWER   Check your labels with Figure 6–10.

ITEM 19   THE PTERYGOPALATINE BRANCHES: THE GREATER PALATINE NERVE

Figure 6–11, a parasagittal section of the lateral nasal wall, shows the greater and lesser palatine nerves.

The greater palatine nerve descends in the palatine canal, emerges through the greater palatine foramen, and extends forward adjacent to the alveolar process of the maxilla to supply mucosa of the hard palate and the lingual gingiva of the maxillary teeth.

The lesser palatine nerves descend in the palatine canal and exit through the lesser palatine foramina to supply the soft palate and palatine tonsil.

In Figure 6–11, the *posterior inferior lateral nasal branches* are given off the greater palatine nerve. These branches extend forward to supply mucosa of the inferior nasal concha.

QUESTION 48

Structures supplied by the greater palatine nerve include mucosa of the _____ _____ and the lingual _____ of the maxillary teeth.

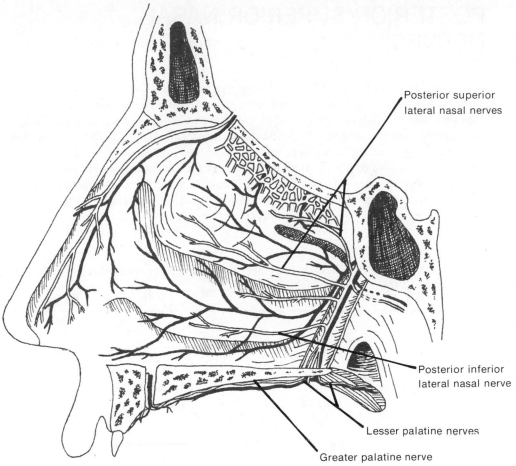

Figure 6–11. Nerves of the lateral nasal wall, seen in a parasagittal section. (Redrawn from Woodburne: Essentials of Human Anatomy. 4th Ed. New York, Oxford University Press.)

hard palate . . . gingiva   *ANSWER*

The nerves which stem from the greater palatine nerve to supply mucosa of the inferior nasal concha are the posterior _____ _____ nasal branches.

QUESTION
49

inferior lateral   *ANSWER*

Lesser palatine nerves supply mucosa of the _____ _____ and the _____ tonsil.

QUESTION
50

soft palate . . . palatine   *ANSWER*

ITEM 20

POSTERIOR SUPERIOR NASAL NERVES

Refer back to Figure 6–11 and note the location of the *posterior superior lateral nasal nerves*. These branches arise from the pterygopalatine ganglion and pass medially through the sphenopalatine foramen to supply mucosa of the middle and superior nasal conchae. Posterior superior lateral nasal branches also supply the superior part of the nasal septum.

It is interesting to note that all the mucosa of the nasal cavity supplied by the maxillary nerve is mucosa overlying bone. Mucosa which overlies cartilage in the anterior portion of the nasal cavity, on the other hand, is supplied by a branch from the ophthalmic division called the *anterior ethmoidal nerve*.

QUESTION 51

Nasal mucosa supplied by branches of the maxillary nerve is mucosa overlying *cartilage/bone* (circle one).

ANSWER

bone

QUESTION 52

Mucosa of the inferior nasal concha is supplied by posterior _____ lateral nasal branches; that of the lateral nasal wall is supplied by posterior _____ lateral nasal branches.

ANSWER

inferior . . . superior

QUESTION 53

En route from the pterygopalatine ganglion to the middle and superior nasal conchae, the posterior superior lateral nasal branches pass through the _____ foramen.

ANSWER

sphenopalatine

ITEM 21

THE NASOPALATINE NERVE

Turn back to Figure 6–10 and locate the remaining sensory branch extending from the pterygopalatine ganglion, the *nasopalatine nerve*. The nasopalatine nerve, like the posterior superior lateral nasal nerve, passes through the sphenopalatine foramen to reach the nasal cavity. It then crosses the roof of the nasal cavity to reach the nasal septum and descends obliquely forward on the septum, supplying mucosa overlying its bony portion. The naso-palatine nerve terminates by passing through the incisive canal to supply both a small area of the hard palate immediately behind the maxillary incisor teeth, and the lingual gingiva of those teeth.

The nasopalatine nerve innervates _____of the nasal cavity; a portion of the _____ palate; and the lingual _____ of the maxillary incisor teeth.

QUESTION 54

mucosa . . . hard . . . gingiva

ANSWER

The nasal mucosa supplied by the nasopalatine nerve is mucosa overlying the *cartilaginous/bony* (circle one) portion of the nasal septum.

QUESTION 55

bony

ANSWER

The foramen through which the nasopalatine nerve passes en route to the nasal cavity is the _____ foramen.

QUESTION 56

sphenopalatine

ANSWER

THE INFRAORBITAL NERVE   ITEM 22

The infraorbital nerve constitutes the forward continuation of the maxillary nerve. The location and branches of the infraorbital nerve are illustrated in Figure 6–12. The infraorbital nerve enters the orbit through the inferior orbital fissure, travels in the infraorbital groove on the floor of the orbit, enters the infraorbital canal, and exits onto the face through the infraorbital foramen. The cutaneous distribution of the terminal branches of the infraorbital nerve were shown in Figure 6–9.

The infraorbital nerve enters the orbit through the _____ _____ fissure and exits from the infraorbital canal through the _____ foramen.

QUESTION 57

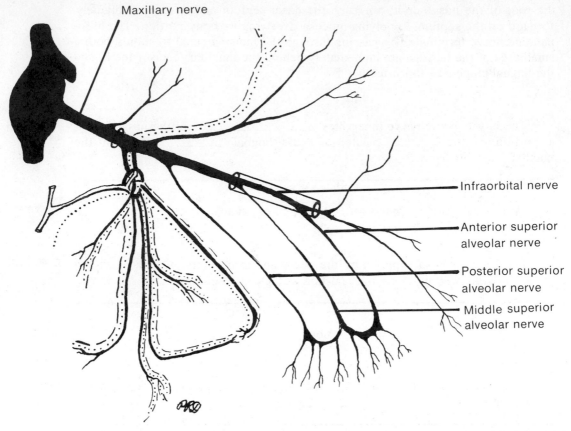

Maxillary nerve

Infraorbital nerve

Anterior superior
alveolar nerve

Posterior superior
alveolar nerve

Middle superior
alveolar nerve

Figure 6–12.   Maxillary division of the trigeminal nerve (V), showing branches of the infraorbital nerve. (Redrawn and modified from Woodburne: Essentials of Human Anatomy. 4th Ed. New York, Oxford University Press.)

ANSWER   inferior orbital . . . infraorbital

QUESTION   While in the orbit, the infraorbital nerve occupies the infraorbital
58   _____ and the infraorbital _____.

ANSWER   groove . . . canal

ITEM 23   THE ANTERIOR SUPERIOR ALVEOLAR NERVE

While within the infraorbital canal, the infraorbital nerve gives off the *anterior superior alveolar nerve*, shown in Figure 6–12. This branch descends through a bony canal in the anterior wall of the maxillary sinus to supply maxillary incisor and canine teeth and adjacent gingiva. Branches of the anterior superior alveolar nerve also distribute to the maxillary sinus.

The anterior superior alveolar nerve branches off the _____ nerve in the infraorbital canal and descends via another canal in the anterior wall of the _____ sinus.

infraorbital . . . maxillary

Branches of the anterior superior alveolar nerve distribute to the maxillary _____ teeth, the maxillary _____ teeth, and to the _____ adjacent to these teeth.

incisor . . . canine . . . gingiva

In addition to the teeth and gingiva it supplies, the anterior superior alveolar nerve also distributes to the _____ sinus.

maxillary

THE MIDDLE SUPERIOR ALVEOLAR NERVE   ITEM 24

Locate the *middle superior alveolar nerve* in Figure 6–12. When present, this nerve branches off from the infraorbital nerve in the infraorbital canal. It descends along a canal in the lateral wall of the maxillary sinus to supply the two maxillary premolar teeth, adjacent gingiva, and the maxillary sinus. In cases where the middle superior alveolar nerve is not present, these areas are innervated by the anterior and posterior superior alveolar nerves.

After branching off the infraorbital nerve, the middle superior alveolar nerve descends in the lateral wall of the _____ sinus.

maxillary

The middle superior alveolar nerve distributes to the maxillary _____ teeth, adjacent _____, and the _____ sinus.

premolar . . . gingiva . . . maxillary

ITEM 25

THE CUTANEOUS BRANCHES OF THE INFRAORBITAL NERVE

Look back to Figure 6–9 and note the cutaneous terminal branches of the infraorbital nerve as they exit onto the face through the infraorbital foramen. *Palpebral branches* supply skin and conjunctiva of the lower eyelid. *External nasal branches* supply skin of the side of the nose. Numerous *superior labial branches* distribute to the skin of the upper lip and to the labial mucosa.

QUESTION
64

In the numbered spaces below write the names of the corresponding numbered structures in the accompanying diagram.

Labels

1. _____ nerve
2. _____ alveolar nerve
3. _____ alveolar nerve
4. _____ alveolar nerve

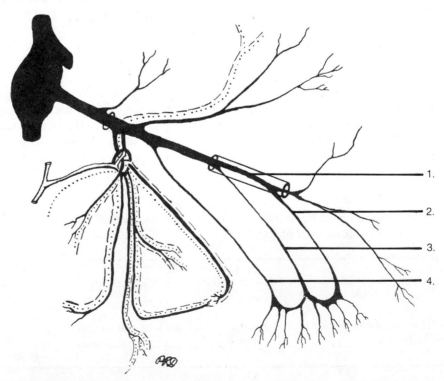

(Redrawn and modified from Woodburne: Essentials of Human Anatomy. 4th Ed. New York, Oxford University Press.)

1. infraorbital
2. anterior superior
3. middle superior
4. posterior superior

The skin and conjunctiva of the eyelid are supplied by the _____ branches of the infraorbital nerve.

palpebral

The skin of the side of the nose receives sensory innervation from external nasal branches of the _____ nerve.

infraorbital

The cutaneous terminal branches of the infraorbital nerve which supply the upper lip and labial mucosa are called the superior _____ branches.

labial

THE MANDIBULAR DIVISION OF THE TRIGEMINAL NERVE

ITEM 26

The mandibular division of the trigeminal nerve, like the ophthalmic and maxillary divisions, contains a large number of general somatic afferent fibers conveying general sensation. The mandibular division, however, differs from the other two divisions in that the mandibular nerve is joined, just after it leaves the foramen ovale, by the *motor root* of the trigeminal nerve.

The mandibular division of the trigeminal nerve contains (circle one) *sensory fibers only/motor fibers only/both sensory and motor fibers.*

both sensory and motor

ITEM
27

THE MANDIBULAR NERVE: SENSORY BRANCHES

The sensory root of the mandibular nerve, along with the motor root, leaves the middle cranial fossa through the foramen ovale. Sensory fibers distribute to four types of structures: (1) skin in the temporal region and overlying the mandible; (2) the lower teeth and gingiva; (3) mucous membranes of the cheek, tongue, and mastoid air cells; and (4) the temporomandibular joint.

QUESTION
69

Both sensory and motor roots of the mandibular nerve exit from the skull at the foramen _____ in the _____ cranial fossa.

ANSWER

ovale . . . middle

QUESTION
70

Besides supplying skin in the temporal region and skin overlying the mandible, the mandibular nerve also supplies the _____ teeth and gingiva and the _____ joint.

ANSWER

mandibular . . . temporomandibular

QUESTION
71

Mucous membranes supplied by sensory branches of the mandibular nerve include those of the _____, of the _____, and of the mastoid _____ _____.

ANSWER

cheek . . . tongue . . . air cells

ITEM
28

THE MANDIBULAR NERVE: THE COMMON SENSORY-MOTOR TRUNK

Figure 6–13 diagrams the branches of the mandibular division of nerve V. Just below the foramen ovale, the sensory and motor roots of the trigeminal nerve unite in a short common trunk. Two small branches, one sensory and one motor, are given off this common trunk. The sensory branch is the *meningeal nerve*, which turns upward to pass through the foramen spinosum to enter the cranium, where it supplies the meninges. The small motor branch supplies the medial pterygoid muscle, the tensor tympani muscle, and the tensor veli palatini muscle.

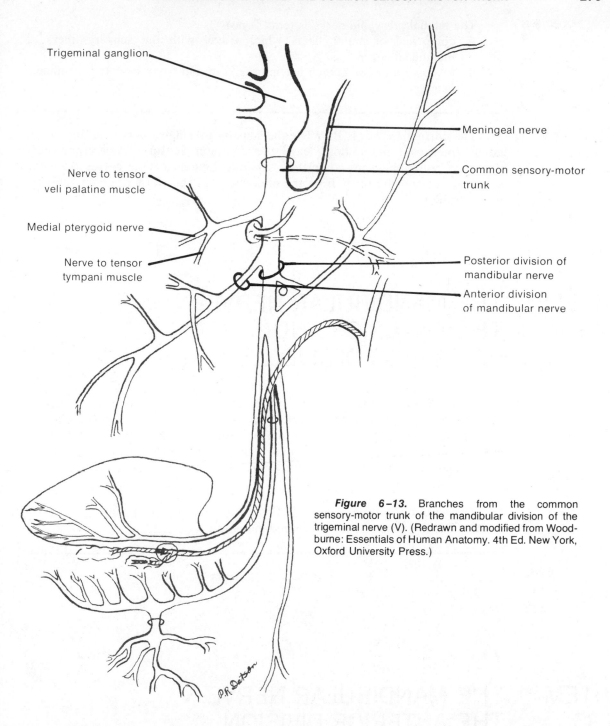

Trigeminal ganglion

Meningeal nerve

Common sensory-motor trunk

Nerve to tensor veli palatine muscle

Medial pterygoid nerve

Nerve to tensor tympani muscle

Posterior division of mandibular nerve

Anterior division of mandibular nerve

Figure 6-13. Branches from the common sensory-motor trunk of the mandibular division of the trigeminal nerve (V). (Redrawn and modified from Woodburne: Essentials of Human Anatomy. 4th Ed. New York, Oxford University Press.)

After branching off the common sensory-motor trunk of the mandibular nerve, the meningeal nerve enters the cranium through the foramen _____ to supply the _____.

QUESTION
72

---

spinosum . . . meninges

ANSWER

QUESTION
73

The medial pterygoid nerve is (circle one)
A. composed of motor fibers which travel with the sensory fibers of meningeal nerve
B. a separate motor branch leaving the common trunk near the meningeal nerve

ANSWER

The correct answer is B. While the sensory meningeal nerve and the motor medial pterygoid nerve both leave the common sensory-motor trunk near the same point, they are completely separate branches. One comes from the sensory root and the other from the motor root in the short common sensory-motor trunk.

ITEM 29   THE MANDIBULAR NERVE: THE ANTERIOR AND POSTERIOR DIVISIONS

After giving off the meningeal nerve and the medial pterygoid nerve, the mandibular nerve bifurcates into anterior and posterior divisions. The anterior division is motor, except for one sensory branch. The posterior division is sensory, except for one motor branch. Anterior and posterior divisions of the mandibular nerve are labeled in Figure 6–13.

QUESTION
74

The anterior division of the mandibular nerve is predominantly _____ in function; the posterior division, predominantly _____.

ANSWER

motor . . . sensory

ITEM 30   THE MANDIBULAR NERVE: THE ANTERIOR DIVISION

Examine Figure 6–14 and observe the four motor branches arising from the anterior division of the mandibular nerve: (1) the *posterior deep temporal nerve;* (2) the *anterior deep temporal nerve;* (3) the *nerve to the masseter muscle;* and (4) the *nerve to the lateral pterygoid muscle.* The anterior division terminates as the *buccal nerve,* the only sensory branch of this division.

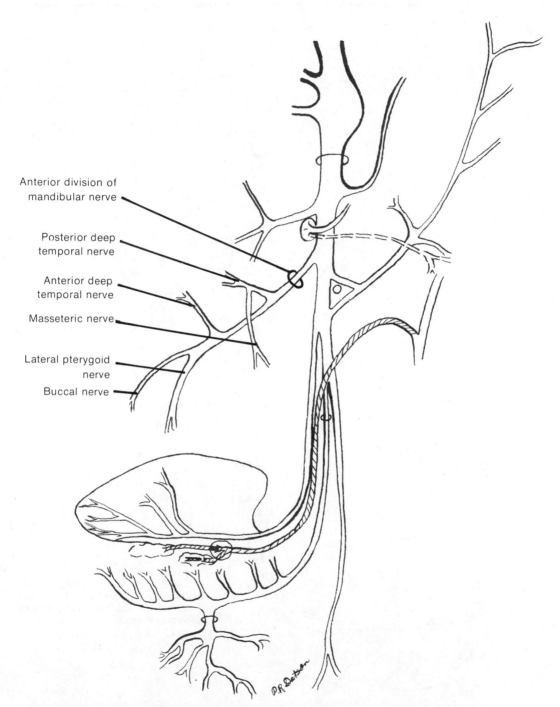

Figure 6–14. Branches of the anterior division of the mandibular nerve. (Redrawn and modified from Woodburne: Essentials of Human Anatomy. 4th Ed. New York, Oxford University Press.)

QUESTION
75
The buccal nerve, the termination of the anterior division of the mandibular nerve, is an *afferent/efferent* (circle one) nerve.

ANSWER

afferent

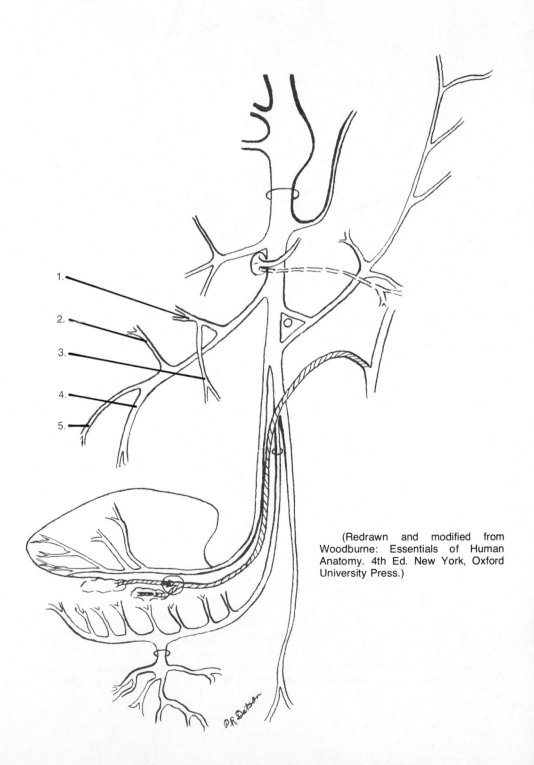

1.

2.

3.

4.

5.

(Redrawn and modified from
Woodburne: Essentials of Human
Anatomy. 4th Ed. New York, Oxford
University Press.)

In the numbered spaces below write the names of the corresponding numbered nerves on the accompanying diagram.

Labels

1. _____ deep temporal nerve
2. _____ deep temporal nerve
3. nerve to the _____ muscle
4. nerve to the _____ _____ muscle
5. _____ nerve

---

1. posterior
2. anterior
3. masseter

4. lateral pterygoid
5. buccal

THE ANTERIOR AND POSTERIOR DEEP TEMPORAL NERVES   ITEM 31

The anterior and posterior deep temporal nerves, seen in Figure 6–14, extend laterally and superiorly around the infratemporal crest of the sphenoid bone to innervate the temporalis muscle. Occasionally a third nerve of this group, a middle deep temporal nerve, may be present.

Anterior and posterior deep temporal nerves ascend over the _____ crest of the sphenoid bone to reach the _____ muscle.

---

infratemporal . . . temporalis

The deep temporal nerve which is occasionally, though not always, present is (circle one)
A. anterior deep temporal nerve
B. middle deep temporal nerve
C. posterior deep temporal nerve

The correct answer is B. Sometimes a middle deep temporal nerve is present, sometimes not.

ITEM 32   NERVE TO THE MASSETER MUSCLE

Locate the nerve to the masseter muscle in Figure 6–14. The masseter muscle is one of the muscles which elevate the mandible. The nerve to this muscle sometimes arises directly from the anterior division of the mandibular nerve; sometimes it appears as a branch of the posterior deep temporal nerve. As the masseteric nerve passes above the lateral pterygoid muscle, it gives off a branch to the temporomandibular joint. It then passes through the mandibular notch to reach the masseter muscle, lateral to the ramus of the mandible.

QUESTION
79

The function of the masseter muscle is to _____ the mandible.

ANSWER

elevate

QUESTION
80

The masseter muscle inserts on the lateral surface of the _____ of the mandible.

ANSWER

ramus

QUESTION
81

On its route to the masseter muscle, the masseteric nerve passes superior to the _____ _____ muscle, gives off a branch to the _____ joint, and then goes through the _____ notch to reach its termination point.

ANSWER

lateral pterygoid . . . temporomandibular . . . mandibular

QUESTION
82

The masseteric nerve originates either directly from the _____ division of the mandibular nerve or as a branch of the posterior _____ _____ nerve.

ANSWER

anterior . . . deep temporal

THE LATERAL PTERYGOID
AND BUCCAL NERVES

Look back to Figure 6–14 and locate the terminal branches of the anterior division of the mandibular nerve: the lateral pterygoid nerve and the buccal nerve. The lateral pterygoid nerve passes anterolaterally to innervate both heads of the lateral pterygoid muscle. This muscle, when contracting bilaterally, protrudes the mandible.

The buccal nerve is the only sensory nerve in the anterior division of the mandibular nerve. It passes between the two heads of the lateral pterygoid muscle and descends anteriorly and inferiorly on the anteromedial surface of the tendon of the temporalis muscle. At this point, branches are given off to buccal gingiva in the molar and premolar region, to buccal mucosa, and to skin of the cheek.

When the lateral pterygoid muscle contracts bilaterally, it _____ the jaw.

protrudes

The buccal nerve is an *afferent/efferent* (circle one) nerve.

Afferent. The buccal nerve is the only afferent nerve in the anterior division of the mandibular nerve.

The buccal nerve, en route to the structures which it innervates, extends laterally through the _____ _____ muscle, then passes anteromedial to the tendon of the _____ muscle.

lateral pterygoid . . . temporalis

The buccal nerve supplies _____ of the cheek as well as buccal _____ and buccal _____.

skin . . . mucosa . . . gingiva

ITEM 34

THE MANDIBULAR NERVE: THE POSTERIOR DIVISION

The posterior division of the mandibular nerve is shown in Figure 6–15. This division gives off one branch, the *auriculotemporal nerve;* then it divides into two terminal branches, the *lingual nerve* and the *inferior alveolar nerve.* Just before the inferior alveolar nerve enters the mandibular foramen, it gives off the *mylohyoid nerve.* At the mental foramen, the inferior alveolar nerve gives off the *mental nerve.* The forward continuation of the inferior alveolar nerve beyond the mental foramen is called the *incisive nerve.*

QUESTION
87

Referring to Figure 6–15, list the names of the six branches which make up the posterior division of the mandibular nerve

1. _____ nerve
2. _____ nerve
3. _____ _____ nerve
4. _____ nerve
5. _____ nerve
6. _____ nerve

ANSWER

1. auriculotemporal
2. lingual
3. inferior alveolar

4. mylohyoid
5. mental
6. incisive

ITEM 35

THE MANDIBULAR DIVISION: CUTANEOUS DISTRIBUTION

Figure 6–16 shows the cutaneous distribution of two branches of the posterior division of the mandibular nerve, the auriculotemporal and mental nerves. After giving off fibers of general sensation to the parotid gland, the auriculotemporal nerve curves laterally to reach skin of the temporal region anterior to the ear.

The mental nerve branches off the inferior alveolar nerve and leaves the bony canal through the mental foramen. Its three terminal branches, seen in Figure 6–16, divide deep to muscle to supply skin of the chin, skin of the lip, and mucous membrane of the lower lip.

QUESTION
88

The auriculotemporal nerve carries general sensation from the skin of the _____ region.

ANSWER

temporal

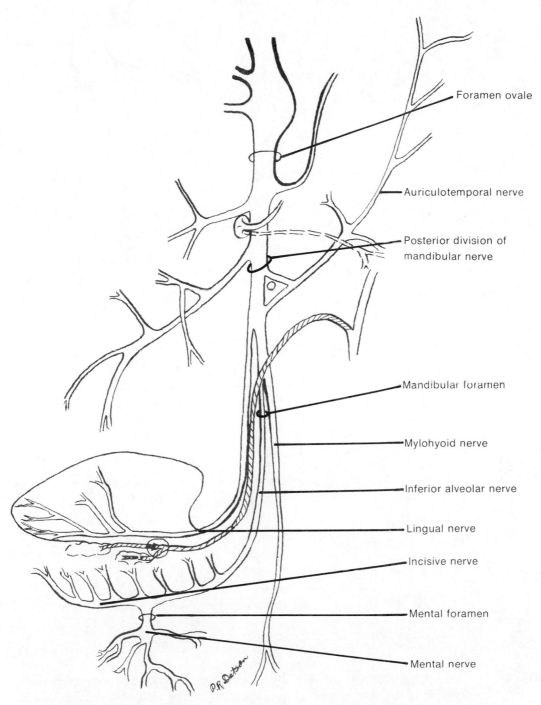

Figure 6-15. Branches of the posterior division of the mandibular nerve. (Redrawn and modified from Woodburne: Essentials of Human Anatomy. 4th Ed. New York, Oxford University Press.)

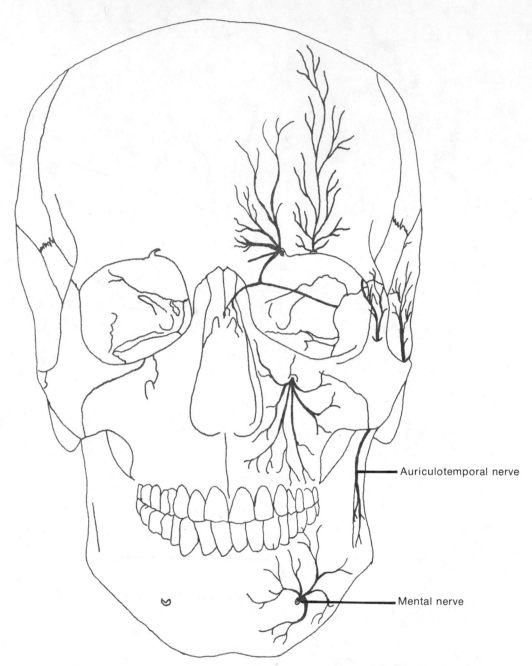

Figure 6–16. Cutaneous nerves of the mandibular division of the trigeminal nerve (V).

QUESTION
89

Branching off the inferior alveolar nerve, the mental nerve provides innervation of the skin of the _____ and _____, as well as to _____ of the lower lip.

ANSWER

chin . . . lip . . . mucosa

THE AURICULOTEMPORAL NERVE: THE PAROTID BRANCH

Examine Figure 6–17 and observe how the auriculotemporal nerve arises in the form of two roots which encircle the middle meningeal artery, then form a single trunk. The trunk passes posterior to the parotid gland, where it gives off a *parotid branch* carrying fibers of general sensation to the parotid gland. Because of various clinical conditions which affect the parotid gland, it is important to recognize that fibers of the trigeminal nerve carry general sensation from this gland.

The nerve which encircles the middle meningeal artery is the _____ nerve.

auriculotemporal

The auriculotemporal nerve carries general sensation from the _____ gland.

parotid

THE MOTOR FIBERS FROM THE OTIC GANGLION

As the auriculotemporal nerve extends toward the parotid gland it is joined by postganglionic neurons from the *otic ganglion,* as shown in Figure 6–17. The otic ganglion, which receives preganglionic fibers from branches of the glosso-pharyngeal nerve, is situated just medial to the trunk of the mandibular nerve. The efferent fibers from this ganglion which travel with the auriculotemporal nerve provide parasympathetic innervation to the parotid gland.

In addition to fibers of general sensation, the auriculotemporal nerve carries postganglionic parasympathetic fibers whose cell bodies are located in the ____ ganglion.

otic

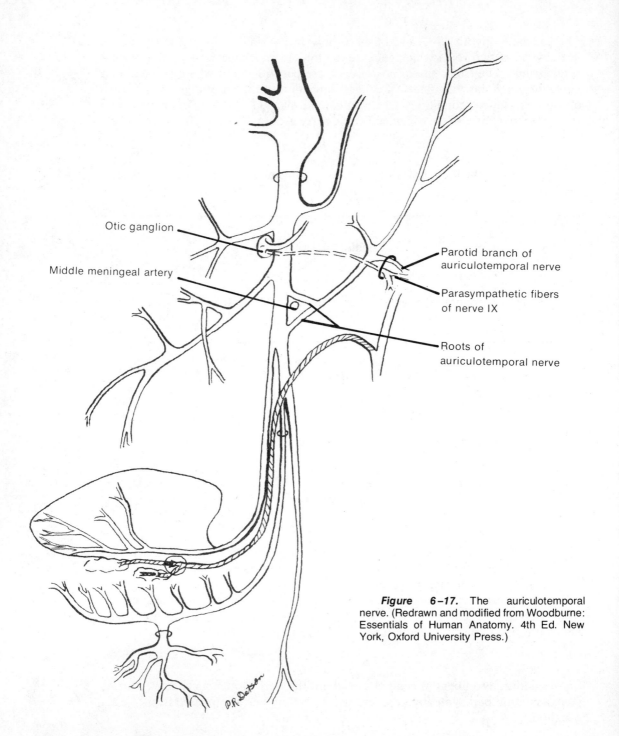

Otic ganglion

Middle meningeal artery

Parotid branch of
auriculotemporal nerve

Parasympathetic fibers
of nerve IX

Roots of
auriculotemporal nerve

Figure 6–17. The auriculotemporal
nerve. (Redrawn and modified from Woodburne:
Essentials of Human Anatomy. 4th Ed. New
York, Oxford University Press.)

Preganglionic fibers received by the otic ganglion are branches of the _____ nerve.

---

glossopharyngeal

MOTOR BRANCHES OF THE POSTERIOR DIVISION: THE MYLOHYOID NERVE

The only motor branches associated with the posterior division of the mandibular nerve are carried in the *mylohyoid nerve*, shown in Figure 6–18. The mylohyoid nerve arises from the inferior alveolar nerve. Take note that before it gives off the mylohyoid nerve, the inferior alveolar nerve is a mixed nerve, carrying both sensory and motor fibers. However, after it gives off the mylohyoid nerve, the continuation of the inferior alveolar nerve is entirely sensory.

The pathway of the mylohyoid nerve pierces the sphenomandibular ligament and runs anteriorly in the mylohyoid groove downward along the medial surface of the ramus of the mandible. The terminal branches of the mylohyoid nerve supply the mylohyoid muscle and the anterior belly of the digastric muscle.

The mylohyoid nerve is the only motor branch of the _____ division of the mandibular nerve, while the buccal nerve is the only sensory branch of the _____ division of the mandibular nerve.

---

posterior . . . anterior

Muscles supplied by the mylohyoid nerve are the _____ muscle and the anterior belly of the _____ muscle.

---

mylohyoid . . . digastric

The mylohyoid nerve originates from the _____ _____ nerve and, after penetrating the sphenomandibular ligament, travels downward in the _____ groove.

---

inferior alveolar . . . mylohyoid

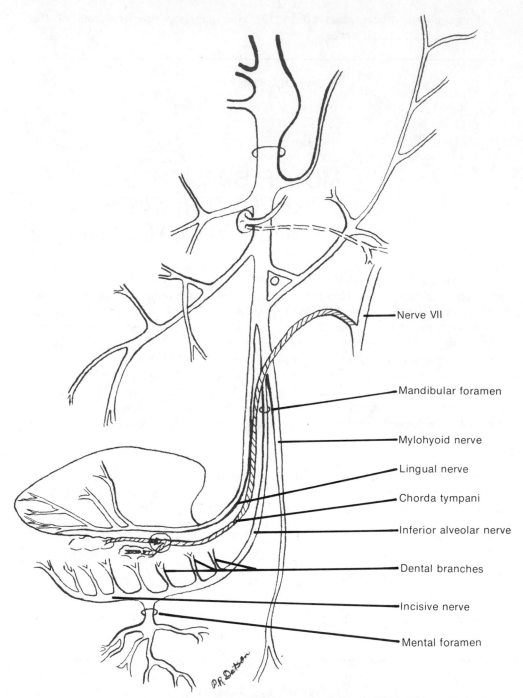

Nerve VII

Mandibular foramen

Mylohyoid nerve

Lingual nerve

Chorda tympani

Inferior alveolar nerve

Dental branches

Incisive nerve

Mental foramen

Figure 6–18.   The mylohyoid, inferior alveolar, lingual, and chorda tympani nerves. (Redrawn and modified from Woodburne: Essentials of Human Anatomy. 4th Ed. New York, Oxford University Press.)

QUESTION
97

The inferior alveolar nerve is entirely *sensory/motor* (circle one) except for the *sensory/motor* (circle one) fibers of the mylohyoid nerve.

_____

ANSWER   sensory . . . motor

THE INFERIOR ALVEOLAR NERVE

ITEM
39

Look at Figure 6–18 and notice the position of the *inferior alveolar nerve*. The inferior alveolar nerve descends behind the lingula and runs between the ramus of the mandible and the sphenomandibular ligament to enter the mandibular canal at the mandibular foramen. The inferior alveolar nerve forms a plexus within the mandibular canal, giving off dental branches to the molar and premolar teeth. The anterior continuation of the inferior alveolar nerve beyond the mental foramen is the incisive nerve, which supplies the lower canine and incisor teeth.

Branches of the inferior alveolar nerve supply the lower _____ and _____ teeth.

QUESTION
98

---

molar . . . premolar

ANSWER

Before entering the mandibular canal, the inferior alveolar nerve passes between the _____ of the mandible and the _____ ligament.

QUESTION
99

---

ramus . . . sphenomandibular

ANSWER

The incisive branch of the inferior alveolar nerve supplies the mandibular _____ and _____ teeth.

QUESTION
100

---

canine . . . incisor

ANSWER

THE LINGUAL NERVE

ITEM
40

The *lingual nerve,* shown in Figure 6–18, leaves the posterior division of the mandibular nerve to extend anteriorly and inferiorly deep to the lateral pterygoid muscle. It then descends between the medial pterygoid muscle and the mandible, and crosses the submandibular triangle to descend laterally across the submandibular duct to enter the tongue.

The lingual nerve is composed of general somatic afferent fibers transmitting general sensation from the anterior two thirds of the tongue, the lingual gingiva of the mandibular teeth, and mucosa of the floor of the mouth.

QUESTION
101

On leaving the posterior division of the mandibular nerve, the lingual nerve runs anteriorly and inferiorly deep to the _____ _____ muscle.

ANSWER

lateral pterygoid

QUESTION
102

After descending between the _____ _____ muscle and the mandible, the lingual nerve descends laterally across the submandibular triangle to the submandibular duct before entering the _____ .

ANSWER

medial pterygoid . . . tongue

QUESTION
103

The areas from which the lingual nerve transmits general sensation include (1) the anterior two thirds of the _____ , (2) lingual _____ of the mandibular teeth, and (3) mucosa of the floor of the _____ .

ANSWER

tongue . . . gingiva . . . mouth

ITEM 41   THE CHORDA TYMPANI

Refer to Figure 6–18 and observe the *chorda tympani* traveling with the lingual nerve. The lingual nerve is joined by the chorda tympani branch of the facial nerve while still in the infratemporal fossa. Fibers of the chorda tympani run with the lingual nerve, supplying parasympathetic innervation to the submandibular and sublingual glands. The chorda tympani also carries special visceral afferent fibers, conveying taste sensations from the anterior two thirds of the tongue.

QUESTION
104

The chorda tympani is a branch of the (circle one)
A. mandibular nerve
B. facial nerve

ANSWER

The correct answer is B. The chorda tympani, a branch of the facial nerve, travels with the lingual branch of the mandibular nerve.

QUESTION
105

The chorda tympani joins the lingual nerve within the _____ fossa.

The chorda tympani carries (circle one)
A. afferent fibers only
B. efferent fibers only
C. both afferent and efferent fibers

QUESTION **106**

The correct answer is C. The chorda tympani carries efferent fibers for parasympathetic innervation of certain salivary glands as well as afferent fibers which transmit the sense of taste.

ANSWER

The functional components of the chorda tympani are _____ _____ efferent and _____ _____ afferent.

QUESTION **107**

---

general visceral . . . special visceral

ANSWER

Special visceral afferent fibers of the chorda tympani nerve convey _____ from the _____ two thirds of the tongue.

QUESTION **108**

---

taste . . . anterior

ANSWER

General visceral efferent fibers of the chorda tympani are parasympathetic to the _____ and _____ salivary glands.

QUESTION **109**

---

sublingual . . . submandibular

ANSWER

TRIGEMINAL PATHWAYS WITHIN THE CENTRAL NERVOUS SYSTEM

ITEM 42

Thus far in this unit we have dealt primarily with the peripheral distribution of branches of the trigeminal nerve. We now need to think about trigeminal pathways within the central nervous system. These connections coordinate and process incoming information so that appropriate motor response can be made. Incoming information includes general sensation and proprioception to the brain and, to a lesser extent, to the spinal cord. Some sensory input reaches conscious levels; a greater amount of input does not. Some motor activity of the efferent fibers is dependent directly on trigeminal input; other aspects of motor activity involve various areas of the brain.

QUESTION
110

The central nervous system coordinates and processes _____ input with _____ output.

ANSWER

sensory . . . motor

QUESTION
111

Incoming information to the brain conveyed over trigeminal pathways includes general _____ and _____.

ANSWER

sensation . . . proprioception

ITEM 43   THE OPHTHALMIC DIVISION: THE GSA FIBERS

Most of the general somatic afferent fibers convey general sensory modalities of pain, temperature, touch, and pressure to the central nervous system. To begin your review of the distribution of divisions of nerve V, note that the ophthalmic division carries only fibers for general sensation, with receptors in skin of the forehead and upper eyelid and in connective tissues of the orbit.

QUESTION
112

Pain, temperature, touch, and pressure are conveyed by (circle one)
A. the ophthalmic division only
B. the maxillary division only
C. the mandibular division only
D. all three divisions

ANSWER

The correct answer is D. All divisions of the trigeminal nerve convey pain, temperature, touch, and pressure.

QUESTION
113

In the ophthalmic division of the trigeminal nerve, receptors for general sensation are located in (1) the skin of the _____, (2) the skin of the upper _____, and (3) connective tissue of the _____.

ANSWER

forehead . . . eyelid . . . orbit

THE MAXILLARY AND MANDIBULAR DIVISIONS: THE GSA FIBERS

ITEM 44

The maxillary division of the trigeminal nerve carries fibers for general sensation from the maxillary teeth; from the skin of the cheek; and from mucosa of the upper lip, palate, gingiva, nasal cavity, and most of the paranasal sinuses.

The mandibular division carries fibers conveying general sensation from the skin of the mandibular region; from the mandibular teeth and gingiva; and from the lower lip, the anterior two thirds of the tongue, and much of the buccal and labial oral mucosa.

In the maxillary division of the trigeminal nerve, receptors for general sensation are found in (1) the skin of the _____, (2) the maxillary teeth and _____, and (3) _____ of the upper lip, palate, nasal cavity, and paranasal sinuses.

QUESTION
114

---

cheek . . . gingiva . . . mucosa

ANSWER

In the mandibular division of the trigeminal nerve, general sensation is received from (1) skin overlying the _____, (2) mandibular teeth and _____, (3) the lower _____, (4) the anterior two thirds of the _____, and (5) buccal and labial oral _____.

QUESTION
115

---

mandible . . . gingiva . . . lip . . . tongue . . . mucosa

ANSWER

THE TRIGEMINAL GANGLION: THE CENTRAL PROCESSES

ITEM 45

Figure 6–19 shows the sensory nuclei of the trigeminal nerve. As you will remember, cell bodies of primary neurons from all three divisions of the trigeminal nerve are located in the trigeminal ganglion, which is totally sensory.

Central processes from cell bodies in the trigeminal ganglion enter the lateral border of the pons where it lies on the clivus in the posterior cranial fossa. As these fibers pass dorsally through the pons, some enter the *spinal tract of the trigeminal nerve,* which extends from the upper pons to the upper cervical levels of the spinal cord. Other fibers ascend to the *principal sensory nucleus* of the trigeminal nerve, which is entirely within the pons.

The trigeminal ganglion is *sensory only/sensory and motor* (circle one).

QUESTION
116

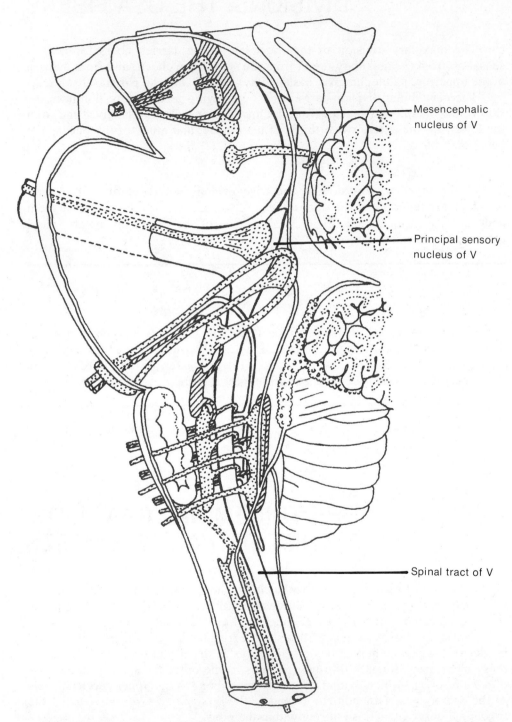

Figure 6–19. Sensory nuclei of the trigeminal nerve (V). (Redrawn from Truex and Carpenter: Human Neuroanatomy. 6th Ed. Baltimore, The Williams & Wilkins Co.)

Mesencephalic nucleus of V

Principal sensory nucleus of V

Spinal tract of V

ANSWER

sensory only

QUESTION
117

Some sensory fibers of the trigeminal nerve coming into the pons enter the _____ tract of nerve V, while other sensory fibers enter the principal _____ nucleus of the nerve.

ANSWER

spinal . . . sensory

QUESTION
118

The span of the spinal tract of nerve V is from the upper _____ down to the upper cervical levels of the _____ _____.

ANSWER

pons . . . spinal cord

THE SPINAL TRACT OF THE TRIGEMINAL NERVE

ITEM 46

Clinical evidence indicates that pain and temperature probably are transmitted to the spinal tract of the trigeminal nerve, whereas proprioception appears to be received in the *mesencephalic nucleus*. Refer to Figure 6–19 for the location of the mesencephalic nucleus.

Lesions in the spinal tract result in diminution or total loss of sensations of pain and temperature from the area where the fibers are distributed. Touch and pressure are less affected, since fibers conveying these modalities terminate in the sensory nucleus.

QUESTION
119

Sensations of pain and temperature appear to be conveyed by fibers in the _____ tract of nerve V; proprioception is transmitted from fibers in the _____ nucleus.

ANSWER

spinal . . . mesencephalic

QUESTION
120

The sensory nucleus of the trigeminal nerve receives sensations of _____ and _____.

ANSWER

touch . . . pressure (in either order)

ITEM
47

THE SPINAL TRACT:
SPATIAL RELATIONSHIPS

Fibers and rami from the three divisions of the trigeminal nerve assume definite spatial relationships within the spinal tract of nerve V. Fibers from the ophthalmic division descend to the lowest portion of the spinal tract, those from the maxillary division terminate in the middle region, and those from the mandibular division terminate in the superior region. Fibers of the spinal tract synapse with cell bodies in the nucleus of the spinal tract. Fibers from these secondary neurons then ascend to the thalamus.

QUESTION
121

Fibers from the opthalmic division descend to the _____ region of the spinal tract of nerve V; those from the maxillary division, to the _____ region; those from the mandibular division, to the _____ region.

ANSWER

lowest . . . middle . . . upper

ITEM
48

THE SPINAL TRACT:
EFFECTS OF LESIONS

There is evidence that sensations of pain and temperature are transmitted by fibers which enter the spinal tract of the trigeminal nerve. Because of the spatial relationships within the tract of the three divisions of nerve V, lesions in the spinal tract of nerve V lead to loss or diminution of the sense of pain and temperature from very specific regions.

Lesions of the lower portion of the spinal tract lead to loss or diminution of pain and temperature sense in those areas supplied by the ophthalmic division; lesions of the middle portion, to loss or diminution of sensation from areas innervated by the maxillary division. Lesions of the upper portion of the spinal tract affect areas supplied by the mandibular division.

QUESTION
122

Lesions of the lower region of the spinal tract of nerve V lead to loss or diminution of pain and temperature sensation in areas supplied by the _____ division of the trigeminal nerve; lesions of the middle region, to loss or diminution in areas supplied by the _____ division; lesions in the superior region, to loss or diminution in areas supplied by the _____ division.

ANSWER

ophthalmic . . . maxillary . . . mandibular

THE SECONDARY PATHWAYS   ITEM 49

Secondary afferent pathways are formed by processes of cells originating in the principal sensory nucleus and spinal nuclei of the trigeminal nerve. Processes of secondary neurons ascend to the thalamus as the *trigeminothalamic tract*. Since trigeminothalamic fibers ascend both contralaterally and ipsilaterally, a lesion affecting one trigeminothalamic tract results in bilateral diminution of sensation instead of causing a unilateral total loss.

The trigeminothalamic tracts are secondary afferent trigeminal fibers from the sensory and spinal nuclei which ascend to the _____.

QUESTION
123

---

thalamus

ANSWER

A lesion affecting the trigeminothalamic tract results in _____ diminution rather than total _____ loss of sensation.

QUESTION
124

---

bilateral . . . unilateral

ANSWER

THE THALAMOCORTICAL PROJECTIONS   ITEM 50

Trigeminothalamic fibers synapse with tertiary neurons in the thalamus. Fibers from these tertiary cells ascend laterally through the posterior limb of the internal capsule to terminate in the lower postcentral gyrus of the cerebral cortex.

While some marginal awareness reaches conscious levels in the thalamus, full awareness and localization of pain, temperature, touch, and pressure sensations require that the impulses reach the sensory area of the cerebral cortex.

Afferent impulses reporting pain, temperature, touch, and pressure achieve marginal awareness at the level of the _____.

QUESTION
125

---

thalamus

ANSWER

QUESTION
126

Afferent impulses reporting pain, temperature, touch, and pressure achieve full consciousness, and localization is perceived, when these impulses reach the _____ _____.

ANSWER

cerebral cortex

QUESTION
127

Fibers from tertiary neurons in the thalamus terminate in _____ gyrus of the cerebral cortex.

ANSWER

postcentral

QUESTION
128

Fibers from tertiary neurons in the thalamus reach their termination in the cerebral cortex via the posterior limb of the _____ _____.

ANSWER

internal capsule

ITEM 51   THE REFLEXES ASSOCIATED WITH THE TRIGEMINAL NUCLEI

Additional fibers arising from the trigeminal nuclei are concerned with various reflexes elicited by stimulation of the following areas: the skin of the face, oral and nasal mucosa, and muscles, tendons, and bones of the face and jaw. Processes from the principal sensory nucleus and the spinal nucleus travel through the reticular formation to the various motor nuclei which carry out the efferent limb of the reflex arc.

The more important of these reflexes include: (1) the corneal reflex, (2) the lacrimal reflex, (3) the vomiting reflex, (4) the salivary reflex, (5) tongue reflexes, and (6) the sucking reflex of the infant. The central connections to the various motor nuclei are, obviously, extremely complex.

QUESTION
129

Areas of stimulation which provoke reflexes associated with the trigeminal nuclei include (1) the skin of the _____, (2) oral and nasal _____, and (3) muscles, tendons, and bones of the _____ and _____.

ANSWER

face . . . mucosa . . . face . . . jaw

In order to complete trigeminal reflex circuits, fibers from sensory nuclei go to various motor nuclei via the _____ formation.

---

reticular

Reflexes associated with the trigeminal nerve include the _____, _____, _____, _____, _____, and _____ reflexes.

---

corneal . . . lacrimal . . . vomiting . . . salivary . . . tongue . . . sucking
(in any order)

PROPRIOCEPTION ITEM 52

Some general somatic afferent fibers of the trigeminal nerve are concerned with proprioception. This particular proprioceptive input apprises the central nervous system of the state of contraction of muscles of mastication and the relative position of the temporomandibular joint.

Proprioceptive impulses carried by GSA fibers of the trigeminal nerve originate from two types of receptors. The first type includes stretch receptors in neuromuscular spindles and tendon spindles within the muscles of mastication and their tendons. The second type of proprioceptive receptor is composed of those concerned with deep or strong pressure. These receptors are found in periodontal ligaments and in the temporomandibular joint.

Sensory input which conveys the position of the temporomandibular joint and the state of contraction of the muscles of mastication is termed _____ _____.

---

proprioception

Stretch receptors consist of _____ within muscles and tendons; proprioceptive receptors in periodontal ligaments and the temporomandibular joint convey sensations of _____ pressure.

---

spindles . . . deep (strong)

ITEM 53   PROPRIOCEPTION AND CONTROL OF THE LOWER JAW

Proprioceptive information is processed in the mesencephalic nucleus. The fibers conveying this information synapse with the motor nucleus of nerve V and, to a lesser extent, with the motor nucleus of the facial nerve (VII). Proprioceptive input brings about control of the efferent impulses to the muscles of mastication which permit the smooth, effective movements of the lower jaw which are necessary for effective speech and mastication, and for facial expression.

QUESTION
134
Proprioceptive impulses from muscles of mastication, periodontal ligaments, and the temporomandibular joint are processed in the _____ nucleus.

ANSWER
mesencephalic

QUESTION
135
Proprioceptive impulses feeding into the motor nuclei of the trigeminal and facial nerves effect smooth and coordinated _____ activity.

ANSWER
muscle

ITEM 54   LESIONS AFFECTING THE MOTOR FIBERS

Lesions affecting the motor fibers of the trigeminal nerve cause atrophy and weakness of the muscles of mastication. The condition can be identified by the absence of contraction of the masseter muscle when the jaws are clenched. When paralysis of the pterygoid muscles occurs, the chin deviates in the direction of the lesion when the mandible is depressed. This deviation occurs because the capacity for the normal action of drawing the mandible toward the midline is lost, and muscles of the other side are unopposed.

QUESTION
136
Atrophy of the muscles of mastication results from lesions affecting _____ fibers of the trigeminal nerve.

ANSWER
motor

The absence of contraction of the _____ muscle is indicative of lesions affecting mandibular motor fibers.

---

masseter

Deviation of the chin in the direction of the lesion occurs with paralysis of the _____ muscles.

---

pterygoid

LESIONS AFFECTING THE SENSORY FIBERS ITEM 55

Trigeminal neuralgia is a disease affecting sensory fibers of the trigeminal nerve. This disease causes paroxysms of excruciating pain in the branches of one or more divisions of the trigeminal nerve. There is usually some trigger zone in which pain sensations may be stimulated with little provocation. Because of the severity of the pain, resection of the sensory nerve involved or sectioning of the sensory roots may be necessary.

The painful disease affecting sensory branches of the trigeminal nerve is called trigeminal _____.

---

neuralgia

The pain resulting from lesion of sensory fibers of the trigeminal nerve may be alleviated by _____ the nerves or their roots.

---

sectioning

SUMMARY OF UNIT SIX

The largest of the cranial nerves, the trigeminal, is of paramount significance in dentistry because of its sensory innervation of the teeth and its motor innervation of the muscles of mastication. The trigeminal nerve branches into three major divisions at the trigeminal ganglion: the ophthalmic (V_1), maxillary (V_2), and mandibular (V_3). The ophthalmic and maxillary divisions are entirely sensory; the mandibular division is both sensory and motor. V_1 exits from the cranium through the superior orbital fissure and supplies the eyes and forehead. V_2 exits through the foramen rotundum and supplies the upper jaw and cheek. V_3 exits through the foramen ovale and supplies sensory innervation to lower jaw and chin, and motor innervation to the muscles of mastication.

THE OPHTHALMIC DIVISION

The ophthalmic division of the trigeminal nerve has three branches, the lacrimal, the frontal, and the nasociliary. The lacrimal nerve supplies the lacrimal gland, conjunctiva, and skin of the lateral upper eyelid. The frontal nerve divides into the supraorbital and supratrochlear nerves. The supraorbital nerve supplies skin of the forehead and anterior scalp, with small branches to the upper eyelid and frontal sinus. The supratrochlear nerve supplies skin of the medial parts of the forehead and upper eyelid. The nasociliary nerve carries long and short ciliary branches which are sensory to the eyeball. Three other branches of the nasociliary nerve are (1) the posterior ethmoidal nerve to mucous membranes of posterior ethmoid air cells and sphenoid sinus; (2) the anterior ethmoidal nerve to anterior ethmoid air cells, nasal mucosa, and skin of the lower half of the nose; and (3) the infratrochlear nerve to skin of the root of the nose and lower eyelid.

THE MAXILLARY DIVISION

The maxillary division of nerve V, after leaving the trigeminal ganglion, gives off a meningeal branch to the dura mater prior to passing through the foramen rotundum. In the pterygopalatine fossa, the maxillary nerve gives off pterygopalatine, posterior superior alveolar, and zygomatic branches.

The zygomatic branch enters the orbit and then passes into the zygomatic bone where it divides into zygomaticofacial and zygomaticotemporal nerves. The former supplies skin overlying the lateral surface of the zygoma; the latter, skin over the anterior fourth of the temporalis muscle.

The posterior superior alveolar nerve, branching off the maxillary nerve, sends one terminal branch to the gingiva of the three posterior molar teeth and two terminal branches to the molar and premolar teeth and to the mucous membrane of the maxillary sinus.

The pterygopalatine branches of the maxillary nerve are trunks which descend into the pterygopalatine ganglion. Intermingled with the GSA fibers of the maxillary nerve are sympathetic fibers and parasympathetic fibers of the facial nerve. The terminal branches of the trigeminal nerve appear to originate in the pterygopalatine ganglion, but actually they merely pass through the ganglion. Postganglionic parasympathetic fibers of the facial nerve emerge from the ganglion together with GSA fibers of the trigeminal nerve. The five sets of branches of the maxillary nerve which appear to arise from the pterygopalatine ganglion are the (1) pharyngeal, (2) lesser palatine, (3) greater palatine, (4) posterior superior lateral nasal, and (5) nasopalatine branches.

Three palatine nerves emerge from the ganglion, the greater and the two lesser palatine branches. The greater palatine branch supplies mucosa of the hard palate and lingual gingiva of the maxillary teeth, giving off inferior nasal branches to mucosa of the inferior nasal conchae.

One of the two lesser palatine nerves supplies mucosa of the soft palate; the other, the soft palate itself and part of the palatine tonsil. Posterior superior lateral nasal branches innervate mucosa of the middle and superior conchae and part of the nasal septum. The nasopalatine nerve supplies mucosa overlying the bony part of the septum, part of the hard palate, and lingual gingiva of the maxillary incisor teeth.

The direct anterior continuation of the maxillary nerve is the infraorbital nerve, which passes through the orbit and exits onto the face. The infraorbital nerve gives off the anterior superior alveolar branch, which supplies upper incisor and canine teeth as well as parts of the maxillary sinus and nasal cavity. Sometimes the infraorbital nerve also gives off a middle superior alveolar nerve, which supplies the two maxillary premolar teeth, adjacent gingiva, and the maxillary sinus. The infraorbital nerve gives off a number of cutaneous branches: palpebral branches to the lower eyelid, external nasal branches to the side of the nose, and labial branches to skin of the upper lip and the labial mucosa.

THE MANDIBULAR DIVISION

The mandibular division of the trigeminal nerve exits from the skull at the foramen ovale. Sensory and motor fibers of the mandibular division join outside the foramen ovale into a very short common trunk which divides into the small anterior and the large posterior parts of the mandibular nerve. The mainly efferent anterior division carries a single afferent branch, the buccal nerve; the mainly afferent posterior division carries a single efferent branch to the mylohyoid muscle and anterior belly of the digastric muscle. Before branching into anterior and posterior divisions, the common trunk gives off the efferent medial pterygoid nerve, which, in turn, sends motor twigs to the tensor tympani and tensor veli palatini muscles, and the afferent meningeal branch.

The anterior division of the mandibular nerve gives off: (1) the anterior and posterior deep temporal nerves, motor to the temporalis muscle; (2) the masseteric nerve, a branch to the masseter muscles; this, in turn, sends a branch to the temporomandibular joint; and (3) the lateral pterygoid nerves, which innervate the two heads of the lateral pterygoid muscle. Since all the motor branches of the trigeminal nerve are branchiomeric, their functional component is special visceral efferent (SVE). In addition, the anterior division contains a single sensory branch, the general somatic afferent buccal nerve supplying skin of the cheek, buccal mucosa, and gingiva of premolar and molar teeth.

The posterior division of the mandibular gives off four sensory branches: (1) the auriculotemporal nerve, which passes through the parotid gland to skin in front of the ear and scalp, and sends branches to the temporomandibular joint and external acoustic meatus; (2) the lingual nerve, which conveys general sensation from the anterior two thirds of the tongue, lingual gingiva of the mandibular teeth, and the floor of the mouth; (3) the inferior alveolar nerve, which conveys sensation from molar and premolar teeth; and (4) the mental nerve, which supplies skin of the chin and lip and mucosa of the lower lip. The continuation of the inferior alveolar nerve within bone is the incisive nerve to the remaining canine and incisor teeth.

The single motor component of the posterior division of the mandibular nerve is the mylohyoid nerve, supplying the mylohyoid muscle and the anterior belly of the digastric muscle.

The proprioceptive GSA fibers of the mandibular division carry sensory impulses from muscle spindles and tendons of the muscles of mastication, as well as from receptors for deep pressure in the periodontal ligaments and temporomandibular joint. The proprioceptive information fed into the mesencephalic nucleus effects control of motor impulses which assures the smooth movements of the lower jaw required for speech and mastication. All other GSA fibers of the trigeminal nerve convey modalities of touch, pressure, pain, and temperature.

THE NUCLEI OF THE TRIGEMINAL NERVE

The trigeminal ganglion contains cell bodies of GSA fibers of the trigeminal nerve. Central processes synapse in the principal sensory nucleus of the trigeminal nerve in the pons, and in the nucleus of the spinal tract of the trigeminal nerve.

From the trigeminal nuclei secondary neurons extend to the thalamus as the trigeminothalamic tract. Tertiary thalamocortical fibers reach the postcentral gyrus of the cerebral cortex.

Additional fibers from trigeminal nuclei are involved in such reflexes as the corneal, lacrimal, vomiting, salivary, sucking, and tongue reflexes. Fibers from sensory nuclei go to various motor nuclei via the reticular formation.

The motor nucleus of the trigeminal nerve is situated in the pons. Accompanying the motor fibers are sensory fibers conveying proprioceptive information about contraction of muscles of mastication to the mesencephalic nucleus.

Lesions of motor fibers of the trigeminal nerve cause atrophy or paralysis of muscles of mastication, indicated, for example, by deviation of the chin to one side when the mandible is depressed. Lesions affecting sensory fibers of the trigeminal nerve produce trigeminal neuralgia, which is characterized by excruciating pain.

QUESTION
141

At the trigeminal ganglion, the trigeminal nerve separates into three main divisions, the _____ division, the _____ division, and the _____ division.

ANSWER

ophthalmic . . . maxillary . . . mandibular (in any order)

QUESTION
142

The division which contains both motor and sensory fibers is the _____ _____ division; the _____ and the _____ divisions contain sensory fibers only.

ANSWER

mandibular . . . ophthalmic . . . maxillary

The three main branches of the ophthalmic division are the _____, _____, and _____ nerves.

QUESTION
143

---

lacrimal . . . frontal . . . nasociliary (in any order)

ANSWER

Branches of the frontal nerve are the _____ and _____ _____.

QUESTION
144

---

supraorbital . . . supratrochlear (in either order)

ANSWER

The posterior and anterior ethmoidal nerves are branches of the _____ _____ nerve, which arises from the _____ division of the trigeminal nerve.

QUESTION
145

---

nasociliary . . . ophthalmic

ANSWER

The nasociliary nerve gives off ciliary branches which are sensory to the _____; the infratrochlear nerve gives off branches to the root of the _____; the _____ ethmoidal nerve, branches sensory to posterior ethmoid air cells and sphenoid sinus; and the _____ ethmoidal nerve, branches sensory to anterior ethmoid air cells and to skin of the lower nose.

QUESTION
146

---

eyeball . . . nose . . . posterior . . . anterior

ANSWER

The pterygopalatine, posterior superior alveolar, and zygomatic nerves are branches of the _____ division of the trigeminal nerve.

QUESTION
147

---

maxillary

ANSWER

The zygomaticotemporal nerve supplies skin over the _____ muscle, while the zygomaticofacial nerve supplies skin over the _____.

QUESTION
148

---

temporalis . . . zygoma

ANSWER

Branches of the posterior superior alveolar nerve supply molar and premolar _____, adjacent _____, and mucous membrane of the _____ sinus.

QUESTION
149

---

teeth . . . gingiva . . . maxillary

ANSWER

QUESTION
150

Pterygopalatine branches containing *afferent/efferent* (circle one) fibers of the maxillary nerve emerge from the pterygopalatine ganglion in company with *afferent/efferent* (circle one) fibers of the facial nerve.

ANSWER

afferent . . . efferent

QUESTION
151

The pharyngeal, palatine, posterior superior lateral nasal, and nasopalatine nerves are afferent branches of the *ophthalmic/maxillary/mandibular* (circle one) division of the trigeminal nerve.

ANSWER

maxillary

QUESTION
152

Match the sensory branch of the maxillary nerve in Column B with the areas of innervation listed in Column A.

Column A	Column B
( ) 1. roof of the pharynx	A. nasopalatine nerve
( ) 2. mucosa of the hard palate	B. posterior superior
( ) 3. mucosa of the soft palate	lateral nasal nerve
( ) 4. nasal conchae	C. greater palatine nerve
( ) 5. mucosa over bony part of	D. lesser palatine nerve
nasal septum	E. pharyngeal nerve

ANSWER

1.—(E); 2.—(C); 3.—(D); 4.—(B); 5.—(A)

QUESTION
153

The infraorbital nerve, a continuation of the _____ nerve, gives off superior _____ branches which are sensory to maxillary incisor, canine, and premolar teeth.

ANSWER

maxillary . . . alveolar

QUESTION
154

Prior to branching into anterior and posterior divisions, the mandibular nerve gives off efferent branches to the medial _____ muscle, the tensor _____ muscle, and the tensor veli _____ muscle.

ANSWER

pterygoid . . . tympani . . . palatini

QUESTION
155

The meningeal nerve is an afferent nerve to the meninges which branches off the *ophthalmic/maxillary/mandibular* (circle one) division.

ANSWER

mandibular

The anterior division of the mandibular nerve is mostly *afferent/efferent* (circle one), while the posterior division is mainly *afferent/efferent* (circle one).

efferent . . . afferent

The efferent branches of the anterior division of the mandibular nerve carry motor impulses to the _____ muscle, the _____ muscle, and the lateral _____ muscle.

temporalis . . . masseter . . . pterygoid

The buccal nerve is a sensory branch of the _____ division of the mandibular nerve which innervates the skin of the _____ and _____ of the premolar and first molar teeth.

anterior . . . cheek . . . gingiva

The auriculotemporal nerve is a sensory branch of the _____ division of the mandibular nerve which innervates skin in front of the _____ and the _____ joint.

posterior . . . ear . . . temporomandibular

General sensation from the anterior two thirds of the tongue is conveyed by the _____ nerve; taste from the anterior two thirds of the tongue by the _____ _____ nerve.

lingual . . . chorda tympani

The inferior alveolar nerve supplies _____ and _____ teeth; the incisive nerve, _____ and _____ teeth.

molar . . . premolar . . . incisor . . . canine

Skin of the chin and the labial mucosa is supplied by the _____ nerve.

mental

QUESTION
163

The afferent branch of the anterior division of the mandibular nerve is the _____ nerve; the efferent branches of the posterior division supply the _____ muscle and the anterior belly of the _____ muscle.

ANSWER

buccal . . . mylohyoid . . . digastric

QUESTION
164

The proprioceptive sensations carried by GSA fibers of the mandibular division convey the state of contraction of muscles of _____ and deep pressure in the _____ ligaments and _____ joint.

ANSWER

mastication . . . periodontal . . . temporomandibular

QUESTION
165

The functional component of all the motor branches of the trigeminal nerve is (circle one)
  A. GSE
  B. GVE
  C. SVE

ANSWER

The correct answer is C, special visceral efferent. All the muscles of mastication innervated by the trigeminal nerve are derived from the second branchial arch and are therefore supplied by branchiomeric, or SVE, fibers.

QUESTION
166

The functional component of all sensory fibers of the trigeminal nerve is _____ _____ _____.

ANSWER

general somatic afferent

QUESTION
167

Lesions of motor fibers of the trigeminal nerve cause atony of the muscles of _____; lesions of sensory fibers cause the painful disease called trigeminal _____.

ANSWER

mastication . . . neuralgia

QUESTION
168

The motor nucleus of the trigeminal nerve is located in the *midbrain/pons/medulla* (circle one).

ANSWER

pons

QUESTION
169

The mesencephalic nucleus of the trigeminal nerve receives fibers conveying _____ impulses.

proprioceptive

General sensation is received in the principal _____ nucleus of the
trigeminal nerve and in the nucleus of the _____ tract of the trigeminal   **170**
nerve.

---

sensory . . . spinal

To convey corneal, lacrimal, vomiting, and tongue reflexes, fibers extend
from sensory nuclei of the trigeminal nerve to motor nuclei by way of the   **171**
_____ formation.

---

reticular

Unit Seven ☐ THE FACIAL NERVE

ITEM 1   THE FACIAL NERVE: ROOTS

Figure 7–1 shows the superficial exit of the facial nerve (cranial nerve VII) at the inferolateral region of the pons. The facial nerve is comprised of a *motor root* and a second root, primarily sensory, called the *nervus intermedius*. The nervus intermedius emerges from the pons lateral to the motor root.

The motor component mainly supplies the muscles of facial expression. The nervus intermedius provides sensory innervation to diverse areas of the head, and also supplies parasympathetic fibers to the lacrimal, submandibular, and sublingual glands.

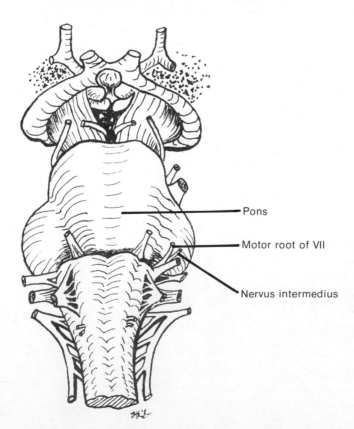

— Pons

— Motor root of VII

— Nervus intermedius

Figure 7–1. Brain stem, ventral aspect, showing roots of the facial nerve. (Redrawn and modified from Truex and Carpenter: Strong and Elwyn's Human Neuroanatomy. 5th Ed. Baltimore, The Williams and Wilkins Co.)

Fibers of the nervus intermedius are (circle one)
A. afferent only
B. efferent only
C. both afferent and efferent

The correct answer is C. Sensory fibers of the nervus intermedius supply various areas of the head, but this root also gives rise to efferent neurons which supply parasympathetic innervation to glands.

The efferent nerves to muscles of facial expression arise from the (circle one)
A. motor root of the facial nerve
B. efferent component of the nervus intermedius

The correct answer is A. If you answered B., remember that the nervus intermedius is *primarily* sensory and that motor fibers which do arise from the nervus intermedius supply glands, not muscles.

THE FACIAL NERVE: FUNCTIONAL COMPONENTS

ITEM
2

The facial nerve is a mixed nerve; it carries several types of functional components. The motor root carries special visceral efferent fibers to muscles of facial expression, and to a few other muscles which, like the facial muscles, are embryonically derived from the second branchial arch.

The nervus intermedius carries four different components, three sensory and one motor. The sensory components of the nervus intermedius are general somatic afferent, or GSA; general visceral afferent, or GVA; and special visceral afferent, or SVA. The motor component is general visceral efferent, or GVE.

Nerves which supply muscles derived from the second branchial arch are *special visceral efferent/general visceral efferent* (circle one).

The correct answer is special visceral efferent. The motor root of the facial nerve (VII) is designated SVE, since the muscles of facial expression which it supplies are derived from the second branchial arch.

The efferent neurons arising from the nervus intermedius are *general visceral efferent/special visceral efferent* (circle one).

The correct answer is general visceral efferent. The functional component of all parasympathetic fibers to glands of the head is general visceral efferent.

ITEM 3

THE NERVUS INTERMEDIUS: AFFERENT COMPONENTS

General somatic afferent fibers from the nervus intermedius primarily innervate the external auditory canal. General visceral afferent fibers supply the mucosa of the most posterior portions of the nasal cavity and palate. Special visceral afferent fibers carry sensations from taste buds on the anterior two thirds of the tongue.

QUESTION 5

Some sensory fibers of the nervus intermedius supply taste buds on the anterior portion of the tongue; the functional component of these fibers is (circle one)

A. GSA
B. GVA
C. SVA

ANSWER

The correct answer is C. Conveying the sensation of taste is a special visceral afferent function.

QUESTION 6

Match the structures listed in Column B with the functional components of the nerves which supply them, listed in Column A.

Column A	Column B
( ) 1. GSA	A. taste buds on the tongue
( ) 2. GVA	B. external auditory canal
( ) 3. SVA	C. mucosa of the nasal cavity and palate

ANSWER

1.—(B); 2.—(C); 3.—(A)

ITEM 4

THE NERVUS INTERMEDIUS: EFFERENT COMPONENT

General visceral efferent fibers of the facial nerve are parasympathetic preganglionic fibers stemming from the nervus intermedius. Preganglionic fibers synapse in the pterygopalatine and submandibular ganglia with postganglionic fibers that supply the submandibular, sublingual, lacrimal, nasal, and palatine glands.

The preganglionic fibers of the nervus intermedius synapse with post-ganglionic fibers in the _____ ganglion and also in the _____ ganglion.

---

pterygopalatine . . . submandibular

Postganglionic fibers of the nervus intermedius supply parasympathetic innervation to the submandibular, sublingual, lacrimal, nasal, and palatine glands. The functional component of these fibers is *GSE/GVE* (circle one).

The correct answer is GVE, general visceral efferent. If you missed this, go back and reread the answer to Question 4.

THE GENICULATE GANGLION   ITEM 5

Cell bodies of afferent fibers of the nervus intermedius are located in the *geniculate ganglion,* a sensory ganglion within the petrous part of the temporal bone. Central processes from the geniculate ganglion continue to the brain as the nervus intermedius. Within the pons, they join with general somatic afferent fibers of the trigeminal nerve and terminate in the trigeminal nucleus.

The geniculate ganglion contains cell bodies of the *sensory/motor* (circle one) component of the nervus intermedius.

---

sensory

THE FACIAL NERVE: THE MOTOR NUCLEUS   ITEM 6

Cell bodies of special visceral efferent fibers of the facial nerve (VII) are located in the *motor nucleus of the facial nerve.* If you will turn to Figure 7–5, you will see this motor nucleus, which is situated in the lateral part of the reticular formation, at the most caudal level of the pons. From the nucleus, fibers pass dorsomedially around the nucleus of the abducens nerve, then laterally and anteriorly to emerge at the extreme lower level of the pons.

QUESTION
10

The motor nucleus of the facial nerve is located in the lateral part of the _____ formation.

ANSWER

reticular

QUESTION
11

Fibers from the motor nucleus pass dorsomedially around the nucleus of the _____ nerve.

ANSWER

abducens

QUESTION
12

Motor fibers emerge at the lower level of the _____.

ANSWER

pons

ITEM 7   THE FACIAL NERVE: PATHWAY

Motor and sensory roots of the facial nerve separately extend through the posterior cranial fossa in a common sheath to enter the internal acoustic meatus. While in the internal acoustic meatus the motor root and the sensory root (nervus intermedius) fuse to form a common trunk, which enters the facial canal in the petrous bone.

QUESTION
13

While in the posterior cranial fossa, the motor and sensory roots of the facial nerve run (circle one)
A. separately in a common sheath
B. together in a common trunk

ANSWER

The correct answer is A. The two roots do not form a common trunk until they leave the posterior cranial fossa.

QUESTION
14

The fusion of the motor and sensory roots of the facial nerve occurs in the *internal acoustic meatus/external acoustic meatus* (circle one).

ANSWER

internal acoustic meatus

THE FACIAL CANAL: PATHWAY   ITEM 8

The intraosseous course of the facial nerve in the facial canal first runs laterally, then makes a sharp bend to run posteriorly. The *geniculate ganglion* is located at this bend. As pointed out in Item 5, the geniculate ganglion is the ganglion for cell bodies of the afferent fibers of the facial nerve (cranial nerve VII).

The facial canal and facial nerve complete their complex course through bone at the *stylomastoid foramen,* where the nerve leaves bone. As it leaves the stylomastoid foramen, the facial nerve is composed almost entirely of special visceral efferent fibers which supply the muscles of facial expression.

The point at which SVE fibers of the facial nerve leave bone to extend to muscles of facial expression is the _____ foramen.

QUESTION 15

---

stylomastoid

ANSWER

The sensory ganglion associated with the facial nerve is the _____ ganglion.

QUESTION 16

---

geniculate

ANSWER

THE FACIAL NERVE: MOTOR BRANCHES   ITEM 9

While still within the petrous bone, the facial nerve gives off a small branch to the stapedius muscle in the middle ear. Emerging from the stylomastoid foramen, the facial nerve bends laterally around the neck of the mandible to enter the parotid gland. Several branches are given off, as shown in Figure 7–2. After leaving the stylomastoid foramen, but before entering the parotid gland, the facial nerve gives off the *posterior auricular branch* and a *branch to the posterior belly of the digastric muscle.* The nerve to the posterior belly of the digastric muscle also supplies the stylohyoid muscle. Locate these branches in Figure 7–2.

The branch of the facial nerve to the stapedius muscle is given off *before/after* (circle one) leaving the stylomastoid foramen.

QUESTION 17

The facial nerve gives off the branch to the stapedius muscle before passing through the stylomastoid foramen.

ANSWER

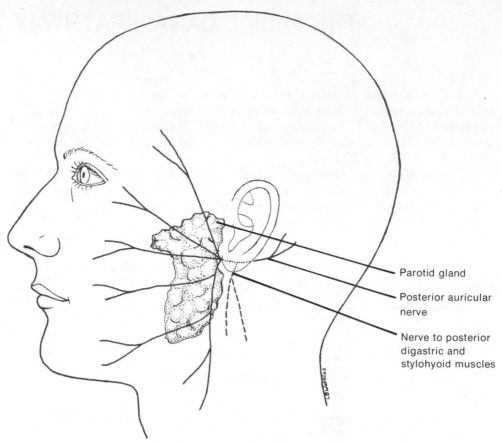

Figure 7–2. Branches of the facial nerve (VII), shown before entering the parotid gland.

QUESTION
18

The branches which the facial nerve gives off after leaving the stylomastoid foramen, but before reaching the parotid gland, are the posterior _____ nerve and the nerve to the _____ and _____ muscles.

ANSWER

auricular . . . digastric . . . stylohyoid

ITEM 10   THE FACIAL NERVE: DIVISIONS

Figure 7–3 illustrates a typical configuration of the special visceral efferent fibers of the facial nerve as it bifurcates into upper and lower divisions. At about the level of the posterior border of the ramus of the mandible, the facial nerve divides into a *temporofacial division* and a *cervicofacial division*. These two portions commonly form a continuous loop, although they may remain distinctly separate with only small anastomoses between them. Despite possible variations, the scheme presented in Figure 7–3 is typical enough to serve as an aid to study.

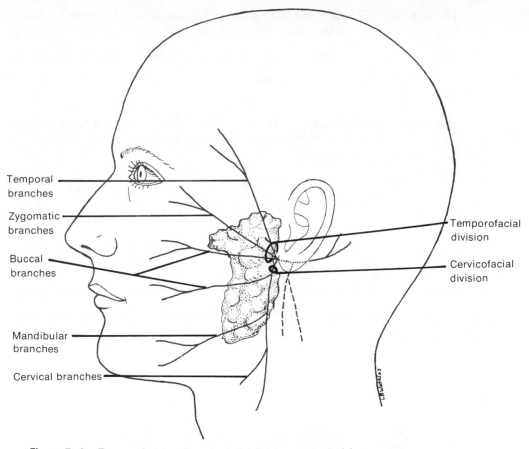

Figure 7–3. Temporofacial and cervicofacial divisions of the facial nerve (VII).

The upper division of the facial nerve is called the _____ division; the lower, the _____ division.

temporofacial . . . cervicofacial

THE FACIAL NERVE: TERMINAL BRANCHES IN THE FACE

Refer to Figure 7–3 to locate the terminal branches of the two divisions of the facial nerve. These branches are generally described in five groups, according to the location of the muscles supplied: *temporal, zygomatic, buccal, mandibular,* and *cervical.* Temporal and zygomatic branches arise primarily from the temporofacial division; mandibular and cervical branches, mainly from the cervicofacial division. Buccal branches arise from both divisions.

QUESTION
20
The terminal branches of the facial nerve are grouped in terms of the locations of the _____ which these branches supply.

ANSWER

muscles

QUESTION
21

The temporofacial division of the facial nerve gives rise to the temporal and _____ branches; the cervicofacial division gives rise to the cervical and _____ branches.

ANSWER

zygomatic . . . mandibular

QUESTION
22

The buccal branches arise from *the temporofacial division/the cervicofacial division/both of the divisions* (circle one).

ANSWER

The buccal branches arise from both the temporofacial and the cervicofacial divisions.

ITEM 12   THE FACIAL NERVE: TEMPORAL AND ZYGOMATIC BRANCHES

Examine Figure 7–3 again and locate the temporal and zygomatic branches of the facial nerve. Temporal branches, primarily from the temporofacial division, supply the anterior auricular muscle, the frontal belly of the epicranius muscle, and the corrugator supercilii muscle.

Zygomatic branches, also mainly from the temporofacial division, ascend obliquely to reach the zygomaticus muscles.

Both temporal and zygomatic branches send motor fibers to the orbicularis oculi muscle.

QUESTION
23

Which muscle receives motor innervation from both the temporal and zygomatic branches of the facial nerve (circle one)?
    A. anterior auricular
    B. epicranius
    C. corrugator supercilii
    D. zygomaticus
    E. orbicularis oculi

ANSWER

The correct answer is E, the orbicularis oculi.

The four principal muscle areas supplied by the temporal branches of the facial nerve are (1) the anterior _____ muscle, (2) the frontal belly of the _____ muscle, (3) the corrugator _____ muscle, and (4) the orbicularis _____ muscle.

QUESTION
24

---

auricular . . . epicranius . . . supercilii . . . oculi

ANSWER

The principal muscles supplied by the zygomatic branch of the facial nerve are the _____ muscles and the orbicularis _____ muscle.

QUESTION
25

---

zygomaticus . . . oculi

ANSWER

THE FACIAL NERVE: THE BUCCAL BRANCHES

ITEM
13

The buccal branches of the facial nerve, as can be seen in Figure 7–3, arise from both the temporofacial and cervicofacial divisions. Buccal branches are commonly involved in anastomoses between the two major divisions. These branches supply all the muscles between the eye and the mouth: the muscles of the infraorbital region, the nose, and the upper lip.

The muscles between the eyes and the mouth which are supplied by buccal branches of the facial nerve include muscles of the _____ region, muscles of the upper _____ and muscles of the _____.

QUESTION
26

---

infraorbital . . . lip . . . nose

ANSWER

THE FACIAL NERVE: MANDIBULAR AND CERVICAL BRANCHES

ITEM
14

Re-examine Figure 7–3 and locate the mandibular and cervical branches of the facial nerve. Mandibular branches, mainly originating in the cervicofacial part of nerve VII, course forward and downward to supply muscles of the lower lip and chin. Cervical branches descend behind the angle of the mandible to supply the platysma muscle.

QUESTION
27

The cervicofacial division of the facial nerve includes the _____ _____ branches and the _____ branches.

ANSWER

mandibular . . . cervical (in either order)

QUESTION
28

The platysma muscle is supplied by the _____ branches; the muscles of the lower lip and chin, by the _____ branches.

ANSWER

cervical . . . mandibular

ITEM 15   THE FACIAL NERVE: THE TASTE FIBERS

Taste sensations from the anterior two thirds of the tongue are carried by the *chorda tympani* branch of the facial nerve. Figure 7–4 shows special visceral afferent fibers of the facial nerve in the chorda tympani leaving the tongue with the lingual nerve, a branch of the mandibular division of the trigeminal nerve. The chorda tympani also carries general visceral efferent fibers for parasympathetic distribution to *submandibular* and *sublingual* glands.

QUESTION
29

On leaving the tongue, peripheral processes of the facial nerve travel with a branch of the _____ nerve.

ANSWER

Trigeminal. Taste fibers from the anterior two thirds of the tongue travel with the general somatic afferent fibers of the lingual nerve. The lingual nerve is a branch of the mandibular division of the trigeminal nerve (V).

QUESTION
30

Besides SVA fibers for taste, the chorda tympani also carries _____ _____ efferent fibers for parasympathetic innervation to sublingual and submandibular glands.

ANSWER

general visceral

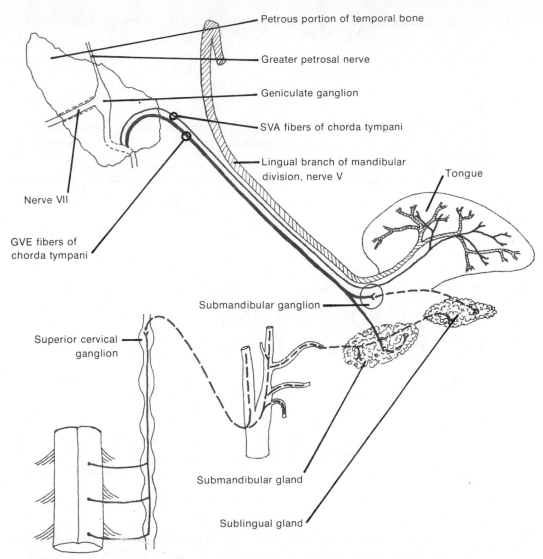

Figure 7–4. Chorda tympani branch of the facial nerve (VII) traveling with the lingual branch of the trigeminal nerve (V). (Redrawn from Woodburne: Essentials of Human Anatomy. 4th Ed. New York, Oxford University Press.)

THE CHORDA TYMPANI: PATHWAY   ITEM 16

The route of the chorda tympani is circuitous. It leaves the lingual branch of the mandibular nerve at the point where the latter passes medial to the lateral pterygoid muscle. The chorda tympani then passes posterolaterally to enter the petrotympanic fissure at its medial end. Thereafter, it follows a complex course through the middle ear. The chorda tympani joins the facial nerve within the petrous portion of the temporal bone, as can be seen in Figure 7–4.

QUESTION
31

The chorda tympani separates from the lingual nerve medial to the _____ _____ muscle.

ANSWER

lateral pterygoid

QUESTION
32

After passing posteriorly and laterally, the chorda tympani enters the medial end of the _____ fissure to join the _____ nerve within the temporal bone.

ANSWER

petrotympanic . . . facial

ITEM 17   THE CHORDA TYMPANI: TERMINATION IN THE CRANIUM

After joining the facial nerve above the stylomastoid foramen, processes of the SVA fibers of the chorda tympani travel in the facial nerve to the geniculate ganglion. Central processes of these neurons which follow the nervus intermedius to enter the brain form part of the *fasciculus solitarius*, which synapses in the nucleus solitarius of the medulla. The fasciculus solitarius can be seen in Figure 7–5. Also in Figure 7–5, notice the *motor nucleus of the facial nerve*, described in Item Six'.

QUESTION
33

Special visceral afferent fibers of the chorda tympani join the facial nerve just above the _____ foramen.

ANSWER

stylomastoid

QUESTION
34

The special visceral afferent fibers of the facial nerve carried in the fasciculus solitarius convey the sensation of _____.

ANSWER

taste

QUESTION
35

Central processes of SVA neurons of the chorda tympani synapse in the nucleus _____.

ANSWER

solitarius

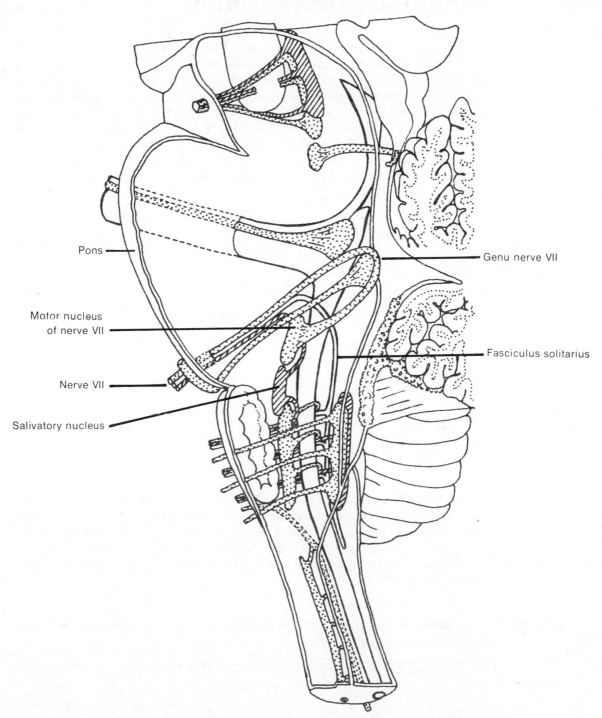

Figure 7–5.   Nuclei of the facial nerve (VII) in the pons, viewed from the medial sagittal surface. (Redrawn from Truex and Carpenter: Human Neuroanatomy. 6th Ed. Baltimore, The Williams and Wilkins Co.)

ITEM 18   THE FACIAL NERVE: THE PARASYMPATHETIC FIBERS

Preganglionic general visceral efferent fibers of the facial nerve have cell bodies in the *salivatory nucleus*. The salivatory nucleus can be seen in Figure 7–5. Some of these GVE preganglionic fibers enter the greater petrosal nerve which synapses in the pterygopalatine ganglion. From this point, parasympathetic post-ganglionic fibers extend to the lacrimal, nasal, and palatine glands. Another group of preganglionic GVE fibers of the facial nerve follows the chorda tympani to synapse in the submandibular ganglion, from which postganglionic fibers distribute to the submandibular and sublingual glands. Re-examine Figure 7–4 and notice the postganglionic fibers of the chorda tympani extending to the submandibular and sublingual glands.

QUESTION 36

Preganglionic fibers of the greater petrosal nerve synapse in the _____ _____ ganglion; those of the chorda tympani synapse in the _____ ganglion.

ANSWER

pterygopalatine . . . submandibular

ITEM 19   LESIONS AFFECTING THE FACIAL NERVE

A lesion affecting the special visceral efferent fibers of the facial nerve is called *Bell's palsy*. The symptomatology depends on the exact site where conduction is interrupted. Branches of the facial nerve are subject to injury during surgical procedures involving the parotid gland. Moreover, the relatively superficial position of branches of the facial nerve within the parotid gland makes them vulnerable to facial lacerations.

QUESTION 37

A lesion of the facial nerve can easily occur during surgery which involves the _____ gland.

ANSWER

parotid

QUESTION 38

A second common cause of injury to the facial nerve is a facial _____ in the area of the _____ gland.

ANSWER

laceration . . . parotid

Malfunction of the facial nerve is termed _____ palsy.

Bell's

PARALYSIS OF THE FACIAL MUSCULATURE   ITEM 20

Lesions in the brain or along the course of the facial nerve may cause complete or partial paralysis of the facial musculature. The effects of such injuries or lesions are very visible, and patients are usually deeply concerned about the resulting strange appearance of the face. The affected muscles lose tone, permitting the lateral angle of the eye to droop, the angle of the mouth may sag so that saliva flows constantly, and the affected side of the face lacks normal expression.

The effect of lesions of the facial nerve is likely to be _____ of the muscles of the face.

paralysis

Distortions of facial expression which may indicate loss of muscle tone due to injury to the facial nerve include drooping of the _____ and sagging of the _____.

eye . . . mouth

LESIONS AT THE STYLOMASTOID FORAMEN   ITEM 21

Complete destruction of the motor fibers at the stylomastoid foramen causes ipsilateral paralysis of all the muscles of the face, with consequent loss of the capacity for facial movement. The palpebral fissure is widened by atony of the orbicularis oculi muscle, which also causes the drooping of the eye mentioned in the preceding Item. However, the sagging of the corner of the mouth, also mentioned in Item 20, results from atony of the levator and zygomatic muscles.

In a patient with lesions of the facial nerve, pain from the cornea is felt, because the sensation of pain is carried by the intact ophthalmic nerve, but the normal corneal reflex is absent, because of the lack of motor innervation to the orbicularis oculi.

QUESTION
42

Drooping of the eye resulting from injury to the facial nerve is due to atony of the _____ _____ muscle, but sagging of the mouth is due to atony of the _____ and the _____ muscles.

ANSWER

orbicularis oculi . . . levator . . . zygomatic

QUESTION
43

The corneal reflex is absent in cases of lesion of the facial nerve because there is no motor supply to the _____ _____ muscle.

ANSWER

orbicularis oculi

QUESTION
44

Despite the fact that the corneal reflex is absent when a lesion of the facial nerve has occurred, pain from the cornea is felt because the _____ nerve remains intact.

ANSWER

ophthalmic

ITEM 22   • LESIONS BELOW THE GENICULATE GANGLION

If the facial nerve is injured or sectioned below the geniculate ganglion, the patient will lose all the motor functions just described, and he will also lose conduction in the fibers of the chorda tympani. Secretion of saliva from the submandibular and sublingual glands will be impaired because preganglionic visceral efferent fibers have been interrupted. *Hyperacusis* (heightened sensitivity to sound) may occur because of loss of innervation to the stapedius muscle in the middle ear, which normally dampens oscillations of the ossicles of the ear. Taste sensation on the anterior two thirds of the tongue will be lost or diminished.

QUESTION
45

Sectioning the facial nerve below the geniculate ganglion produces loss of conduction in the fibers of the _____ _____.

ANSWER

chorda tympani

QUESTION
46

Hyperacusis means *increased/decreased* (circle one) sensitivity to sound.

The correct answer is "increased". The prefix *hyper-* connotes increase, as its opposite, *hypo-,* connotes decrease.

ANSWER

Hyperacusis results from loss of motor innervation to the _____ muscle, which ordinarily reduces sensitivity to sound by reducing oscillations of the small _____ of the middle ear.

QUESTION
47

stapedius . . . bones

ANSWER

Impairment of salivary secretion results from a lesion of the facial nerve below the geniculate ganglion, which causes interruption of *preganglionic/postganglionic* (circle one) GVE fibers.

QUESTION
48

preganglionic

ANSWER

In addition to suffering facial paralysis, impairment of salivation, and hyperacusis, a patient with lesions of the facial nerve will also suffer loss or diminution of the sense of _____.

QUESTION
49

taste

ANSWER

LESIONS PROXIMAL TO THE GENICULATE GANGLION

ITEM 23

Lesions proximal to the geniculate ganglion cause motor paralysis, cessation of salivation from the sublingual and submandibular glands, loss of taste, and hyperacusis. In addition, preganglionic general visceral efferent fibers to the lacrimal gland lose conduction. The resulting inability to produce tears may lead to secondary eye inflammations.

Lesions of the facial nerve proximal to the geniculate ganglion involve all the effects of lesions below the geniculate ganglion, including, (1) paralysis of _____ muscles, (2) loss of _____ from submandibular and sublingual glands, (3) loss of _____ from the anterior two thirds of the tongue, and (4) increased sensitivity to _____.

QUESTION
50

facial . . . salivation . . . taste . . . sound

ANSWER

QUESTION
51

Besides the effects mentioned in Question 50, a lesion of the facial nerve proximal to the geniculate ganglion also causes loss of conduction in preganglionic GVE fibers to the _____ gland, often leading to secondary eye infections caused by the absence of _____ .

ANSWER

lacrimal . . . tears

ITEM 24   LESIONS AFFECTING NUCLEI OF THE FACIAL NERVE

Central lesions affecting the nuclei or fibers of the facial nerve cause one or more of a variety of symptoms, depending on the extent of the lesion. Interruption of fibers from the cortex which eventually terminate on the facial nucleus may cause paresis of the muscles of the lower part of the face. Because these cortical fibers are crossed, the paresis will be contralateral. Muscles of the forehead, on the other hand, may remain unaffected by this type of lesion because cortical fibers projecting to these neurons are distributed bilaterally.

QUESTION
52

Lesions affecting nuclei of the facial nerve may result in contralateral paresis of the muscles of the _____ part of the face.

ANSWER

lower

QUESTION
53

Interruption of cortical fibers terminating in the facial nucleus may leave muscles of the _____ able to function because of the bilateral distribution of cortical fibers.

ANSWER

forehead

ITEM 25   THE TYPES OF FACIAL PARESIS

Patients with facial paralysis caused by disruption of the cortical fibers lose voluntary control of the lower facial muscles, but involuntary motion elicited by emotional states may be preserved. Thus two types of facial paresis are recognized: loss of voluntary control and loss of involuntary movement. Various clinical cases have produced firm eivdence that voluntary and involuntary emotional control of the facial muscles are handled by two separate and distinct neural mechanisms. Although the route for involuntary motor fibers is not definitely known, it has been suggested that the globus pallidus and the thalamus may be involved in the mechanism of involuntary facial expression.

Disruption of cortical fibers causes loss of _____ control of lower facial muscles, but does not affect _____ motion resulting from emotional states.

QUESTION 54

---

voluntary . . . involuntary

ANSWER

Two structures of the brain which possibly may be involved in emotion related involuntary movement of lower facial muscles are the _____ _____ and the _____.

QUESTION 55

---

globus pallidus . . . thalamus

ANSWER

SUMMARY OF UNIT SEVEN

The facial nerve is a mixed nerve carrying five functional components, three sensory and two motor. The facial nerve has a motor root and a second root, primarily sensory, called the nervus intermedius. Fibers originating from the motor root are special visceral efferent, supplying the branchiomeric muscles of facial expression. The motor fibers of the nervus intermedius provide parasympathetic supply to the lacrimal, sublingual, and submandibular glands. The sensory fibers of the facial nerve are GSA, GVA, and SVA.

PATHWAY OF THE FACIAL NERVE

The motor and sensory roots of the facial nerve arise in the pons and enter the internal acoustic meatus. A common motor and sensory trunk runs in the facial canal of the petrous bone to the external genu of the nerve where the geniculate ganglion is located. The geniculate ganglion contains cell bodies of afferent neurons of the facial nerve. Fibers which are mostly efferent leave the bone through the stylomastoid foramen and course through the parotid gland, where the SVE fibers distribute to various muscles.

After leaving bone, but before entering the parotid gland, the facial nerve gives off the posterior auricular nerve to the posterior and superior auricular muscles and to the occipital belly of the epicranius muscle. A second nerve goes to the posterior belly of the digastric muscle and to the stylohyoid muscle.

On entering the parotid gland, the facial nerve divides into two parts, an upper temporofacial part and a lower cervicofacial part. Temporal and zygomatic muscles are supplied by the temporofacial division; mandibular and cervical muscles, by the cervicofacial division; buccal muscles, by both divisions.

Sensory fibers of the nervus intermedius carry three functional components: GSA, GVA, and SVA. General somatic afferent fibers carry sensations of pain, temperature, touch, and pressure from the external acoustic meatus. These fibers, whose cell bodies are contained in the geniculate ganglion, have central processes which go to the pons. Here they join GSA fibers of the trigeminal nerve to terminate in the trigeminal nucleus. Special visceral afferent fibers, with cell bodies in the geniculate ganglion, convey taste from the anterior two thirds of the tongue.

THE CHORDA TYMPANI

The chorda tympani is a branch of the facial nerve which carries sensory fibers for taste as well as motor fibers for parasympathetic innervation to submandibular and sublingual glands. Leaving the tongue, the chorda tympani travels with the lingual branch of the trigeminal nerve past the lateral pterygoid muscle, and then makes its way separately through the petrotympanic fissure to join the facial nerve in the facial canal above the stylomastoid foramen. The chorda tympani runs in the facial nerve to the geniculate ganglion. From this point, central processes which form part of the fasciculus solitarius enter the brain to synapse in the nucleus solitarius of the dorsal medulla.

General visceral efferent fibers to various glands have cell bodies of preganglionic fibers in the superior salivatory nucleus of the pons. These parasympathetic fibers divide at the genu of the facial nerve in the petrous bone.

One group of fibers, constituting the greater petrosal nerve, synapses in the pterygopalatine ganglion. From the pterygopalatine ganglion, postganglionic fibers distribute to the lacrimal, nasal, and palatine glands. The other group of preganglionic fibers follows the chorda tympani to synapse in the submandibular ganglion, from which postganglionic fibers distribute to the submandibular and sublingual glands.

LESIONS AFFECTING THE FACIAL NERVE

Lesions affecting the facial nerve may occur in the brain or along the course of the nerve. Lesions at the stylomastoid foramen result in atony of muscles of facial expression. Denervation of the orbicularis oculi muscle causes drooping of the eye; denervation of the levator and zygomatic muscles causes sagging of the corner of the mouth. Lesions below the geniculate ganglion have the additional effects of impairing salivation, impairing taste from the anterior two thirds of the tongue, and causing hyperacusis (increased sensitivity to sound). If a lesion is proximal to the geniculate ganglion, the aforementioned consequences will be accompanied by an inability to produce tears, with a consequent danger of secondary eye infection.

Finally, central lesions affecting nuclei or fibers of the facial nerve may cause a contralateral paresis of muscles of the lower part of the face. When voluntary control of these facial muscles is lost, involuntary movement elicited by emotional states may be preserved, since the voluntary and involuntary movements of facial muscles apparently are handled by two separate neural mechanisms.

The functional component of motor fibers of the facial nerve which supply muscles of facial expression is _____ visceral efferent, while the component of fibers which supply various glands is _____ visceral efferent.

QUESTION 56

---

special . . . general

ANSWER

The geniculate ganglion is located at the _____ of the facial nerve within the _____ bone.

QUESTION 57

---

genu . . . petrous

ANSWER

Special visceral efferent fibers of the facial nerve travel from the stylomastoid foramen to the _____ gland, from which point they distribute to muscles of _____ _____.

QUESTION 58

---

parotid . . . facial expression

ANSWER

The geniculate ganglion is a *motor/sensory* (circle one) ganglion.

QUESTION 59

ANSWER
sensory

QUESTION
60

Before entering the parotid gland, motor fibers of the facial nerve send branches to (1) the _____ muscle of the middle ear, (2) the posterior and superior _____ muscles, (3) the occipital belly of the _____ muscle, (4) the posterior belly of the _____ muscle, and to (5) the stylo-hyoid muscle.

ANSWER
stapedius . . . auricular . . . epicranius . . . digastric

QUESTION
61

General somatic afferent fibers of the facial nerve convey sensations of pain, temperature, touch, and pressure from the external _____ meatus.

ANSWER
acoustic

QUESTION
62

Cell bodies of GSA fibers of the facial nerve are located in the _____ ganglion, with central processes terminating in the _____ nucleus in the pons.

ANSWER
geniculate . . . trigeminal

QUESTION
63

The sensation of taste is conveyed from the anterior portion of the tongue by _____ _____ afferent fibers of the facial nerve.

ANSWER
special visceral

QUESTION
64

The chorda tympani nerve carries afferent fibers for the sensation of _____ and efferent fibers to the _____ and the _____ glands.

ANSWER
taste . . . submandibular . . . sublingual

QUESTION
65

On leaving the tongue, the chorda tympani travels with the lingual branch of the _____ nerve.

ANSWER
trigeminal

QUESTION
66

After separating from the lingual nerve, the chorda tympani courses through the _____ fissure before entering the facial canal.

ANSWER
petrotympanic

Preganglionic parasympathetic fibers of the greater petrosal nerve synapse in the _____ ganglion.

pterygopalatine

Glands to which postganglionic fibers of the greater petrosal nerve distribute include the _____, _____, and _____ glands.

lacrimal . . . nasal . . . palatine (in any order)

Preganglionic parasympathetic fibers of the facial nerve carrying impulses destined for the salivary glands synapse in the _____ ganglion.

submandibular

Lesions of the facial nerve at the stylomastoid foramen result in atony of muscles of _____ _____.

facial expression

Lesions of the facial nerve below the geniculate ganglion have the additional effects of impairing _____ and _____, as well as of heightening sensitivity to _____.

salivation . . . taste . . . sound

Interruption of preganglionic fibers to the lacrimal gland, with consequent absence of tears, occurs with lesions of the facial nerve proximal to the _____ ganglion.

geniculate

Contralateral paresis of the muscles of the _____ part of the face results from central lesions of the nuclei or fibers of the facial nerve.

lower

Even when voluntary control of facial muscles is lost through lesions of the facial nerve, involuntary movement stemming from states of _____ may still occur.

emotion

Unit Eight □ THE GLOSSO-PHARYNGEAL AND VAGUS NERVES

ITEM 1

THE GLOSSOPHARYNGEAL NERVE: FUNCTIONAL COMPONENTS

The glossopharyngeal nerve, cranial nerve IX, primarily supplies the tongue and pharynx. Like the facial and vagus nerves, the glossopharyngeal nerve carries five functional components, three afferent and two efferent. General somatic afferent fibers convey cutaneous sensation from skin of the ear. General visceral afferent fibers convey sensation from mucous membranes of the pharynx, middle ear, and posterior third of the tongue. GVA fibers also transmit sensation from the parotid gland and carry afferent input concerning blood pressure. Special visceral afferent fibers carry taste from the posterior third of the tongue.

General visceral efferent fibers of the glossopharyngeal nerve are parasympathetic to the parotid gland. Special visceral efferent fibers supply motor innervation to the stylopharyngeus muscle.

QUESTION 1

Motor fibers of the glossopharyngeal nerve provide parasympathetic innervation to the _____ gland and supply the _____ muscle.

ANSWER

parotid . . . stylopharyngeus

QUESTION 2

The types of sensation carried by sensory fibers of the glossopharyngeal nerve include _____, _____, and _____ sensations.

ANSWER

cutaneous . . . visceral . . . taste (in any order)

QUESTION 3

Match the items in column B with the related functional components of the glossopharyngeal nerve listed in column A.

Column A		Column B
(	) 1. SVE	A. taste
(	) 2. GVE	B. innervation of stylopharyngeus muscle
(	) 3. GVA	C. cutaneous sensation
(	) 4. SVA	D. secretion of the parotid gland
(	) 5. GSA	E. visceral sensation

1.—(B); 2.—(D); 3.—(E); 4.—(A); 5.—(C)   *ANSWER*

THE GLOSSOPHARYNGEAL NERVE: PATHWAY

ITEM 2

The superficial exit of the rootlets of the glossopharyngeal nerve is a sulcus on the ventrolateral surface of the superior medulla. Examine Figure 8–1 and notice the emergence of the glossopharyngeal nerve from the medulla in line with the vagus and accessory nerves. The glossopharyngeal nerve, like the vagus and accessory nerves, exits from the skull at the jugular foramen, along with the internal

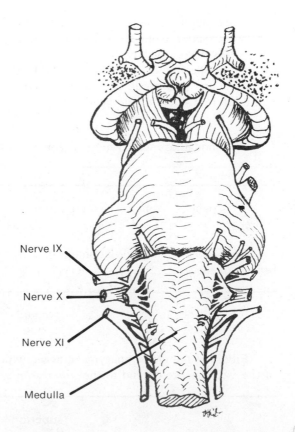

Figure 8–1. Brain stem, ventral aspect, showing exit of the glossopharyngeal, vagus, and accessory nerves. (Redrawn and modified from Truex and Carpenter: Strong and Elwyn's Human Neuroanatomy. 5th Ed. Baltimore, The Williams and Wilkins Co.)

Nerve IX

Nerve X

Nerve XI

Medulla

jugular vein. Outside the skull, the glossopharyngeal nerve descends between the internal carotid artery and the internal jugular vein.

QUESTION
4

The glossopharyngeal nerve exits from the medulla in line with the _____ ____ and _____ nerves.

ANSWER

vagus . . . accessory

QUESTION
5

Cranial nerves IX, X, and XI exit from the skull through the _____ foramen.

ANSWER

jugular

ITEM 3   THE GLOSSOPHARYNGEAL NERVE: GSA FIBERS

The general somatic afferent component of the glossopharyngeal nerve carries general sensation from a small area of skin posterior to the ear. Peripheral processes travel with the auricular branch of the vagus nerve to the *superior ganglion* located in the jugular foramen. Central processes from the superior ganglion terminate and synapse in the spinal nucleus of the trigeminal nerve, as do all somatic afferent fibers of the head.

QUESTION
6

The modalities which general somatic afferent fibers convey are those of _____, _____, _____, and _____.

ANSWER

pain . . . touch . . . temperature . . . pressure (in any order)

QUESTION
7

GSA fibers of the glossopharyngeal nerve are included with the auricular branch of the _____ nerve.

ANSWER

vagus

QUESTION
8

Fibers of the glossopharyngeal nerve which travel with the auricular branch of the vagus nerve extend to the *superior/inferior* (circle one) ganglion.

ANSWER

superior

GSA fibers of the head synapse in the spinal nucleus of the _____
nerve.

QUESTION
9

trigeminal

ANSWER

GVA FIBERS FROM THE MUCOSA OF THE MIDDLE EAR

ITEM 4

General visceral afferent fibers of the glossopharyngeal nerve carry visceral sensation from several regions: from mucosa of the middle ear, from the carotid sinus, from the posterior third of the tongue, and from the pharyngeal mucosa.

Examine Figure 8–2. Notice the *tympanic plexus,* an extensive plexus in the mucosa of the middle ear formed by afferent fibers from the middle ear, the auditory tube, and the mastoid air cells. Notice how the fibers of this plexus converge to form the *tympanic nerve,* which passes downward through bone to enter the sensory inferior ganglion of the glossopharyngeal nerve. Central processes from the inferior ganglion join the tractus solitarius and terminate in its nucleus.

GVA fibers of the glossopharyngeal nerve supply the following areas: (1) mucosa of the _____ ear, (2) mucosa of the _____, (3) the _____ sinus, and (4) the posterior third of the _____.

QUESTION
10

middle . . . pharynx . . . carotid . . . tongue

ANSWER

The plexus located in the middle ear is called the _____ plexus.

QUESTION
11

tympanic

ANSWER

Fibers of the tympanic plexus form the _____ nerve.

QUESTION
12

tympanic

ANSWER

Cell bodies of peripheral processes of the fibers of the tympanic plexus are located in the _____ ganglion of the glossopharyngeal nerve.

QUESTION
13

inferior

ANSWER

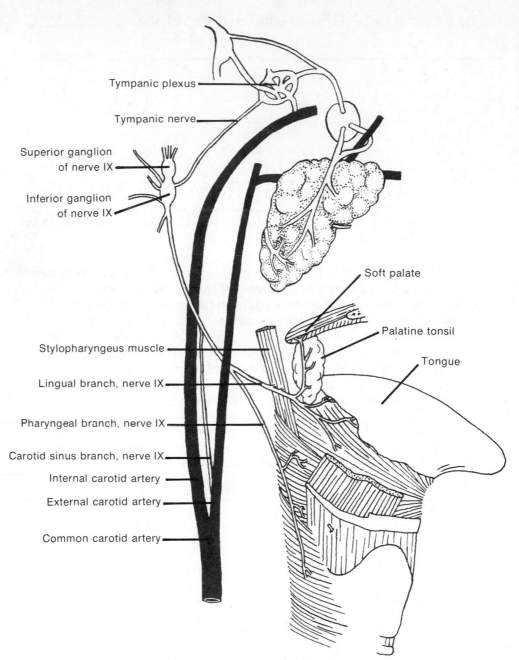

Figure 8–2. Branches of the glossopharyngeal nerve (IX) with cell bodies in the inferior ganglion. (Modified from Woodburne: Essentials of Human Anatomy. 4th Ed. New York, Oxford University Press.)

QUESTION
14

Central processes from the inferior ganglion of the glossopharyngeal nerve terminate in the nucleus of the tractus _____.

ANSWER   solitarius

GVA FIBERS FROM THE TONGUE, THE PHARYNGEAL MUCOSA, AND THE CAROTID SINUS

ITEM
5

Refer to Figure 8–2 and observe the *lingual, pharyngeal,* and *carotid sinus branches* which ascend with the main trunk of the glossopharyngeal nerve. These branches carry general visceral afferent fibers from the tongue, pharyngeal mucosa, and carotid sinus, respectively. From their cell bodies in the inferior ganglion, these GVA fibers also send central processes to the nucleus of the tractus solitarius.

QUESTION
15

In addition to GVA fibers from the middle ear, the nucleus solitarius also receives GVA fibers from the _____, from mucosa of the _____, and from the _____ sinus.

ANSWER

tongue . . . pharynx . . . carotid

THE CAROTID SINUS NERVE

ITEM
6

Locate the *carotid sinus nerve* in Figure 8–2. Notice the GVA fibers which constitute this nerve leaving the main trunk of the glossopharyngeal nerve to reach the bifurcation of the common carotid artery. The carotid sinus nerve carries afferent impulses from chemoreceptors of the carotid body and from pressoreceptors of the carotid sinus. Chemoreceptors are sensitive to blood carbon dioxide levels; pressoreceptors are sensitive to changes in blood pressure.

QUESTION
16

The carotid sinus nerve monitors levels of _____ _____ in the blood, and changes in blood _____.

ANSWER

carbon dioxide . . . pressure

QUESTION
17

Receptors sensitive to carbon dioxide are termed _____.

ANSWER

chemoreceptors

QUESTION
18

Receptors sensitive to blood pressure are termed _____.

ANSWER

pressoreceptors

ITEM 7   THE GLOSSOPHARYNGEAL NERVE: THE SVA FIBERS

Taste sensations from the posterior third of the tongue and adjacent pharyngeal wall are carried by the special visceral afferent component of the glossopharyngeal nerve. Again refer to Figure 8–2 and observe the route of these SVA fibers. Peripheral processes follow the main trunk of the nerve as it ascends on the lateral surface of the stylopharyngeus muscle, then between the external and internal carotid arteries, to the jugular foramen. Cell bodies of these afferent neurons are located in the inferior ganglion. Central processes enter the medulla to terminate in the nucleus of the tractus solitarius.

QUESTION
19

Special visceral afferent fibers of the glossopharyngeal nerve convey the sensation of taste from the *anterior/posterior* (circle one) *third/two thirds* (circle one) of the tongue.

ANSWER

posterior . . . third

QUESTION
20

The main trunk of the glossopharyngeal nerve ascends on the lateral surface of the _____ muscle.

ANSWER

stylopharyngeus

QUESTION
21

On its way to the skull, the main trunk of the glossopharyngeal nerve ascends between the _____ and _____ carotid arteries.

ANSWER

external . . . internal

QUESTION
22

The glossopharyngeal nerve enters the skull at the _____ foramen.

ANSWER

jugular

Central processes of the ninth cranial nerve terminate in the nucleus of the tractus _____.

solitarius

THE GLOSSOPHARYNGEAL NERVE: THE GVE FIBERS

General visceral efferent fibers of the glossopharyngeal nerve are parasympathetic nerves to the parotid gland. Locate these branches on Figure 8–3.

Cell bodies of preganglionic neurons are located in the inferior salivatory nucleus in the medulla. Axons follow the path described for the rootlets of the nerve, course through the superior and inferior ganglia without synapse, and enter the tympanic nerve just below the jugular foramen. The tympanic nerve enters the tympanic cavity through a small bone canal between the jugular foramen and the carotid canal. Fibers of the tympanic nerve form the tympanic plexus on the medial wall of the middle ear. The continuation of preganglionic fibers beyond the tympanic plexus is known as the *lesser petrosal nerve*.

The inferior salivatory nucleus in the medulla contains cell bodies of neurons which supply the _____ gland.

parotid

General visceral efferent preganglionic fibers of the glossopharyngeal nerve travel with the _____ nerve to the tympanic plexus, then form the lesser _____ nerve.

tympanic . . . petrosal

THE LESSER PETROSAL NERVE

At the point where the tympanic nerve forms the tympanic plexus within the middle ear, the general visceral efferent fibers pass through, leaving the tympanic plexus as the *lesser petrosal nerve*. The lesser petrosal nerve passes through the anterior wall of the petrous portion of the temporal bone to enter the middle cranial fossa. The nerve sometimes exits from the middle fossa through a fissure

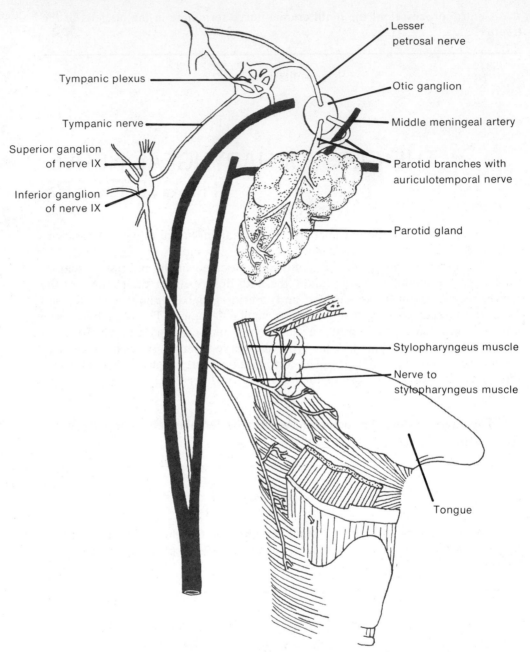

Figure 8-3. Efferent branches of the glossopharyngeal nerve (IX). (Modified from Woodburne: Essentials of Human Anatomy. 4th Ed. New York, Oxford University Press.)

between the petrous part of the temporal bone and the greater wing of the sphenoid bone, and sometimes through the foramen ovale. It synapses with postganglionic cell bodies in the *otic ganglion*. Re-examine Figure 8–3 and note the position where the tympanic nerve becomes the lesser petrosal nerve.

When GVE fibers of the glossopharyngeal nerve leave the tympanic plexus they are called the _____ _____ nerve.

QUESTION 26

---

lesser petrosal

ANSWER

GVE fibers of the glossopharyngeal nerve enter the middle cranial fossa through the _____ portion of the _____ bone.

QUESTION 27

---

petrous . . . temporal

ANSWER

The lesser petrosal nerve leaves the middle cranial fossa through either of two exits: (1) through a fissure between the _____ part of the _____ bone and the greater wing of the sphenoid bone, or (2) through the foramen _____ _____.

QUESTION 28

---

petrous . . . temporal . . . ovale

ANSWER

Postganglionic cell bodies of the GVE fibers of the glossopharyngeal nerve are located in the _____ ganglion.

QUESTION 29

---

otic

ANSWER

THE OTIC GANGLION ITEM 10

The *otic ganglion,* shown in Figure 8–3, is located just medial to the trunk of the mandibular nerve as the latter exits through the foramen ovale. The general visceral efferent fibers contained in the lesser petrosal nerve terminate in the otic ganglion by synapsing with postganglionic fibers, axons of which distribute to the parotid gland with the auriculotemporal branch of the mandibular nerve.

The location of the otic ganglion is medial to the _____ nerve at the foramen _____.

QUESTION 30

---

mandibular . . . ovale

ANSWER

QUESTION
31

Postganglionic fibers of the glossopharyngeal nerve which leave the otic ganglion distribute with the _____ branch of the mandibular nerve.

ANSWER

auriculotemporal

QUESTION
32

GVE fibers of the glossopharyngeal nerve supply the _____ gland.

ANSWER

parotid

ITEM 11   THE GLOSSOPHARYNGEAL NERVE: THE SVE FIBERS

The only special visceral efferent component of the glossopharyngeal nerve is the *nerve to the stylopharyngeus muscle,* shown in Figure 8–3. Cell bodies of SVE fibers of the glossopharyngeal nerve are contained in the cephalic region of the nucleus ambiguus, in the medulla. Along with the main body of the glossopharyngeal nerve, these fibers exit at the jugular foramen. Outside the skull, the glossopharyngeal nerve extends to the lateral surface of the stylopharyngeus muscle after descending between the internal and external carotid arteries.

QUESTION
33

Cell bodies of SVE fibers of the glossopharyngeal nerve are located in the nucleus _____ in the medulla.

ANSWER

ambiguus

QUESTION
34

SVE fibers of the glossopharyngeal nerve exit from the skull through the _____ foramen.

ANSWER

jugular

QUESTION
35

The nerve to the stylopharyngeus muscle approaches the muscle from its _____ side.

ANSWER

lateral

LESIONS AFFECTING THE GLOSSOPHARYNGEAL NERVE

Lesions confined to the glossopharyngeal nerve occur infrequently. When they do occur, their major symptoms include loss of the gag reflex, alteration in the cardiovascular reflex mediated by the carotid sinus nerve, and loss or diminution of taste sensation in the posterior third of the tongue.

In some patients, particularly in elderly patients with arteriosclerosis, the carotid sinus reflex may be hyperactive. A slight increase in blood pressure, or pressure applied externally to the region under the angle of the mandible, may bring forth a fullblown pressoreceptor response. Such a pressoreceptor response includes bradycardia (slowing of the heartbeat), syncope, and sometimes convulsions and loss of consciousness. This hypersensitive response to pressure is termed *carotid sinus syndrome*.

Two symptoms which would indicate a lesion of the glossopharyngeal nerve are a loss of the _____ reflex and an alteration of the _____ reflex.

QUESTION 36

gag . . . pressoreceptor

ANSWER

Lesion of the glossopharyngeal nerve brings on diminution of the sensation of _____ emanating from the _____ third of the tongue.

QUESTION 37

taste . . . posterior

ANSWER

Symptomatology sometimes found in cases of hypersensitive carotid sinus reflex includes _____, _____, _____, and _____.

QUESTION 38

bradycardia . . . syncope . . . convulsions . . . loss of consciousness (in any order)

ANSWER

Patients particularly susceptible to carotid sinus syndrome are those suffering from _____.

QUESTION 39

arteriosclerosis

ANSWER

ITEM 13

GLOSSOPHARYNGEAL NEURALGIA

Occasionally a patient will show extreme sensitivity to pain in the region of distribution of sensory fibers of the glossopharyngeal nerve. Attacks may be initiated by any stimulus to the wall of the pharynx, even coughing or swallowing. Excruciating pain may radiate from the pharynx to the auditory tube, the middle ear, and the region behind the ear. This hyperalgesia (extreme sensitivity to pain) of sensory fibers of the ninth cranial nerve is termed *glossopharyngeal neuralgia*.

QUESTION 40

Extreme sensitivity to pain is termed _____.

ANSWER

hyperalgesia

QUESTION 41

Attacks of extreme pain along the distribution route of the ninth cranial nerve is termed _____ _____.

ANSWER

glossopharyngeal neuralgia

QUESTION 42

Unprovoked attacks of extreme pain along the distribution of the glossopharyngeal nerve may be brought on simply from _____ or _____.

ANSWER

coughing . . . swallowing (in either order)

ITEM 14

THE VAGUS NERVE

The vagus nerve, cranial nerve X, is a mixed nerve composed of the same functional components as are found in the facial and glossopharyngeal nerves: three afferent components and two efferent. The afferent components are general somatic, general visceral, and special visceral; the efferent components are general visceral and special visceral. The vagus nerve is the most widely distributed of the cranial nerves, supplying not only the pharynx and larynx but also smooth muscles of the thoracic and abdominal viscera.

The two principal areas innervated by the vagus nerve are (1) the _____ and the _____, and (2) viscera of the _____ and of the _____.

---

pharynx . . . larynx . . . thorax . . . abdomen

The sensory components of the vagus nerve are
    1. _____ _____ afferent
    2. _____ _____ afferent
    3. _____ _____ afferent

---

    1. general somatic
    2. general visceral
    3. special visceral

The motor components of the vagus nerve are
    1. _____ _____ efferent
    2. _____ _____ efferent

---

    1. general visceral
    2. special visceral

THE VAGUS NERVE: ITEM
ORIGIN IN THE MEDULLA 15

The vagus nerve arises from the side of the medulla as a series of rootlets in line with and between those of the glossopharyngeal nerve cranially and those of the cranial root of the accessory nerve caudally. These rootlets unite to form a single trunk which enters the jugular foramen. Re-examine Figure 8–1 to observe the superficial exit of the vagus nerve from the brain stem.

The rootlets of the vagus nerve arise in the (circle one)
A. pons
B. midbrain
C. medulla

ANSWER   The correct answer is C. The rootlets arising from the side of the medulla are those of the glossopharyngeal, vagus, and accessory nerves.

QUESTION
47

The rootlets of the vagus nerve are situated between those of the cranial root of the _____ nerve caudally and those of the _____ _____ nerve cranially.

ANSWER   accessory . . . glossopharyngeal

QUESTION
48

After its rootlets unite to form a single trunk, the vagus nerve enters the _____ foramen.

ANSWER   jugular

ITEM 16   THE VAGUS NERVE: SUPERIOR AND INFERIOR GANGLIA

In Figure 8–4, observe the position of the superior and inferior ganglia of the vagus nerve relative to the jugular foramen. As the vagus nerve passes through the jugular foramen the small ganglion known as the *superior ganglion* frequently, but not always, appears. Just after the nerve emerges from the jugular foramen, a second, larger ganglion appears. It is called the *inferior ganglion*. Both of these ganglia contain cell bodies of the afferent neurons of the vagus nerve.

As the vagus nerve leaves the jugular foramen, it is joined by the cranial portion of the accessory nerve, which distributes together with branches of the vagus nerve.

QUESTION
49

The larger of the two ganglia of the vagus nerve is the *superior/inferior* (circle one) ganglion, which appears *before/after* (circle one) the vagus nerve emerges from the jugular foramen.

ANSWER   inferior . . . after

QUESTION
50

Branches of the cranial part of the spinal accessory nerve are distributed with branches of the _____ nerve.

ANSWER   vagus

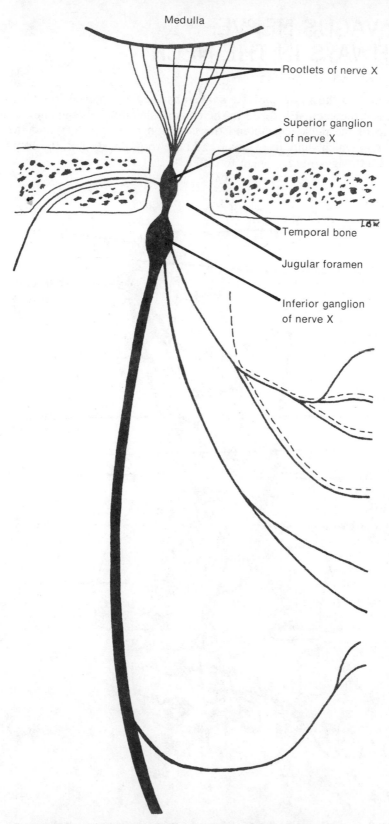

Figure 8–4. Superior and inferior ganglia of the vagus nerve (X).

ITEM 17   THE VAGUS NERVE: PATHWAYS IN THE NECK

Figure 8–5 shows the pathways taken by the vagus nerve down the right and left sides of the neck. Enclosed in the carotid sheath, the vagus nerve descends each side of the neck just behind the common carotid artery and the internal jugular vein, which share its enclosure. At the root of the neck, the courses of the right and left vagus nerves begin to differ.

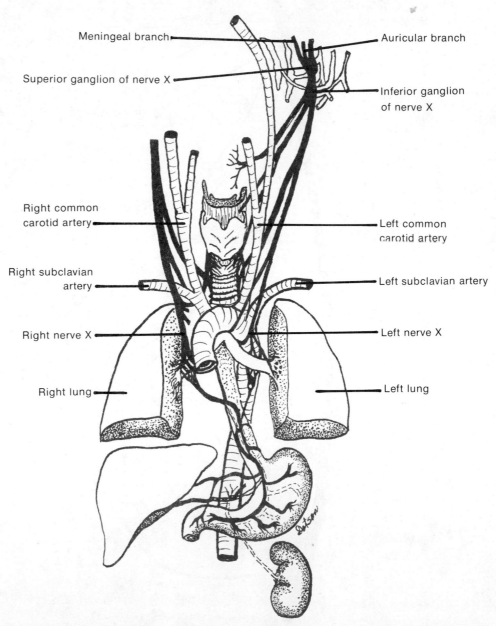

Meningeal branch

Superior ganglion of nerve X

Auricular branch

Inferior ganglion of nerve X

Right common carotid artery

Left common carotid artery

Right subclavian artery

Left subclavian artery

Right nerve X

Left nerve X

Right lung

Left lung

Figure 8–5.   Routes of the right and left vagus nerves (X). (Redrawn from Woodburne: Essentials of Human Anatomy. 4th Ed. New York, Oxford University Press.)

The vagus nerve descends in the neck in company with the common _____ artery and the internal _____ vein.

carotid . . . jugular

Structures enclosed in the carotid sheath include the _____ _____ artery, the _____ _____ vein, and the _____ nerve.

common carotid . . . internal jugular . . . vagus

THE RIGHT AND LEFT VAGUS NERVES: PATHWAYS ITEM 18

Examine Figure 8–5 again and notice the divergent routes by which the right and left vagus nerves travel to the roots of the lungs. The right vagus nerve passes anterior to the first part of the right subclavian artery and then swings obliquely to a dorsal position as it enters the thorax to reach the trachea and the root of the right lung.

The left vagus nerve descends into the thorax between the common carotid artery and the internal jugular vein. It crosses in front of the root of the left subclavian artery and the arch of the aorta to reach the root of the left lung.

The right vagus nerve travels anterior, then dorsal, to the right _____ artery.

subclavian

Descending into the thorax, the left vagus nerve passes between the _____ _____ artery and the _____ _____ vein.

common carotid . . . internal jugular

To reach the root of the left lung, the left vagus nerve passes anterior to the left _____ artery and the arch of the _____.

subclavian . . . aorta

ITEM 19

THE VAGUS NERVE: THE GSA FIBERS

As you can see in Figure 8–5, the general somatic afferent fibers of the vagus nerve have cell bodies in the superior or the inferior ganglion. Central processes of these fibers terminate in the spinal nucleus of the trigeminal nerve. Peripheral processes form two small branches, the *auricular* and the *meningeal,* which leave the vagus nerve at the superior ganglion within the jugular foramen. These branches are also shown in Figure 8–5. The auricular branch supplies the external acoustic meatus and posterior portion of the external ear. The meningeal branch supplies dura around the sigmoid sinus.

QUESTION 56

The termination point of the central processes of GSA fibers of the vagus nerve is the _____ nucleus of the _____ nerve.

ANSWER

spinal . . . trigeminal

QUESTION 57

The branches formed by peripheral processes of GSA fibers of the vagus nerve are the _____ and _____ branches.

ANSWER

auricular . . . meningeal

QUESTION 58

The external acoustic meatus and the posterior part of the external ear are supplied by GSA fibers of the vagus nerve carried in the _____ branch.

ANSWER

auricular

QUESTION 59

The area supplied by the meningeal branch of the vagus nerve is the dura around the _____ sinus.

ANSWER

sigmoid

ITEM 20

THE VAGUS NERVE: THE GVA FIBERS

General visceral afferent fibers are clearly present in the pharyngeal and superior laryngeal branches of the vagus nerve. GVA fibers are undoubtedly also present in the thoracic and abdominal distribution of the vagus nerve, but many details of their distribution have not yet been confirmed.

Cell bodies of the general visceral afferent neurons of the vagus nerve are found mainly in the inferior ganglion, and their central processes terminate primarily in the nucleus of the tractus solitarius.

Cell bodies of GVA neurons of the vagus nerve are mainly located in the _____ ganglion.

QUESTION
60

inferior

ANSWER

The termination point of central processes of GVA neurons of the vagus nerve is the nucleus of the tractus _____.

QUESTION
61

solitarius

ANSWER

THE VAGUS NERVE: PHARYNGEAL BRANCHES AND PHARYNGEAL PLEXUS

ITEM 21

Peripheral processes of afferent neurons distribute to the pharynx by way of two or three *pharyngeal branches* from each vagus nerve. Figure 8–6 shows the pharyngeal branches from the left vagus nerve. At the pharynx, these afferent neurons enter a *pharyngeal plexus* where they join similar fibers of the glossopharyngeal nerve. Branches from the pharyngeal plexus are sensory to the mucosa of the pharynx and soft palate.

The pharyngeal plexus contains fibers of afferent neurons of the _____ _____ nerve and the _____ nerve.

QUESTION
62

vagus . . . glossopharyngeal (in either order)

ANSWER

The pharyngeal plexus supplies mucosa of the _____ and of the _____ _____.

QUESTION
63

pharynx . . . soft palate

ANSWER

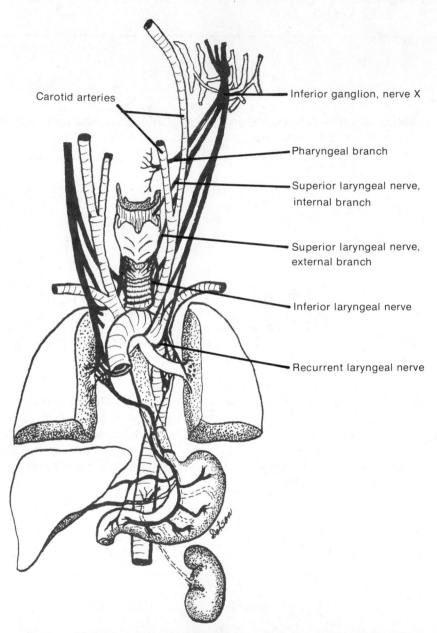

Carotid arteries

Inferior ganglion, nerve X

Pharyngeal branch

Superior laryngeal nerve,
internal branch

Superior laryngeal nerve,
external branch

Inferior laryngeal nerve

Recurrent laryngeal nerve

Figure 8-6.   Pharyngeal and laryngeal branches of the vagus nerve (X). (Redrawn from Woodburne: Essentials of Human Anatomy. 4th Ed. New York, Oxford University Press.)

THE SUPERIOR AND INFERIOR LARYNGEAL NERVES

Figure 8–6 shows the *superior laryngeal nerve* and the *inferior laryngeal nerve,* which is the continuation of the *recurrent laryngeal nerve.* Although these nerves are not purely sensory, they do carry general visceral afferent fibers.

The superior laryngeal nerve arises from the inferior ganglion and passes posterior to the carotid arteries to reach the larynx. There it divides into a larger *internal branch* and a smaller *external branch.* The internal branch carries GVA fibers to the mucosa of the larynx as far down as the level of the true vocal folds. It also carries sensory fibers to the mucosa of the epiglottis and to part of the base of the tongue.

The inferior laryngeal nerve carries sensory fibers which innervate the mucosa of the larynx below the true vocal folds.

The laryngeal nerves carry (circle one)
A. sensory fibers only
B. motor fibers only
C. both sensory and motor fibers

QUESTION 64

The correct answer is C. Both general visceral afferent fibers and efferent fibers comprise the laryngeal nerves.

ANSWER

The superior laryngeal nerve arises from the *superior/inferior* (circle one) ganglion.

QUESTION 65

---

inferior

ANSWER

GVA fibers to the mucosa of the larynx are carried by the *external/internal* (circle one) branch of the superior laryngeal nerve.

QUESTION 66

---

internal

ANSWER

The internal branch of the superior laryngeal nerve supplies sensory innervation to mucosa of the _____, mucosa of the _____, and to the base of the _____.

QUESTION 67

---

larynx . . . epiglottis . . . tongue

ANSWER

The continuation of the recurrent laryngeal nerve is called the *superior/inferior* (circle one) laryngeal nerve.

QUESTION 68

ANSWER   inferior

QUESTION
69

Sensory innervation of the part of the mucosa of the larynx above the true vocal folds is supplied by the _____ laryngeal nerve; innervation of the mucosa below the true vocal folds, by the _____ laryngeal nerve.

ANSWER   superior . . . inferior

ITEM
23

THE VAGUS NERVE:
THE SVA FIBERS

Special visceral afferent fibers conveying taste in the vagus nerve are distributed to a small area at the base of the tongue and in the epiglottic region. Cell bodies of these neurons are in the inferior ganglion. Their central processes join the tractus solitarius and terminate in the medulla in the nucleus of the tractus solitarius. Peripheral processes of the special visceral afferent fibers reach the base of the tongue and the epiglottis by way of the superior laryngeal nerve and its internal branch.

QUESTION
70

SVA fibers of the vagus nerve convey the sensation of taste from the _____ of the tongue and from the _____.

ANSWER   base . . . epiglottis

QUESTION
71

Cell bodies of SVA fibers of the vagus nerve are in the *superior/inferior* (circle one) ganglion.

ANSWER   inferior

QUESTION
72

Central processes of SVA fibers of the vagus nerve join the tractus _____ ____ and terminate in the nucleus of the tractus _____.

ANSWER   solitarius . . . solitarius

QUESTION
73

SVA fibers of the vagus nerve supply the base of the tongue and the epiglottis by way of the _____ branch of the superior laryngeal nerve.

ANSWER   internal

THE VAGUS NERVE: THE SVE FIBERS

ITEM 24

The special visceral efferent fibers of the vagus nerve supply the muscles of the pharynx, soft palate, and larynx. Motor impulses to pharynx and soft palate travel via pharyngeal branches; motor impulses to the larynx, via the inferior and superior laryngeal nerves. SVE fibers of the vagus nerve, like those of the glossopharyngeal nerve and the cranial part of the accessory nerve, have cell bodies in the nucleus ambiguus of the medulla.

Motor innervation to muscles of the soft palate and pharynx is carried by _____ branches of the vagus nerve; that to the larynx, by external branches of the _____ nerves.

---

pharyngeal . . . laryngeal

The location of the cell bodies of SVE fibers of the vagus nerve is in the nucleus _____ of the medulla.

---

ambiguus

SVE FIBERS TO THE PHARYNX AND SOFT PALATE

ITEM 25

Axons of special visceral efferent neurons of the vagus nerve destined for muscles of the pharynx and soft palate are shown in Figure 8–7. These axons pass out of the vagus nerve as the _pharyngeal branches_ and distribute through the _pharyngeal plexus_. These SVE fibers supply all the muscles of the pharynx except the stylopharyngeus muscle, which is supplied by the glossopharyngeal nerve. They also supply all muscles of the soft palate except the tensor veli palatini muscle, which is supplied by a branch of the mandibular division of the trigeminal nerve.

Muscles of the pharynx and soft palate are innervated by _____ _____ efferent fibers from the _____ plexus.

---

special visceral . . . pharyngeal

The only muscle of the pharynx to which the vagus nerve does not send efferent fibers is the _____ muscle.

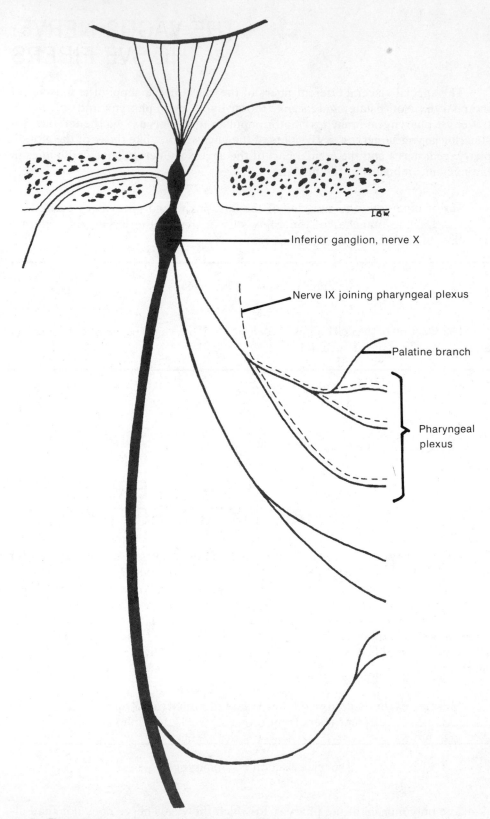

Figure 8-7. Pharyngeal branches of the vagus nerve (X) and pharyngeal plexus.

stylopharyngeus

The only muscle of the soft palate to which the vagus nerve does not send motor fibers is the _____ _____ palatini muscle.
78

---

tensor veli

SVE FIBERS TO THE LARYNX   ITEM 26

With the exception of the cricothyroid muscle, all muscles of the larynx are supplied by the inferior laryngeal nerve. Axons of special visceral efferent neurons follow the vagus nerve into the thorax, enter the recurrent laryngeal nerve, and continue in the inferior laryngeal nerve to reach the muscles of the larynx. Axons of other SVE neurons form the external branch of the superior laryngeal nerve, which supplies the cricothyroid muscle of the larynx.

All muscles of the larynx except the cricothyroid muscle are supplied by the *superior/inferior* (circle one) laryngeal nerve.
79

---

inferior

The *external/internal* (circle one) branch of the *superior/inferior* (circle one) laryngeal nerve supplis the cricothyroid muscle.
80

---

external . . . superior

THE VAGUS NERVE: GVE FIBERS   ITEM 27

General visceral efferent fibers of the vagus nerve have their cell bodies located in the dorsal motor nucleus of the nerve. These GVE fibers are para-sympathetic preganglionic fibers which synapse with postganglionic fibers to supply smooth muscle and glands of the thoracic and abdominal viscera, as well as cardiac muscle. They also innervate involuntary striated muscle of the esophagus.

These GVE fibers, which are presumed to be accompanied by some GVA fibers, make up the principal distribution of the vagus nerve in the thorax and abdomen. GVE fibers of the vagus nerve have little or no distribution within the head and neck.

QUESTION 81   Cell bodies of GVE fibers of the vagus nerve are located in the _____ motor nucleus of the _____ nerve.

ANSWER   dorsal . . . vagus

QUESTION 82   GVE fibers of the vagus nerve supply parasympathetic innervation to _____ muscles, to _____ muscles, and to _____.

ANSWER   cardiac . . . smooth . . . glands

SUMMARY OF UNIT EIGHT

THE GLOSSOPHARYNGEAL NERVE

The glossopharyngeal nerve distributes primarily to the tongue and pharynx. It contains five functional components: GSA, GVA, SVA, GVE, and SVE. The general somatic afferent fibers of the glossopharyngeal nerve carry general sensation from the skin of the ear. Peripheral processes travel with the auricular branch of the vagus nerve to synapse eventually in the trigeminal nucleus. General visceral afferent fibers distribute to the mucosa of the middle ear, the carotid sinus, the posterior third of the tongue, and the pharyngeal mucosa. Peripheral processes travel with the main trunk of the ninth cranial nerve and with the tympanic nerve to terminate in the brain in the nucleus of the tractus solitarius. Special visceral afferent fibers carry the sensation of taste from the posterior third of the tongue and adjacent pharyngeal mucosa. Cell bodies of these neurons are located in the inferior ganglion of the glossopharyngeal nerve; central processes terminate in the nucleus of the tractus solitarius.

Motor fibers of the glossopharyngeal nerve are general visceral efferent and special visceral efferent. General visceral efferent fibers are parasympathetic to the parotid gland. Preganglionic cell bodies are located in the inferior salivatory nucleus. Axons of these neurons extend through the tympanic nerve and synapse with postganglionic cell bodies in the otic ganglion near the foramen ovale. Postganglionic axons travel with the auriculotemporal nerve to the parotid gland. Special visceral efferent cell bodies are located in the nucleus ambiguus in the medulla. These SVE fibers innervate the stylopharyngeus muscle.

Lesions of the glossopharyngeal nerve involve loss of the gag reflex, alteration in the carotid sinus reflex concerned with blood pressure, and diminution of taste in the posterior third of the tongue. An occasional patient will exhibit an excruciatingly painful hyperesthesia along the route of the glossopharyngeal nerve, a phenomenon known as glossopharyngeal neuralgia.

THE VAGUS NERVE

The vagus nerve, like the glossopharyngeal nerve, has five functional components: GSA, GVA, SVA, GVE, and SVE. The vagus nerve arises from the ventral surface of the medulla and exits from the skull through the jugular foramen. At the jugular foramen, cell bodies of the afferent components of the vagus nerve form a superior and an inferior ganglion.

Peripheral processes of the two vagi distribute differently in the root of the neck. The right vagus nerve passes anterior to the proximal part of the subclavian artery and then moves dorsally to reach the thorax posterior to the root of the right lung. As the right vagus nerve passes the right subclavian artery, a branch known as the recurrent laryngeal nerve turns posteriorly and upward, encircling the artery to ascend in a groove between the trachea and esophagus to the pharynx. The left vagus nerve descends in the thorax between the common carotid artery and internal jugular vein. It crosses anterior to the subclavian artery and lateral to the arch of the aorta. It then moves dorsally to descend posterior to the root of the left lung.

General somatic afferent fibers of the vagus nerve distribute to skin of the ear and to the meninges. General visceral afferent fibers from the pharynx and larynx and from thoracic and abdominal viscera terminate in the nucleus of the tractus solitarius. These GVA fibers are carried in the inferior and superior laryngeal nerves, the inferior laryngeal nerve being a continuation of the recurrent laryngeal nerve. The superior laryngeal nerve divides into a large internal branch and a smaller external branch. The large internal branch carries GVA fibers to the mucosa of the larynx and epiglottis and to the base of the tongue. Special visceral afferent fibers convey the sensation of taste from a small area at the base of the tongue and epiglottis. Peripheral processes run with the internal branch of the superior laryngeal nerve to cell bodies located in the inferior ganglion. Central processes terminate in the nucleus of the tractus solitarius in the medulla.

Special visceral efferent fibers convey motor impulses to muscles of the pharynx, soft palate, and larynx. Axons of these neurons are in the pharyngeal branches of the vagus nerve to the pharynx and in the inferior and superior laryngeal branches to the larynx. Cell bodies of the SVE fibers of the vagus nerve, like those of the glossopharyngeal and accessory nerves, are located in the nucleus ambiguus.

General visceral efferent fibers of the vagus nerve are parasympathetic to the thorax and abdomen. Preganglionic cell bodies are located in the dorsal motor nucleus of the vagus nerve. Postganglionic cell bodies are located close to the viscera supplied. Terminal processes distribute to cardiac muscle, to involuntary striated muscle of the esophagus, and smooth muscle and glands of thoracic and abdominal viscera.

QUESTION
83

The name of the glossopharyngeal nerve indicates that this ninth cranial nerve distributes primarily to the _____ and _____.

ANSWER

tongue . . . pharynx

QUESTION
84

The five functional components of the glossopharyngeal nerve are
1. _____ _____ afferent
2. _____ _____ afferent
3. _____ _____ afferent
4. _____ _____ efferent
5. _____ _____ efferent

ANSWER

1. general somatic
2. general visceral
3. special visceral
4. general visceral
5. special visceral

QUESTION
85

General sensation from part of the skin of the ear is carried in the glossopharyngeal nerve by fibers with a general _____ _____ component.

---

somatic afferent

ANSWER

GSA fibers of the glossopharyngeal nerve travel with the _____ branch of the vagus nerve.

QUESTION
86

auricular

ANSWER

Fibers of the glossopharyngeal nerve which convey sensation from mucosa of the middle ear, the carotid sinus, and pharyngeal mucosa carry a _____ _____ afferent functional component.

QUESTION
87

general visceral

ANSWER

GVA fibers of the glossopharyngeal nerve terminate in the brain in the nucleus of the _____ _____.

QUESTION
88

tractus solitarius

ANSWER

The component of the glossopharyngeal nerve which carries parasympathetic fibers to the parotid gland is the _____ _____ _____ component.

QUESTION
89

general visceral efferent

ANSWER

GVE preganglionic cell bodies of the glossopharyngeal nerve are in the inferior _____ nucleus.

QUESTION
90

salivatory

ANSWER

GVE postganglionic cell bodies of the glossopharyngeal nerve are located in the _____ ganglion.

QUESTION
91

otic

ANSWER

Sensation of taste from the posterior third of the tongue and adjacent pharyngeal mucosa are carried by the _____ _____ _____ component of the glossopharyngeal nerve.

QUESTION
92

special visceral afferent

ANSWER

QUESTION 93

SVA fibers of the glossopharyngeal nerve eventually terminate in the nucleus of the _____ _____.

ANSWER

tractus solitarius

QUESTION 94

The functional component which is motor to the stylopharyngeus muscle is the _____ _____ _____ component.

ANSWER

special visceral efferent

QUESTION 95

Cell bodies of the SVE fibers of the glossopharyngeal nerve are located in the nucleus _____.

ANSWER

ambiguus

QUESTION 96

Absence of the gag reflex, alteration in the carotid sinus reflex, and diminution of taste in the posterior third of the tongue may indicate a lesion of the _____ nerve.

ANSWER

glossopharyngeal

QUESTION 97

A condition characterized by hyperesthesia along the route of the glossopharyngeal nerve is termed glossopharyngeal _____.

ANSWER

neuralgia

QUESTION 98

The vagus nerve, like the glossopharyngeal nerve, has five functional components; they are

1. _____ _____ afferent
2. _____ _____ afferent
3. _____ _____ afferent
4. _____ _____ efferent
5. _____ _____ efferent

ANSWER

1. general somatic
2. general visceral
3. special visceral
4. general visceral
5. special visceral

The vagus nerve exits from the skull through the _____ foramen.

jugular

SVA fibers of the vagus nerve convey sensations of _____ from the base of the tongue and the epiglottis.

taste

The superior laryngeal nerve divides into two branches, the _____ branch and the _____ branch.

internal . . . external (in either order)

The inferior laryngeal nerve is a continuation of the _____ _____ nerve.

recurrent laryngeal

The functional component of the vagus nerve which is motor to muscles of the pharynx, soft palate, and larynx is the _____ _____ _____ component.

special visceral efferent

Cell bodies of the SVE component of the vagus nerve, like those of the glosso-pharyngeal and accessory nerves, are located in the _____ _____.

nucleus ambiguus

The parasympathetic fibers of the vagus nerve which distribute to the thorax and abdomen are termed the _____ _____ _____ component.

general visceral efferent

Preganglionic cell bodies of GVE fibers of the vagus nerve are located in the _____ _____ nucleus of the vagus nerve.

ANSWER   dorsal motor

QUESTION   GVE postganglionic cell bodies of the vagus nerve are located close to the
107   _____ supplied by these cell bodies.

ANSWER   viscera

QUESTION   GVE fibers of the vagus nerve distribute to _____ muscles, to
108   _____ muscles, and to _____.

ANSWER   cardiac . . . smooth . . . glands

Unit Nine ☐ AUTONOMIC NERVES TO THE HEAD AND NECK

THE AUTONOMIC NERVOUS SYSTEM: GENERAL CONSIDERATIONS

ITEM 1

The autonomic nervous system is concerned with the regulation of visceral activity. Specifically, visceral activity is controlled by nerve stimulation of smooth muscle, cardiac muscle, and glands.

This unit will deal primarily with autonomic pathways in the head. It should be remembered, however, that the autonomic nervous system as a whole also regulates the functioning of thoracic, abdominal, and pelvic viscera.

The autonomic nervous system is the mechanism by which the body controls _____ activity.

QUESTION 1

visceral

ANSWER

Structures directly controlled by the autonomic nervous system include _____ muscle, _____ muscle, and _____.

QUESTION 2

smooth . . . cardiac . . . glands

ANSWER

INITIATION OF VISCERAL CHANGE

ITEM 2

Changes in visceral activity are for the most part initiated by receptors within the particular organs involved. From these receptors, impulses travel by way of general visceral afferent fibers to the spinal cord and brain. However, general somatic afferent fibers with receptors located in the body wall can also initiate changes in visceral activity.

Both GSA and GVA fibers have cell bodies in cranial and spinal ganglia, and central processes which synapse in the brain and spinal cord. Clearly, then, there is no rigid line of distinction between the function of autonomic neurons and the function of the nervous system as a whole.

QUESTION
3

Sensory impulses which initiate changes in visceral activity are carried to the spinal cord and brain by way of (circle one)
    A. GVA fibers only
    B. GSA fibers only
    C. GVA and GSA fibers

ANSWER

The correct answer is C. Although most afferent impulses which trigger changes in visceral activity are carried by way of general visceral afferent fibers, some impulses originate from receptors in the body wall and are carried by general somatic afferent fibers.

QUESTION
4

Receptors which originate visceral change are mostly located in *particular organs/the body wall* (circle one).

ANSWER

particular organs

ITEM 3   INNERVATION OF SMOOTH MUSCLE, CARDIAC MUSCLE, AND GLANDS

Skeletal muscle is innervated by neurons which have cell bodies in the brain and spinal cord. Smooth muscle, cardiac muscle, and glands receive innervation through efferent pathways which involve preganglionic neurons whose cell bodies are located in the central nervous system. Peripheral processes of these preganglionic neurons synapse with postganglionic neurons in sympathetic chain ganglia, in collateral ganglia, or in peripheral ganglia. From these various points of synapse, postganglionic fibers in turn extend to the various organs innervated.

QUESTION
5

The two types of neurons included in an autonomic pathway are termed _____ and _____.

ANSWER

preganglionic . . . postganglionic (in either order)

QUESTION
6

In the ganglia of the autonomic nervous system, peripheral processes of _____ neurons synapse with cell bodies of _____ neurons.

ANSWER

preganglionic . . . postganglionic

THE AUTONOMIC NERVOUS SYSTEM: THE SYMPATHETIC DIVISION

ITEM 4

Figure 9–1 shows the general topography of the autonomic nervous system. That part of the autonomic nervous system which has preganglionic neurons in the thoracic and lumbar regions of the spinal cord is termed the *sympathetic* or *thoracolumbar division*. Preganglionic fibers of the sympathetic division synapse with postganglionic neurons located in the sympathetic chain ganglia or in collateral ganglia in the neck, thorax, abdomen, or pelvis. The sympathetic division is shown on the left side of Figure 9–1. Preganglionic fibers are shown as solid lines; postganglionic fibers, as broken lines.

QUESTION
7

Preganglionic neurons of the sympathetic division of the autonomic nervous system are located in _____ and _____ regions.

ANSWER

thoracic . . . lumbar (in either order)

QUESTION
8

Sites of synapse of preganglionic neurons of the sympathetic nervous system are in _____ ganglia in the thorax, abdomen, and pelvis, and in sympathetic _____ ganglia.

ANSWER

collateral . . . chain

THE AUTONOMIC NERVOUS SYSTEM: PARASYMPATHETIC DIVISION

ITEM 5

That part of the autonomic nervous system which has preganglionic cell bodies in the brain and sacral region is termed the *parasympathetic division,* or *craniosacral* outflow. The parasympathetic outflow is shown on the right side of Figure 9–1. Preganglionic fibers are indicated by solid lines; postganglionic fibers, by broken lines. Ganglia associated with the parasympathetic division in the thorax and abdomen are located distally, frequently within the organ innervated.

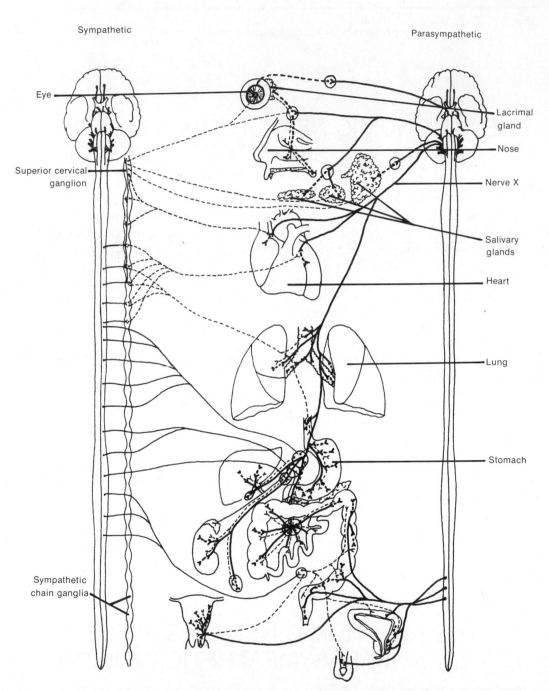

Sympathetic

Parasympathetic

Eye

Superior cervical
ganglion

Sympathetic
chain ganglia

Lacrimal
gland

Nose

Nerve X

Salivary
glands

Heart

Lung

Stomach

Figure 9–1. Topography of the autonomic nervous system. (Modified from Woodburne: Essentials of Human Anatomy. 4th Ed. New York, Oxford University Press.)

In Figure 9–1, notice that the vagus nerve supplies parasympathetic innervation to thoracic and abdominal viscera. Observe also that most viscera are
supplied by both sympathetic and parasympathetic fibers. Because each division of
the autonomic system reacts differently, both physiologically and pharma-
cologically, the net effect is dual control of visceral function, with the sympathetic
reaction usually opposite to that of the parasympathetic reaction.

Preganglionic neurons of the parasympathetic division of the autonomic
nervous system are located in the _____ and in the _____
region.

QUESTION
9

brain . . . sacral

ANSWER

The vagus nerve supplies *sympathetic/parasympathetic* (circle one) innervation to viscera of the thorax and abdomen.

QUESTION
10

parasympathetic

ANSWER

In the dual control of visceral activity by the autonomic nervous system,
the effect of the _____ division is often opposite to that of the
_____ division.

QUESTION
11

sympathetic . . . parasympathetic (in either order)

ANSWER

THE SYMPATHETIC NERVE SUPPLY TO THE HEAD

ITEM 6

Observe the sympathetic nerve supply to the head, shown in Figure 9–1.
Preganglionic neurons from the upper thoracic region synapse with postganglionic
neurons in the superior cervical sympathetic ganglion. Postganglionic fibers
distribute with adjacent cranial nerves or form plexuses which surround, and
travel with, branches of the internal and external carotid arteries. Notice that
sympathetic fibers innervate smooth muscles of the eye, and extend to the lacrimal
gland, to glands of the oral and nasal mucosa, and to the salivary glands.

Preganglionic sympathetic neurons in the upper thoracic region synapse
with postganglionic neurons in the _____ _____ sympathetic
ganglion.

QUESTION
12

superior cervical

ANSWER

QUESTION
13

The plexuses of postganglionic sympathetic fibers surround branches of the _____ and _____ _____ arteries.

ANSWER

internal . . . external carotid

QUESTION
14

Glands of the head innervated by sympathetic fibers include the _____ gland, the _____ glands, and glands of the oral and nasal _____.

ANSWER

lacrimal . . . salivary . . . mucosa

QUESTION
15

Postganglionic sympathetic fibers which do not form plexuses surrounding blood vessels travel with adjacent _____ nerves.

ANSWER

cranial

ITEM 7　SYMPATHETIC CONTROL OF THE DIAMETER OF BLOOD VESSELS

Sympathetic stimulation of glands of the head is for the most part exerted by controlling the diameter of the blood vessels supplying these glands. A normal sympathetic tone transmitted to smooth muscle in the blood vessels maintains the lumen in a partially constricted state. A decreased sympathetic tone, therefore, allows the blood vessels to dilate; an increased sympathetic impulse causes the vessels to constrict.

Besides controlling the caliber of blood vessels, sympathetic fibers also innervate myoepithelial cells associated with the stroma and duct systems of the glands.

QUESTION
16

Sympathetic nerves regulate glandular function by controlling the _____ of blood vessels to glands and by innervation of myoepithelial cells associated with glandular _____ and _____ systems.

ANSWER

diameter . . . stroma . . . duct

QUESTION
17

Dilatation of blood vessels accompanies *increased/decreased* (circle one) sympathetic impulses; constriction accompanies *increased/decreased* (circle one) sympathetic stimulation.

ANSWER

decreased . . . increased

THE PARASYMPATHETIC NERVE SUPPLY TO THE HEAD

ITEM 8

Figure 9–2 shows the parasympathetic nerve supply to the head. It originates in the form of preganglionic fibers of the oculomotor, facial, and glossopharyngeal nerves.

Take note of the ganglia in which the preganglionic fibers of the third, seventh, and ninth cranial nerves synapse. Those of the oculomotor nerve (III) synapse in the *ciliary ganglion,* from which postganglionic fibers distribute to smooth muscles of the eye. Preganglionic fibers associated with the facial nerve (VII) synapse in the *pterygopalatine ganglion* and in the *submandibular ganglion.* Postganglionic fibers from the pterygopalatine ganglion distribute to the lacrimal and nasal glands, among others; postganglionic fibers from the submandibular ganglion distribute to the submandibular and sublingual glands. Preganglionic parasympathetic fibers of the glossopharyngeal nerve (IX) synapse in the *otic ganglion,* from which postganglionic fibers extend to the parotid gland.

Parasympathetic neurons of the oculomotor nerve synapse in the _____ ganglion; those of the facial nerve, in the _____ ganglion and the _____ ganglion; those of the glossopharyngeal nerve, in the _____ ganglion.

QUESTION 18

---

ciliary . . . pterygopalatine . . . submandibular . . . otic

ANSWER

THE OCULOMOTOR NERVE: THE GVE FIBERS

ITEM 9

Look at Figure 9–3 to see the origin of the general visceral efferent fibers of the oculomotor nerve (III), represented as crosshatched lines. Cell bodies of these neurons are located in the *visceral nucleus of the oculomotor nerve* in the midbrain. Peripheral processes of the GVE fibers travel with the other fibers of the oculomotor nerve to leave the ventral surface of the midbrain near its midline junction with the pons.

The visceral nucleus of the oculomotor nerve is located in the *midbrain/pons/medulla* (circle one).

QUESTION 19

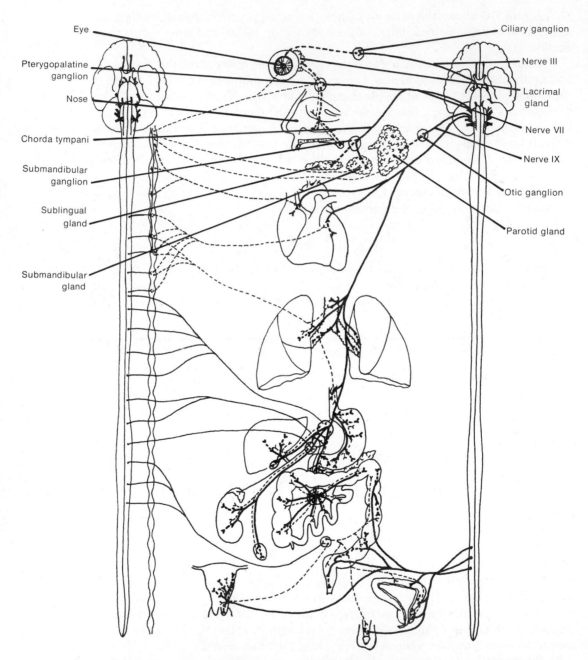

Figure 9–2.   Parasympathetic nerve supply to the head. (Modified from Woodburne: Essentials of Human Anatomy. 4th Ed. New York, Oxford University Press.)

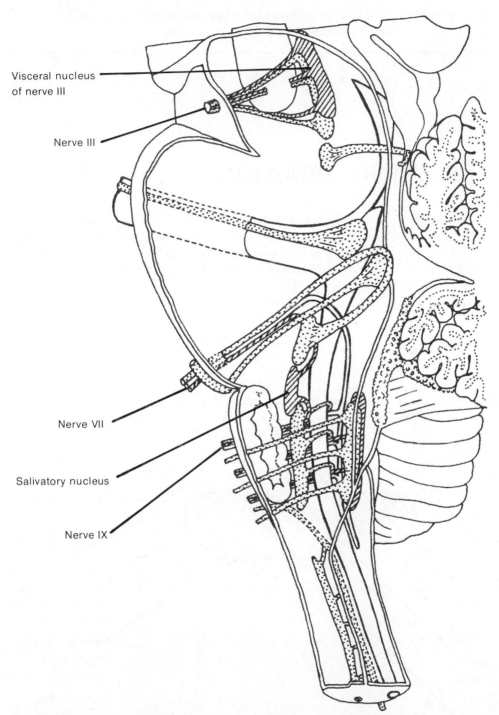

Figure 9–3. Visceral nuclei of the oculomotor (III), facial (VII), and glossopharyngeal (IX) nerves viewed from the median sagittal surface of the brain stem. (Redrawn from Truex and Carpenter: Human Neuroanatomy. 6th Ed. Baltimore, The Williams and Wilkins Co.)

ANSWER   midbrain

QUESTION
20
GVE fibers of the oculomotor nerve leave the ventral surface of the
_____ near its junction with the _____.

ANSWER   midbrain . . . pons

ITEM 10   THE CILIARY GANGLION

Figure 9–4 shows the general visceral efferent component of the oculomotor nerve in the orbit. Having entered the orbit through the superior orbital fissure, these GVE processes synapse with postganglionic cell bodies in the *ciliary ganglion*. Locate the ciliary ganglion in Figure 9–4. It is near the posterior wall of the orbit, lateral to the optic nerve (II).

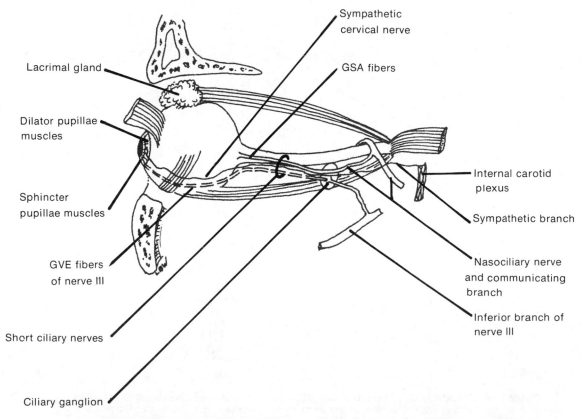

Figure 9–4. The ciliary ganglion and its important connections. (Modified from Woodburne: Essentials of Human Anatomy. 4th Ed. New York, Oxford University Press.)

The opening through which GVE fibers of the oculomotor nerve enter the orbit is the _____ _____ fissure.

QUESTION
21

superior orbital

ANSWER

Preganglionic fibers of the oculomotor nerve synapse in the ciliary ganglion (circle one)
A. within the orbit
B. outside the orbit

QUESTION
22

The correct answer is A. The ciliary ganglion is within the orbit.

ANSWER

THE PUPIL OF THE EYE: GVE SUPPLY   ITEM 11

Look at Figure 9–4 again, and notice the *short ciliary nerves*. Contained within the short ciliary nerves are parasympathetic postganglionic fibers which have synapsed in the ciliary ganglion with preganglionic GVE fibers of the *inferior branch* of the oculomotor nerve. The postganglionic GVE fibers from the ciliary ganglion distribute to the *sphincter pupillae muscle* to provide parasympathetic stimulation which constricts the pupil and adjusts the lens for near vision.

The short ciliary nerves which supply the sphincter pupillae muscle are postganglionic fibers of the _____ nerve.

QUESTION
23

oculomotor

ANSWER

GVE fibers of the oculomotor nerve provide *sympathetic/parasympathetic* (circle one) stimulation of smooth muscles of the eye.

QUESTION
24

parasympathetic

ANSWER

Parasympathetic stimulation of smooth muscles of the eye *dilates/constricts* (circle one) the pupil.

ANSWER   constricts

ITEM 12

THE PUPIL OF THE EYE: SYMPATHETIC INNERVATION

Postganglionic sympathetic fibers, whose cell bodies synapse in the superior cervical sympathetic ganglion, reach the orbit by way of the *internal carotid plexus* of nerves on the ophthalmic artery. Locate the internal carotid plexus in Figure 9–4. These postganglionic sympathetic fibers extend through the ciliary ganglion without synapse and continue with the short ciliary nerves to the *dilator pupillae muscle*. Whereas parasympathetic stimulation constricts the pupil, sympathetic stimulation of the dilator pupillae muscle dilates the pupil.

Sympathetic fibers to the dilator pupillae muscle synapse in the (circle one)
A. ciliary ganglion
B. superior cervical sympathetic ganglion

ANSWER
The correct answer is B. Although postganglionic sympathetic fibers to the dilator pupillae muscle do not synapse in the ciliary ganglion, they do pass through this ganglion without synapse.

The short ciliary nerves to the dilator pupillae muscle are branches of (circle one)
A. the oculomotor nerve
B. cervical nerves

ANSWER
The correct answer is B. The short ciliary nerves contain both sympathetic postganglionic fibers to the dilator pupillae muscle and parasympathetic postganglionic fibers to the sphincter pupillae muscle. The sympathetic fibers are branches of cervical nerves, while the parasympathetic fibers are branches of the oculomotor (third cranial) nerve.

Dilation of the pupil of the eye results from *sympathetic/parasympathetic* (circle one) stimulation of smooth muscle.

ANSWER   sympathetic

SENSORY FIBERS IN THE SHORT CILIARY NERVES

ITEM 13

In addition to fibers to the sphincter pupillae and dilator pupillae muscles, general somatic afferent fibers which are sensory to the eyeball are also included in the short ciliary nerves. These GSA fibers course through the ciliary ganglion without synapse and join the *nasociliary nerve,* a branch of the ophthalmic division of the trigeminal nerve. Locate the nasociliary nerve and the communicating branch to the ciliary ganglion in Figure 9–4.

The short ciliary nerves which convey general sensation from the eyeball (circle one)
  A. synapse within the ciliary ganglion
  B. pass through the ciliary ganglion without synapse
  C. do not pass through the ciliary ganglion

QUESTION
29

The correct answer is B.

ANSWER

The GSA fibers which are sensory to the eyeball travel within the _____ _____ branch of the ophthalmic nerve.

QUESTION
30

---

nasociliary

ANSWER

THE FACIAL NERVE: THE PARASYMPATHETIC FIBERS

ITEM 14

Preganglionic parasympathetic fibers associated with the facial nerve (VII) synapse in two ganglia: the pterygopalatine ganglion and the submandibular ganglion. Postganglionic fibers from the pterygopalatine ganglion supply the lacrimal gland and glands of the nasal, palatine, and upper pharyngeal mucosa.
Postganglionic fibers of the chorda tympani nerve synapse in the submandibular ganglion and supply the submandibular and sublingual salivary glands.

The ganglia in which parasympathetic neurons of the facial nerve synapse are the _____ ganglion and the _____ ganglion.

QUESTION
31

---

pterygopalatine . . . submandibular (in either order)

ANSWER

QUESTION
32

The lacrimal gland and glands of the nasal, palatine, and upper pharyngeal mucosa are innervated by _____ postganglionic fibers of the facial nerve.

ANSWER

parasympathetic

QUESTION
33

Postganglionic cell bodies with fibers which supply the lacrimal and various mucosal glands are located in the _____ ganglion.

ANSWER

pterygopalatine

QUESTION
34

Submandibular and sublingual salivary glands receive parasympathetic innervation from the _____ _____ nerve, a branch of the facial nerve.

ANSWER

chorda tympani

ITEM 15   THE FACIAL NERVE: ORIGIN OF THE GVE FIBERS

Cell bodies of parasympathetic preganglionic neurons of the facial nerve are located in the salivatory nucleus. Refer to Figure 9–3, where the salivatory nucleus appears as a striped area in the lower pons and upper medulla. Observe the peripheral processes of these neurons as they ascend to join other components of the facial nerve.

QUESTION
35

Preganglionic neurons of the facial nerve whose fibers supply the salivary glands have their cell bodies in the _____ nucleus.

ANSWER

salivatory

QUESTION
36

The salivatory nucleus is located in the brain stem at the juncture of the _____ and _____.

ANSWER

pons . . . medulla (in either order)

THE FACIAL NERVE: PATHWAY OF THE GVE FIBERS

ITEM 16

Leaving the brain at the inferior border of the pons, GVE fibers of the facial nerve form part of the nervus intermedius. The facial nerve enters the petrous part of the temporal bone at the internal acoustic meatus. Within bone, the *greater petrosal nerve,* carrying GVE fibers, branches off the main trunk to enter the middle cranial fossa at the hiatus of the facial canal.

The point of entry of the facial nerve into the temporal bone is the internal _____ _____.

QUESTION 37

---

acoustic meatus

ANSWER

The greater petrosal nerve consists of general _____ _____ fibers of the _____ nerve.

QUESTION 38

---

visceral efferent . . . facial

ANSWER

THE NERVE TO THE PTERYGOID CANAL: THE GVE FIBERS

ITEM 17

Extending through the middle cranial fossa, deep to the trigeminal ganglion, the *greater petrosal nerve* joins the *deep petrosal nerve,* which carries sympathetic fibers from the internal carotid plexus. Combined fibers of the greater and deep petrosal nerves enter the pterygoid canal as the *nerve to the pterygoid canal.* The pterygoid canal extends from the anterior wall of the foramen lacerum anteriorly to the pterygopalatine fossa.

The nerve to the pterygoid canal is composed of general visceral _____ fibers of both the _____ petrosal nerve and the _____ petrosal nerve.

QUESTION 39

---

efferent . . . greater . . . deep

ANSWER

The canal which runs forward from the foramen lacerum to the pterygopalatine fossa is called the _____ canal.

QUESTION 40

---

pterygoid

ANSWER

QUESTION
41

The deep petrosal nerve carries *sympathetic/parasympathetic* (circle one) fibers from the internal carotid plexus.

ANSWER

Sympathetic. If you missed this one, you should reread Item 6. Postganglionic sympathetic fibers form plexuses which surround the internal and external carotid arteries.

ITEM
18

THE PTERYGOPALATINE GANGLION

Examine Figure 9–5, and observe the greater petrosal branch of the facial nerve as it approaches the *pterygopalatine ganglion*. Notice also the deep petrosal nerve carrying sympathetic fibers from the internal carotid plexus. Fibers of the greater petrosal nerve synapse with postganglionic neurons in the pterygopalatine ganglion, while fibers of the deep petrosal nerve course through the ganglion without synapse. Also passing through the pterygopalatine ganglion without synapse are general somatic afferent fibers of the maxillary division of the trigeminal nerve, which reach their cell bodies in the trigeminal ganglion. Fibers of both the greater and deep petrosal nerves distribute beyond the pterygopalatine ganglion with branches of the maxillary division. Fibers of the greater and deep petrosal nerves extend to the lacrimal gland and to glands of the nasal, palatine, and upper pharyngeal mucosa.

QUESTION
42

Fibers of the greater petrosal nerve
A. synapse in the pterygopalatine ganglion
B. pass through the pterygopalatine ganglion without synapse

ANSWER

The correct answer is A. Although sympathetic fibers of the deep petrosal nerve as well as afferent fibers of branches of the maxillary nerve pass through the pterygopalatine ganglion without synapse, the parasympathetic preganglionic fibers of the greater petrosal branch of the facial nerve do synapse in the ganglion.

QUESTION
43

Fibers of the deep petrosal nerve (circle one)
A. synapse in the pterygopalatine ganglion
B. pass through the pterygopalatine ganglion without synapse

ANSWER

The correct answer is B.

QUESTION
44

After emerging from the pterygopalatine ganglion, fibers of the greater and deep petrosal nerves travel with the _____ divison of the _____ nerve.

ANSWER

maxillary . . . trigeminal

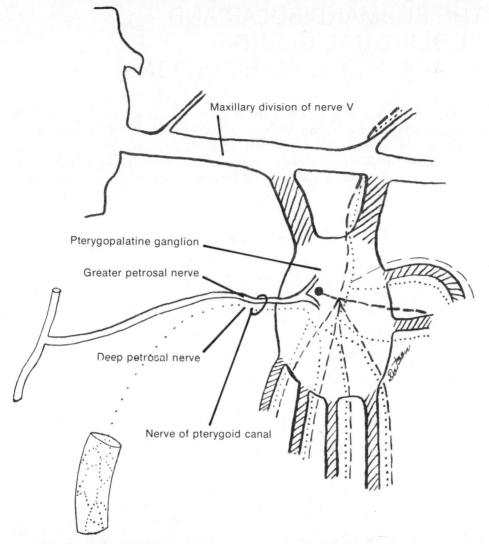

Figure 9-5. The pterygopalatine ganglion, showing relationship of greater and deep petrosal nerves to branches of the maxillary division of the trigeminal nerve (V). Dotted lines represent sympathetic nerves; dashed lines, parasympathetic nerves; crosshatched areas, GSA fibers of branches of the maxillary nerve. (Modified from Woodburne: Essentials of Human Anatomy. 4th Ed. New York, Oxford University Press.)

Fibers which pass through the pterygopalatine ganglion without synapse include those of (circle one)

    A. the greater petrosal nerve
    B. the deep petrosal nerve
    C. the maxillary division
    D. both the greater and the deep petrosal nerves
    E. both the deep petrosal nerve and the maxillary division

The correct answer is E. Although parasympathetic fibers of the greater petrosal nerve do synapse in the pterygopalatine ganglion, the sympathetic fibers of the deep petrosal nerve and the sensory fibers of the maxillary division simply pass through the ganglion without synapse.

ITEM 19   THE SUBMANDIBULAR AND SUBLINGUAL GLANDS: SYMPATHETIC INNERVATION

Figure 9–6 illustrates the sympathetic innervation of the submandibular and sublingual salivary glands. Sympathetic fibers are distributed to these glands through plexuses which follow branches of the facial artery. Observe the sympathetic supply originating in the upper thoracic spinal cord, synapsing in the superior cervical sympathetic ganglion, and distributing with the facial artery. Sym-

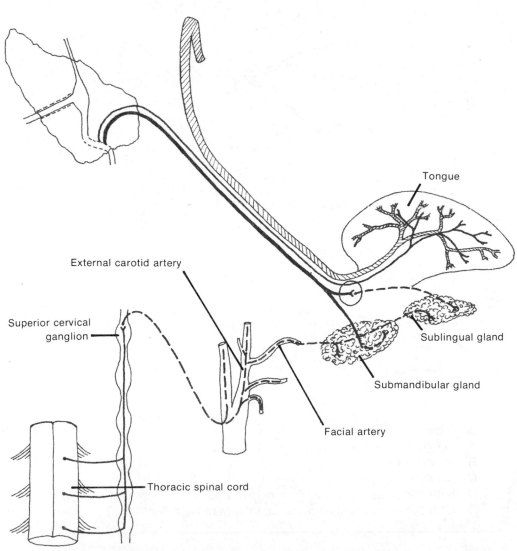

Figure 9-6. Sympathetic innervation of the submandibular and sublingual glands. (Redrawn from Woodburne: Essentials of Human Anatomy. 4th Ed. New York, Oxford University Press.)

pathetic stimulation of the submandibular and sublingual glands reduces salivary secretion.

Preganglionic fibers supplying the submandibular and sublingual glands synapse in the _____ _____ ganglion; postganglionic fibers distribute by way of plexuses surrounding the _____ artery.

superior cervical . . . facial

THE SUBMANDIBULAR AND SUBLINGUAL GLANDS: PARASYMPATHETIC INNERVATION

Parasympathetic impulses sent to the submandibular and sublingual glands increase salivary secretion. Parasympathetic supply is provided by GVE fibers which form part of the chorda tympani branch of the facial nerve. The distribution of the chorda tympani is shown in Figure 9–7.

Besides carrying GVE fibers to the submandibular and sublingual glands, the chorda tympani includes special visceral afferent fibers which convey sensations of taste from the anterior two thirds of the tongue. Taste fibers as well as preganglionic parasympathetic fibers travel with the lingual branch of the mandibular division of the trigeminal nerve (V). The preganglionic parasympathetic fibers leave the lingual nerve at the submandibular ganglion, from which postganglionic fibers distribute to the submandibular and sublingual glands.

Sympathetic stimulation of the submandibular and sublingual glands *increases/reduces* (circle one) salivary secretion; parasympathetic stimulation *increases/reduces* (circle one) salivary secretion.

reduces . . . increases

The functional component of the chorda tympani nerve which carries the sensation of taste is _____ _____ afferent.

special visceral

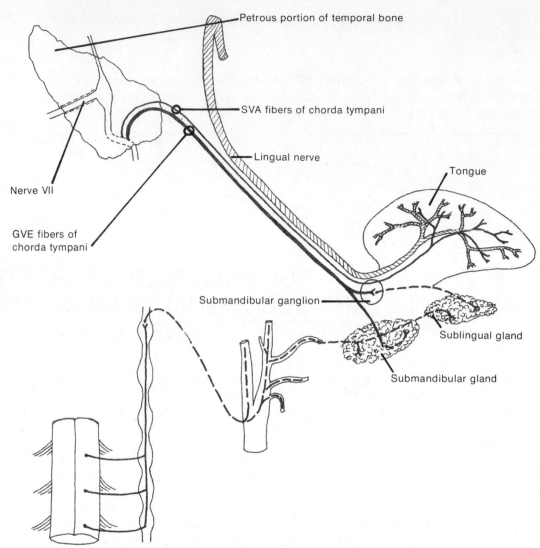

Figure 9-7.   Distribution of the chorda tympani. (Redrawn from Woodburne: Essentials of Human Anatomy. 4th Ed. New York, Oxford University Press.)

QUESTION
49

The functional component of the chorda tympani which provides parasympathetic supply to the submandibular and sublingual glands is _____ _____ efferent.

ANSWER

general visceral

QUESTION
50

SVA and GVE fibers of the chorda tympani run with the _____ branch of the _____ division of the trigeminal nerve.

ANSWER

lingual . . . mandibular

THE CHORDA TYMPANI NERVE: THE PATHWAY

The chorda tympani leaves the petrous portion of the temporal bone through the petrotympanic fissure. It then extends forward medial to the spine of the sphenoid bone and joins the lingual nerve high in the infratemporal fossa. Taste fibers remain with the lingual nerve as it courses downward to the tongue. Parasympathetic preganglionic fibers also run with the lingual nerve through the infratemporal fossa, but leave the lingual nerve at the submandibular ganglion. This ganglion is located on the hyoglossus muscle near the posterior border of the mylohyoid muscle. Postganglionic neurons with cell bodies in the submandibular ganglion distribute to the sublingual and submandibular glands as well as to lesser lingual glands. Some fibers of the chorda tympani extend through the submandibular ganglion to synapse with postganglionic neurons contained within the stroma of the submandibular gland.

The opening through which the chorda tympani exits from the petrous portion of the temporal bone is the _____ fissure.

petrotympanic

The site at which the chorda tympani joins the lingual branch of the mandibular nerve is the _____ fossa.

infratemporal

The location of the submandibular ganglion is on the _____ muscle near the posterior border of the _____ muscle.

hyoglossus . . . mylohyoid

THE GLOSSOPHARYNGEAL NERVE: THE GVE FIBERS

Fibers of the glossopharyngeal nerve (IX) leave the brain at the ventral surface of the medulla, as can be seen by re-examining Figure 9–3. Cell bodies of these GVE neurons are, like the preganglionic cell bodies of the facial nerve, located in the salivatory nucleus at the junction of pons and medulla. General visceral efferent fibers leave the inferior ganglion of the glossopharyngeal nerve just as the main trunk descends through the jugular foramen.

QUESTION
54

Cell bodies of parasympathetic preganglionic neurons of the glossopharyngeal nerve are located in the _____ nucleus in the brain stem.

ANSWER

salivatory

QUESTION
55

GVE fibers leave the inferior ganglion of the glossopharyngeal nerve at the _____ foramen.

ANSWER

jugular

ITEM 23

THE LESSER PETROSAL NERVE

In Figure 9–8, general visceral efferent fibers of the glossopharyngeal nerve can be seen ascending as part of the tympanic nerve. These fibers enter the tympanic cavity through a small canal, form the tympanic plexus within the petrous part of the temporal bone, and then branch off to form the *lesser petrosal nerve*.

QUESTION
56

GVE fibers of the glossopharyngeal nerve enter the tympanic cavity as part of the _____ nerve.

ANSWER

tympanic

QUESTION
57

The lesser petrosal nerve consists of _____ _____ efferent fibers which leave the _____ plexus in the petrous part of the temporal bone.

ANSWER

general visceral . . . tympanic

ITEM 24

THE LESSER PETROSAL NERVE: THE PATHWAY

The lesser petrosal nerve leaves the tympanic cavity to enter the middle cranial fossa by way of a small foramen lateral to the hiatus of the facial canal. It leaves the middle cranial fossa to reach the otic ganglion through a fissure in the petrosquamous suture. The otic ganglion is located medial to the mandibular division of the trigeminal nerve a short distance beyond the point where the latter emerges from the foramen ovale.

The lesser petrosal nerve enters the middle cranial fossa through a foramen lateral to the hiatus of the _____ canal and leaves the middle cranial fossa through a fissure in the _____ suture.

QUESTION
58

facial . . . petrosquamous

ANSWER

The location of the otic ganglion is medial to the _____ nerve at a point just beyond the exit of this nerve through the foramen _____.

QUESTION
59

mandibular . . . ovale

ANSWER

THE PAROTID GLAND: PARASYMPATHETIC INNERVATION

ITEM 25

The preganglionic fibers which constitute the lesser petrosal nerve originate as part of the glossopharyngeal nerve and carry parasympathetic impulses to the parotid gland. Examine Figure 9–8 again and observe the general visceral efferent fibers of the lesser petrosal nerve as they synapse in the otic ganglion. Postganglionic fibers from the otic ganglion distribute with the auriculotemporal branch of the mandibular nerve to the parotid gland, the largest of the salivary glands.

The otic ganglion is the site where preganglionic parasympathetic fibers of the _____ _____ nerve synapse with postganglionic neurons.

QUESTION
60

lesser petrosal

ANSWER

Postganglionic neurons with cell bodies in the otic ganglion travel to the parotid gland in the company of the _____ branch of the mandibular nerve.

QUESTION
61

auriculotemporal

ANSWER

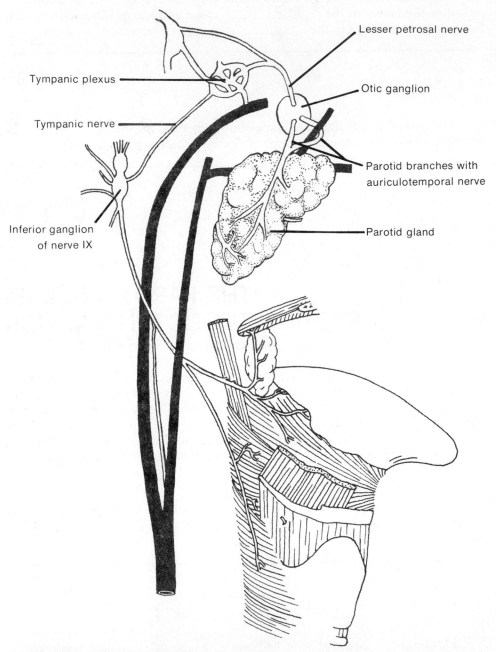

Figure 9-8.   General visceral efferent supply of the glossopharyngeal nerve (IX). (Modified from Woodburne: Essentials of Human Anatomy. 4th Ed. New York, Oxford University Press.)

Sympathetic stimulation supplied to the parotid gland originates from preganglionic fibers which synapse in the superior cervical ganglion. Postganglionic sympathetic fibers supplying the parotid gland arrive by way of plexuses surrounding the maxillary artery. As is the case with the sublingual and submandibular glands, the two divisions of the autonomic nervous system exert opposite forms of control over parotid gland secretion. An increase in sympathetic impulses decreases secretion by causing constriction of blood vessels supplying the parotid and other salivary glands. An increase in parasympathetic impulses to salivary glands results in increased secretion.

Sympathetic fibers which supply the parotid gland follow plexuses surrounding the _____ artery.

QUESTION
62

---

maxillary

ANSWER

Increased secretion of the salivary glands accompanies increase in *parasympathetic/sympathetic* (circle one) stimulation; decreased secretion follows increase in *parasympathetic/sympathetic* (circle one) stimulation.

QUESTION
63

---

parasympathetic . . . sympathetic

ANSWER

Decreased secretion of salivary glands results from _____ of blood vessels supplying those glands.

QUESTION
64

---

constriction

ANSWER

SUMMARY OF UNIT NINE

GENERAL CONSIDERATIONS

The function of the autonomic nervous system is to regulate visceral activity through stimulation of smooth muscle, cardiac muscle, and glands. Sensory impulses initiating visceral change travel to the brain and spinal cord from receptors in the organs involved or, less frequently, from receptors in the body wall. The motor impulses effecting visceral change travel over an autonomic pathway involving two neurons, one preganglionic and one postganglionic. Preganglionic and postganglionic neurons synapse in various ganglia.

The autonomic nervous system is composed of two divisions, the sympathetic and the parasympathetic, which usually act on the structures innervated in opposite ways. In the thoracic and lumbar regions of the spinal cord, the sympathetic division has preganglionic fibers which synapse with postganglionic neurons in sympathetic chain ganglia or in collateral ganglia in the thorax, abdomen, and pelvis. The parasympathetic division has preganglionic cell bodies in the brain and sacral region. Peripheral processes of these neurons synapse with postganglionic neurons in peripheral ganglia.

The sympathetic nerve supply to the head innervates smooth muscles of the eye, the lacrimal gland, the salivary glands, and glands of oral and nasal mucosa. Postganglionic fibers from superior cervical sympathetic ganglia distribute by forming plexuses around the internal and external carotid arteries or by traveling with adjacent cranial nerves. Sympathetic influence on glands of the head is effected largely through control of the diameter of blood vessels. Decreased sympathetic stimulation permits the vessels to dilate; increased stimulation causes the vessels to constrict.

Parasympathetic supply to the head includes preganglionic fibers of the oculomotor, facial, glossopharyngeal, and vagus nerves. Preganglionic fibers of the oculomotor nerve synapse with postganglionic neurons in the ciliary ganglion; fibers of the facial nerve synapse in the pterygopalatine and submandibular ganglia; fibers of the glossopharyngeal nerve synapse in the otic ganglion.

THE OCULOMOTOR NERVE: THE AUTONOMIC FIBERS

Originating in the visceral nucleus of the oculomotor nerve in the midbrain, parasympathetic preganglionic fibers of the third cranial nerve synapse within the orbit in the ciliary ganglion. Postganglionic fibers then distribute as short ciliary nerves to the sphincter pupillae muscle, which constricts the pupil of the eye. Other short ciliary nerves, passing through the ciliary ganglion without synapse, include postganglionic sympathetic fibers to the dilator pupillae muscle, which dilates the pupil. Afferent fibers which are sensory to the eyeball also pass through the ciliary ganglion without synapse.

THE FACIAL NERVE: THE AUTONOMIC FIBERS

Preganglionic parasympathetic fibers of the facial nerve have cell bodies in the salivatory nucleus near the junction of the pons and medulla. Within the temporal bone, parasympathetic fibers forming the greater petrosal nerve leave the main trunk of the facial nerve, extend through the middle cranial fossa, and join sympathetic fibers of the deep petrosal nerve. The parasympathetic fibers of the greater petrosal and the sympathetic fibers of the deep petrosal travel together through the pterygoid canal and make their way to the pterygopalatine ganglion. The greater petrosal nerve synapses in the pterygopalatine ganglion with post-ganglionic neurons which supply the lacrimal gland. The sympathetic fibers of the deep petrosal nerve pass through the ganglion without synapse, as do sensory fibers of the maxillary division of the trigeminal nerve. Traveling with the maxillary division, parasympathetic and sympathetic postganglionic fibers extend to the lacrimal gland and to glands of nasal, palatine, and upper pharyngeal mucosa.

Other parasympathetic fibers of the facial nerve are contained in the chorda tympani along with sensory fibers for taste. The parasympathetic preganglionic fibers of the chorda tympani travel with the lingual nerve as far as the submandibular ganglion. Some GVE fibers of the chorda tympani synapse in the submandibular ganglion with postganglionic neurons which supply the sublingual gland; other fibers pass through the submandibular ganglion and synapse with postganglionic neurons in the stroma of the submandibular gland.

Sympathetic supply to sublingual and submandibular glands distributes by way of plexuses which travel with branches of the facial artery.

THE GLOSSOPHARYNGEAL NERVE: THE AUTONOMIC FIBERS

Preganglionic parasympathetic fibers of the glossopharyngeal nerve have cell bodies in the salivatory nucleus. These GVE fibers branch off in the tympanic cavity as the lesser petrosal nerve, which exits from the middle cranial fossa through a fissure in the petrosquamous suture. The lesser petrosal nerve synapses in the otic ganglion, which lies medial to the mandibular division of the trigeminal nerve just beyond the foramen ovale. Traveling with the auriculotemporal branch of the mandibular nerve, postganglionic fibers from the otic ganglion supply parasympathetic impulses to the parotid gland.

Sympathetic fibers to the parotid gland travel with the maxillary artery. The effect of parasympathetic impulses on the parotid and other salivary glands is to increase secretion; the effect of sympathetic impulses is to decrease secretion.

The parasympathetic and sympathetic divisions of the autonomic nervous system act as dual and opposite controls of _____ activity.

QUESTION 65

---

visceral

ANSWER

Structures affected by the autonomic nervous system include _____ muscle, _____ muscle, and _____.

QUESTION 66

---

smooth . . . cardiac . . . glands

ANSWER

The two types of neurons in an autonomic pathway are _____ neurons and _____ neurons.

QUESTION 67

ANSWER
preganglionic . . . postganglionic (in either order)

QUESTION
68
Sensations which trigger autonomic responses travel from the sensory receptors to the _____ and to the _____.

ANSWER
spinal cord . . . brain (in either order)

QUESTION
69
Preganglionic sympathetic fibers synapse in sympathetic _____ ganglia or in _____ ganglia.

ANSWER
chain . . . collateral

QUESTION
70
Increased sympathetic stimulation causes blood vessels to _____; decreased stimulation causes blood vessels to _____.

ANSWER
constrict . . . dilate

QUESTION
71
Match the letters of the nerves listed in Column B with the numbers of the ganglia in Column A in which they synapse.

Column A	Column B
( ) 1. pterygopalatine ganglion	A. oculomotor nerve
( ) 2. otic ganglion	B. facial nerve
( ) 3. ciliary ganglion	C. glossopharyngeal nerve
( ) 4. submandibular ganglion	

ANSWER
1.—(B); 2.—(C); 3.—(A); 4—(B)

QUESTION
72
Postganglionic fibers which distribute by forming plexuses around blood vessels are *sympathetic/parasympathetic* (circle one).

ANSWER
sympathetic

QUESTION
73
Preganglionic sympathetic fibers to structures of the head synpase with postganglionic neurons in superior _____ sympathetic ganglia.

ANSWER
cervical

QUESTION
74
Located in the brain and sacral region are cell bodies of preganglionic *sympathetic/parasympathetic* (circle one) fibers.

parasympathetic

Parasympathetic short ciliary nerves innervate the ＿＿＿＿＿＿＿＿ pupillae *QUESTION* **75** muscle to constrict the pupil of the eye; sympathetic short ciliary nerves supply the ＿＿＿＿＿＿＿＿ pupillae muscle to dilate the pupil.

---

sphincter . . . dilator   *ANSWER*

Parasympathetic fibers of the facial nerve which synapse in the pterygo- *QUESTION* **76** palatine ganglion form the ＿＿＿＿＿＿＿ ＿＿＿＿＿＿＿＿ nerve; those which synapse in the submandibular ganglion are part of the ＿＿＿＿＿＿＿ ＿＿＿＿＿＿＿ nerve.

---

greater petrosal . . . chorda tympani   *ANSWER*

Parasympathetic supply to the lacrimal gland and to glands of the nasal, pala- *QUESTION* **77** tine, and upper pharyngeal mucosa is provided by postganglionic neurons which synapse with preganglionic fibers of the ＿＿＿＿＿＿＿ ＿＿＿＿＿＿＿ nerve; sympathetic supply to these glands is provided by the ＿＿＿＿ ＿＿＿＿＿＿＿ nerve.

---

greater petrosal . . . deep petrosal   *ANSWER*

Sympathetic and parasympathetic postganglionic fibers to the lacrimal gland *QUESTION* **78** and to glands of the nasal, palatine, and upper pharyngeal mucosa travel with afferent fibers of the ＿＿＿＿＿＿＿ division of the trigeminal nerve.

---

maxillary   *ANSWER*

In addition to special visceral afferent fibers for taste, the chorda tympani *QUESTION* **79** carries general visceral efferent fibers which provide parasympathetic supply to the ＿＿＿＿＿＿＿＿ and ＿＿＿＿＿＿＿ glands.

---

submandibular . . . sublingual (in either order)   *ANSWER*

Plexuses bringing sympathetic supply to the submandibular and sublingual *QUESTION* **80** glands travel with the ＿＿＿＿＿＿＿ artery.

---

facial   *ANSWER*

QUESTION
81

Located in the salivatory nucleus are cell bodies of preganglionic parasympathetic fibers of the _____ nerve and the _____ nerve.

ANSWER

facial . . . glossopharyngeal (in either order)

QUESTION
82

Preganglionic parasympathetic fibers which branch off from the glossopharyngeal nerve constitute the _____ _____ nerve, which synapses in the _____ ganglion.

ANSWER

lesser petrosal . . . otic

QUESTION
83

The lesser petrosal nerve contains preganglionic fibers which synapse in the _____ ganglion with postganglionic fibers which innervate the _____ gland.

ANSWER

otic . . . parotid

QUESTION
84

Preganglionic fibers of the lesser petrosal nerve branch off from the glossopharyngeal nerve in the _____ cavity and exit from the _____ cranial fossa through a fissure in the petrosquamous suture.

ANSWER

tympanic . . . middle

QUESTION
85

Plexuses which follow the maxillary artery provide sympathetic supply to the _____ gland.

ANSWER

parotid

QUESTION
86

Increased secretion of the salivary glands is caused by increased _____ stimulation; decreased secretion, by increased _____ stimulation.

ANSWER

parasympathetic . . . sympathetic

Unit Ten □ THE MENINGES AND THE VENOUS DURAL SINUSES

THE MENINGES ITEM 1

The *meninges* are connective tissue coverings which enclose the brain and spinal cord and provide a shock absorber filled with cerebrospinal fluid between the central nervous system and bone. In addition, the meninges enclose and protect major arteries to the brain as well as venous channels called the *venous dural sinuses*. Figure 10–1 shows the meninges as they appear in a coronal section just under the midline of the skull. The three layers of meninges, reading from outside

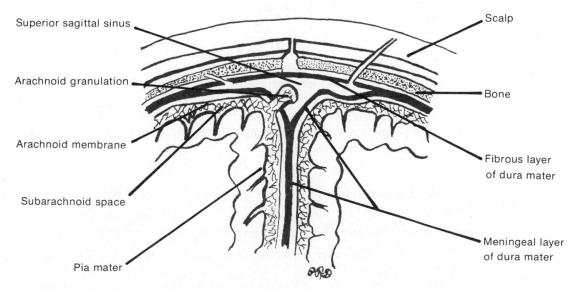

Figure 10–1. Layers of the meninges, seen in a coronal section. (Modified from Leeson and Leeson: Human Structure. Philadelphia, W. B. Saunders Co.)

to inside, are called the *dura mater,* the *arachnoid,* and the *pia mater.* Locate these three layers in Figure 10–1.

QUESTION
1

The meninges protect the _____ and the _____ _____ with coverings of connective tissue.

ANSWER

brain . . . spinal cord

QUESTION
2

The meninges and their cerebrospinal fluid act as a shock absorber between bone and the _____ _____ _____.

ANSWER

central nervous system

QUESTION
3

Match the terms in Column A with their definitions from Column B.

Column A	Column B
( ) 1. arachnoid	A. the outer layer of meninges
( ) 2. pia mater	B. the middle layer of meninges
( ) 3. dura mater	C. the inner layer of meninges

ANSWER

1.—(B); 2.—(C); 3.—(A)

ITEM 2   THE DURA MATER

Re-examine Figure 10–1 and notice that the outer layer of the meninges, the dura mater, is a dense connective tissue membrane composed of two layers. The outer layer of dura, the *fibrous dura,* adheres closely to bone and has the same structure as the connective tissue covering of bone referred to as *periosteum.* The inner layer of dura is the *meningeal layer.*

QUESTION
4

The fibrous connective tissue layer of dura mater is the (circle one) *outer/ inner* layer.

ANSWER

The outer fibrous layer adheres to bone.

QUESTION
5

The inner layer of dura mater is the (circle one) *periosteal/meningeal* layer.

ANSWER

The inner meningeal layer is farthest away from bone.

THE DURA MATER: THE INNER LAYER   ITEM 3

The inner meningeal layer of dura mater folds into a doubled partition in several regions of bone. Four membranes formed from folding of dura mater can be seen in a sagittal section in Figure 10–2. This fold of the inner layer of dura mater between the cerebral hemispheres is called the *falx cerebri*. A similar fold between the cerebellar hemispheres is called the *falx cerebelli*. The doubled partition between the cerebrum and the cerebellum is the *tentorium cerebelli*. A double layer above the hypophysis (pituitary gland) is the *diaphragma sellae*.

The falx cerebri is a fold of the _____ layer of the dura mater between the _____ hemispheres.

QUESTION 6

meningeal (inner) . . . cerebral

ANSWER

The fold of the meningeal layer of dura mater between the two cerebellar hemispheres is called the _____ _____.

QUESTION 7

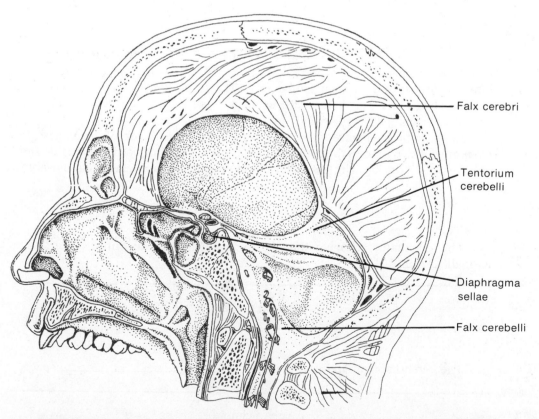

Falx cerebri

Tentorium cerebelli

Diaphragma sellae

Falx cerebelli

Figure 10–2. Sagittal section showing the four membranes formed from enfolding of dura mater. (Redrawn from Wolf-Heidegger: Atlas of Systematic Human Anatomy. Vol. III. Basel, S. Karger AG.)

ANSWER   falx cerebelli

QUESTION   The tentorium cerebelli is located between the _____ and the
8   _____.

ANSWER   cerebrum . . . cerebellum

QUESTION   The diaphragma sellae overlies the _____.
9

ANSWER   hypophysis (pituitary gland)

ITEM 4   THE ARACHNOID MEMBRANE AND THE PIA MATER

The *arachnoid membrane,* which is shown in Figure 10–1, is the delicate middle layer of meninges which, like the dura, bridges the sulci, but also dips into the major fissures such as the falx. The trabeculated space between the arachnoid and the pia mater, also seen in Figure 10–1, is the *subarachnoid space,* containing cerebrospinal fluid.

Look back to Figure 10–1 and notice the inner layer of meninges, the *pia mater,* which follows the contours of the brain and spinal cord. It dips into sulci and fissures, carrying with it smaller blood vessels and applying them closely to tissue.

QUESTION   The pia mater, clinging directly to brain and spinal cord, carries with
10   it small _____ _____.

ANSWER   blood vessels

QUESTION   The cerebrospinal fluid is contained in the _____ space.
11

ANSWER   subarachnoid

CLINICAL CONSIDERATIONS OF THE POTENTIAL SPACES: HEMATOMAS

ITEM 5

Potential spaces between the layers of meninges enclose blood vessels or cerebrospinal fluid. The *extradural space* between bone and the fibrous layer of dura contains meningeal arteries. If these vessels are torn when head injuries occur, bleeding may be profuse enough effectively to tear the fibrous dura loose from its bony attachment. An accumulation of blood outside the fibrous dura is called an *extradural hematoma*. An accumulation of blood within or under the dura is called a *subdural hematoma*.

The potential space between bone and the fibrous layer of dura is called _____ space.

QUESTION 12

---

extradural

ANSWER

An extradural hematoma is an accumulation of blood between _____ _____ and _____.

QUESTION 13

---

dura mater . . . bone

ANSWER

An accumulation of blood below the dura is a _____ hematoma.

QUESTION 14

---

subdural

ANSWER

CLINICAL CONSIDERATIONS OF THE POTENTIAL SPACES: SUBARACHNOID HEMORRHAGE

ITEM 6

The *subarachnoid space* is the area under the arachnoid membrane. Within this space are located branches of major arteries to the brain. The subarachnoid space is continuous around the brain and spinal cord and is in communication with the ventricles, the fluid filled cavities of the brain. In cases of subarachnoid hemorrhage, blood mixes with cerebrospinal fluid; therefore, subarachnoid hemorrhage can be readily detected by withdrawing cerebrospinal fluid by a procedure called a *lumbar puncture*.

QUESTION
15

Subarachnoid space, as part of the route of circulation of _____ _____, is in communication with the _____ of the brain and is continuous around the brain and spinal cord.

ANSWER

cerebrospinal fluid . . . ventricles

QUESTION
16

A subarachnoid hemorrhage will be detected if a lumbar puncture reveals _____ mixed with _____ fluid.

ANSWER

blood . . . cerebrospinal

ITEM 7   THE CHOROID PLEXUSES

Cerebrospinal fluid is elaborated from blood at the *choroid plexuses*. A choroid plexus is a membranous partition extending into the cavity of each of the ventricles, forming a semipermeable filtering partition between arterial blood and cerebrospinal fluid. The circulation route of cerebrospinal fluid, then, begins with the choroid pelxuses.

QUESTION
17

The semipermeable membranes separating arterial blood from cerebrospinal fluid are called the _____ _____.

ANSWER

choroid plexus

QUESTION
18

The membranous partitions separating arterial blood from cerebrospinal fluid extend into the _____ of the brain.

ANSWER

ventricles

CEREBROSPINAL FLUID: THE CIRCULATION

ITEM 8

Figure 10–3 shows the details of the ventricular system of the brain. Remember that this is a fluid filled system, rather than a solid structure. Cerebrospinal fluid circulates through the ventricles and the subarachnoid spaces around the brain and spinal cord. From the right and left *lateral ventricles,* fluid flows through *interventricular foramina* into the *third ventricle;* from the third ventricle, fluid flows through the *cerebral aqueduct* into the *fourth ventricle.* From the fourth ventricle, it flows through a *medial* and two *lateral recesses* to circulate in subarachnoid space around the brain and spinal cord.

The communication between the lateral and third ventricles is the _____ foramen.

QUESTION 19

---

interventricular

ANSWER

The communication between the third and fourth ventricles is the cerebral _____.

QUESTION 20

---

aqueduct

ANSWER

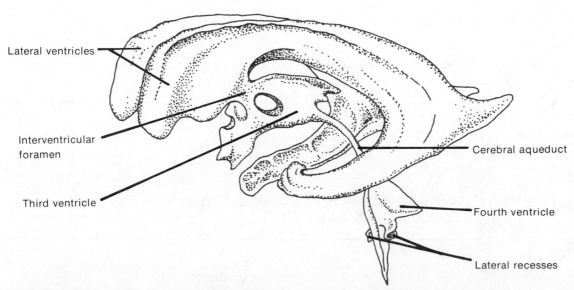

Figure 10–3. Ventricles of the brain, lateral aspect. (Redrawn from Wolf-Heidegger: Atlas of Systematic Human Anatomy. Vol. III. Basel, S. Karger AG.)

QUESTION
21

Foramina which drain the fourth ventricle are called the _____ and _____ recesses.

ANSWER

medial . . . lateral (in either order)

ITEM 9   CEREBROSPINAL FLUID: RETURN TO VENOUS CIRCULATION

Cerebrospinal fluid, which is essentially a filtrate of blood, returns to the venous system through small membranous villi called *arachnoid granulations*. These arachnoid granulations, seen in Figure 10–1, occur along the course of a large venous sinus, the *superior sagittal sinus*, which extends from front to back under the midline of the skull. The superior sagittal sinus appears in a coronal section in Figure 10–1. The flow of cerebrospinal fluid is unidirectional because of the pressure gradient between its sources, arterial blood, and its termination, venous blood.

QUESTION
22

Cerebrospinal fluid returns to blood by way of small villi called _____ _____.

ANSWER

arachnoid granulations

QUESTION
23

Arachnoid granulations are located along the course of the superior _____ sinus.

ANSWER

sagittal

QUESTION
24

Cerebrospinal fluid flows in a single direction because of _____ _____ of blood.

ANSWER

pressure gradients

THE VENOUS DURAL SINUSES

ITEM 10

Drainage of blood from the brain takes place through a system of sinuses which empty into the internal jugular veins. These *venous dural sinuses* are epithelially lined spaces, or channels, between the two layers of dura. Dural sinuses receive blood from three sources: primarily, from (1) *cerebral veins,* but also from (2) *diploic veins* between layers of the skull, and from (3) *emissary veins* connecting extracranial with intracranial veins.

The venous dural sinuses, situated between the two layers of _____, are lined with _____.

QUESTION 25

---

dura . . . epithelium

ANSWER

Blood which drains through the venous dural sinuses empties into the _____ _____ veins.

QUESTION 26

---

internal jugular

ANSWER

Blood enters the venous dural sinuses mainly from _____ veins, but also from _____ veins and _____ veins.

QUESTION 27

---

cerebral . . . diploic . . . emissary

ANSWER

THE VENOUS DURAL SINUSES: CLINICAL SIGNIFICANCE

ITEM 11

Because of the fibrous nature of their walls, the venous dural sinuses have little tendency to collapse as most other veins of the body do. The fibrous structure has an advantage in that the vessels tend to stay filled with blood against the forces of gravity. An obvious clinical disadvantage, however, is that profuse bleeding ensues if one of the sinuses is ruptured by a fragment of bone, as may happen if the head is injured.

A clinical advantage of the fibrous walls of the venous dural sinuses is their tendency to remain filled against the force of _____; a clinical dis-

QUESTION 28

advantage is the likelihood of profuse _____ in case of a rupture of one of these vessels.

ANSWER

gravity . . . bleeding

ITEM 12   THE UNPAIRED DURAL SINUSES

Three of the dural sinuses are unpaired, and lie in the midline associated with the falx cerebri. Figure 10–4 shows these three unpaired sinuses: (1) the *superior sagittal sinus,* (2) the *inferior sagittal sinus,* and (3) the *straight sinus.* Also shown in Figure 10–4, a sagittal section through the skull and meninges, is the extent of the falx cerebri as it dips down into the longitudinal fissure.

QUESTION
29

The three unpaired dural sinuses are the _____ _____ sinus, the _____ _____ sinus, and the _____ sinus.

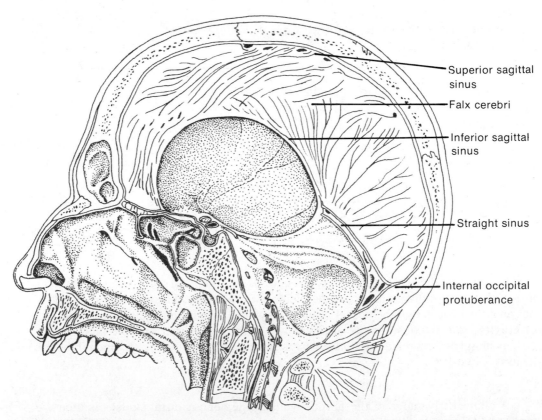

Superior sagittal sinus

Falx cerebri

Inferior sagittal sinus

Straight sinus

Internal occipital protuberance

Figure 10–4. Sagittal section showing the unpaired dural sinuses. (Redrawn from Wolf-Heidegger: Atlas of Systematic Human Anatomy. Vol. III. Basel, S. Karger AG.)

superior sagittal . . . inferior sagittal . . . straight

THE UNPAIRED DURAL SINUSES: LOCATION

ITEM 13

You will remember from Item 3 that the falx cerebri is formed by folds of the meningeal layer of dura. Look back to Figure 10–1 and notice how the superior sagittal sinus occupies the traingular space between the meningeal layer and the fibrous layer of the dura. Now re-examine Figure 10–4 and observe the inferior sagittal sinus in the lower fold of the meningeal layer. Also notice the straight sinus extending from the posterior limit of the inferior sagittal sinus back to the *internal occipital protuberance* in the falx cerebelli.

In the numbered spaces below write the names of the corresponding numbered structures in the accompanying diagram.

QUESTION
30

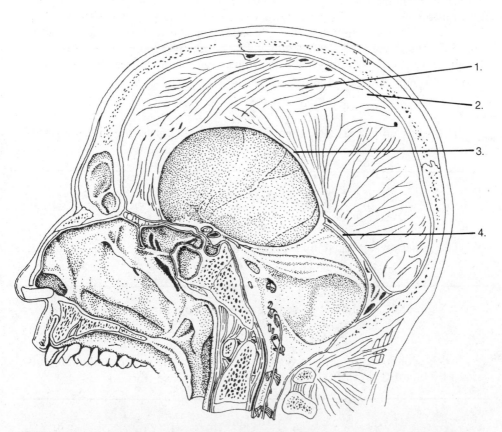

(Redrawn from Wolf-Heidegger: Atlas of Systematic Human Anatomy. Vol. III. Basel, S. Karger AG.)

Labels
1. _____
2. _____ sinus
3. _____ sinus
4. _____ sinus

ANSWER

1. falx cerebri   3. inferior sagittal
2. superior sagittal 4. straight

ITEM 14   THE SUPERIOR SAGITTAL SINUS

In Figure 10–5, locate the first of the three unpaired dural sinuses, the *superior sagittal sinus*. The superior sagittal sinus begins as a continuation of a nasal vein at the *foramen cecum*. Along its course, it receives blood from cerebral, diploic, meningeal, and emissary veins, as well as cerebrospinal fluid from arachnoid granulations. Notice how the superior sagittal sinus extends along the midline from its anterior attachment to the *crista galli* to its posterior termination at the *confluens of sinuses*. The straight sinus also terminates at the confluens of sinuses, where blood from the superior sagittal sinus is joined by blood from the straight sinus. The confluens of sinuses is located in the triangular space at the site of the internal occipital protuberance, between the fibrous dura and the enfolded meningeal dura.

QUESTION 31

The sinus which extends from the foramen cecum to the internal occipital protuberance is the _____ _____ sinus.

ANSWER

superior sagittal

QUESTION 32

The superior sagittal sinus receives blood from _____, _____, _____, and _____ veins.

ANSWER

cerebral . . . diploic . . . meningeal . . . emissary (in any order)

QUESTION 33

At the confluens of sinuses, venous blood from the superior sagittal sinus is joined by blood from the _____ sinus.

ANSWER

straight

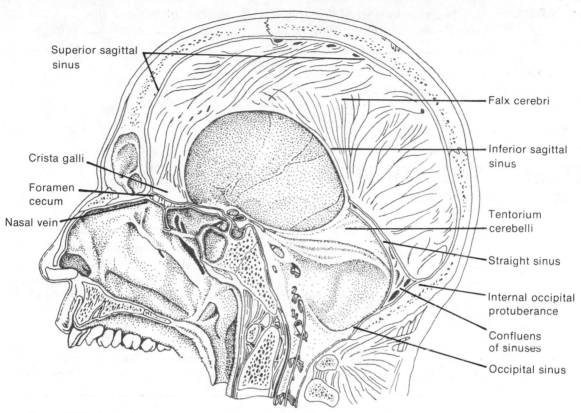

Figure 10–5. Sagittal section showing the unpaired sinuses in relationship to the confluens of sinuses and the occipital sinus. (Redrawn from Wolf-Heidegger: Atlas of Systematic Human Anatomy. Vol. III. Basel, S. Karger AG.)

THE INFERIOR SAGITTAL SINUS   ITEM 15

Figure 10–5 shows the inferior sagittal sinus occupying the lower margin of the falx cerebri and extending posteriorly within its meningeal fold. The inferior sagittal sinus receives blood from veins on the medial surface of the brain. Also notice the point where the inferior sagittal sinus joins the beginning of the straight sinus. At this point, the straight sinus receives blood from the posteriorly directed great cerebral vein, which drains deeper areas of brain tissue.

.

The sinus which occupies the lower free margin of the falx cerebri is the _____ _____ sinus.

QUESTION
34

---

inferior sagittal

ANSWER

QUESTION
35
The anterior part of the straight sinus receives blood from the _____ sagittal sinus as well as from the _____ _____ vein.

ANSWER

inferior . . . great cerebral

ITEM 16   THE STRAIGHT SINUS AND THE OCCIPITAL SINUS

The straight sinus occupies the area between the falx cerebri above, and the transversely directed tentorium cerebelli below. At its posterior, inferior limit, the straight sinus receives the *occipital sinus,* which drains blood from below. In Figure 10–5, notice the location of the occipital sinus, from which blood flows upward into the straight sinus.

QUESTION
36
The straight sinus joins the superior sagittal sinus at the _____ of sinuses, where blood is also received from the _____ sinus below.

ANSWER

confluens . . . occipital

ITEM 17   THE TRANSVERSE SINUSES

The position of the *transverse sinuses* in relation to the other dural sinuses may be studied in Figure 10–6. On the right side of this horizontal section, the tentorium cerebelli has been removed, as have all portions of the falx cerebri except its anterior and posterior attachments.

The transverse sinuses are paired channels. They extend laterally in a groove of the skull which runs from the end of the straight sinus at the point of the internal occipital protuberance to the petrous portion of the temporal bone. The transverse sinuses, like the superior sagittal sinus, occupy the triangular space between the fibrous dura and the fold of the meningeal dura. They traverse the length of the tentorium cerebelli, as the superior sagittal sinus traverses the bony attachment of the falx cerebri.

Figure 10–6 also illustrates the positions of the superior and inferior sagittal sinuses, the straight sinus, the occipital sinus, and the confluens of sinuses.

QUESTION
37
The superior sagittal sinus runs the length of the bony attachment of the _____ cerebri, while the transverse sinus runs the length of the bony attachment of the _____ cerebelli.

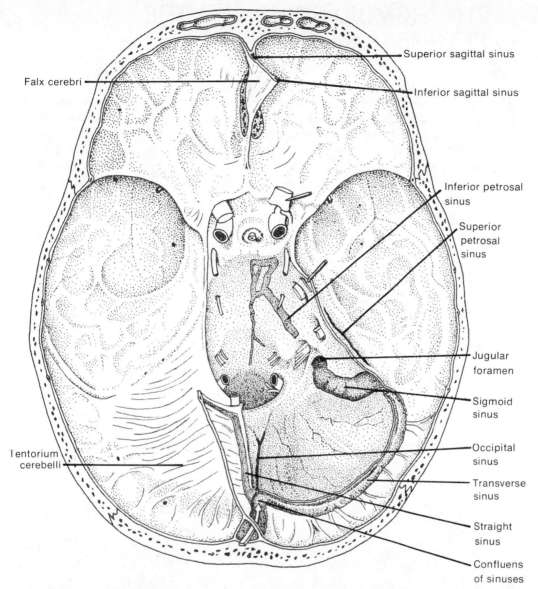

Falx cerebri

Superior sagittal sinus

Inferior sagittal sinus

Inferior petrosal sinus

Superior petrosal sinus

Jugular foramen

Sigmoid sinus

Occipital sinus

Transverse sinus

Straight sinus

Confluens of sinuses

Tentorium cerebelli

Figure 10–6. Horizontal section showing transverse, sigmoid, and petrosal sinuses. (Redrawn from Wolf-Heidegger: Atlas of Systematic Human Anatomy. Vol. III. Basel, S. Karger AG.)

falx . . . tentorium   *ANSWER*

The transverse sinuses extend bilaterally from the ＿＿＿＿＿＿ of sinuses   QUESTION
to the posterior end of the ＿＿＿＿＿＿ part of the ＿＿＿＿＿＿ bone.   **38**

confluens . . . petrous . . . temporal   *ANSWER*

ITEM 18

THE SIGMOID SINUS AND THE PETROSAL SINUSES

Refer back to Figure 10–6. Notice how the *sigmoid sinus,* which in effect is a continuation of the transverse sinuses, takes an S-shaped course toward the jugular foramen. Extending between the petrous and mastoid parts of the temporal bone, the sigmoid sinus continues over the occipital bone to terminate in the internal jugular vein. Along its course, the sigmoid sinus receives blood from the lower cerebrum, from the cerebellum, and from local emissary veins. The *superior* and *inferior petrosal sinuses,* shown in Figure 10–6, also drain into the sigmoid sinus.

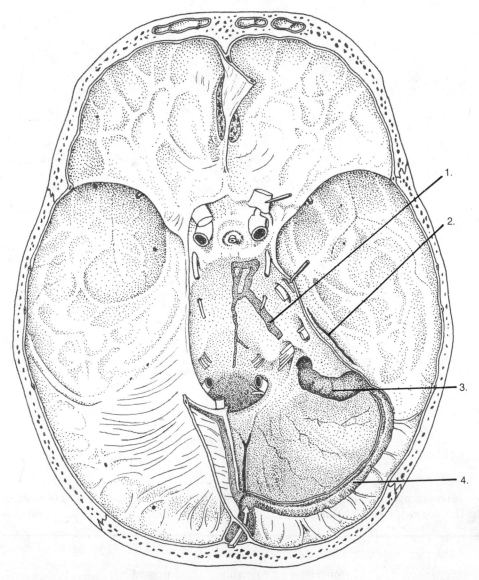

1.

2.

3.

4.

(Redrawn from Wolf-Heidegger: Atlas of Systematic Human Anatomy. Vol. III. Basel, S. Karger AG.)

In the numbered spaces below, write the names of the corresponding numbered structures in the accompanying diagram.

Labels

1. inferior _____sinus
2. superior _____ sinus
3. _____ sinus
4. _____ sinus

1. petrosal   2. petrosal   3. sigmoid   4. transverse   *ANSWER*

At its beginning, the sigmoid sinus is a continuation of the _____ sinus; at its termination, it becomes the _____ _____ vein.

transverse . . . internal jugular   *ANSWER*

The sigmoid sinus receives blood from three other sinuses: the _____ sinus, the superior _____ sinus, and the _____ _____ sinus.

transverse . . . petrosal . . . inferior petrosal   *ANSWER*

THE CAVERNOUS SINUSES   ITEM 19

The remaining sinuses are interconnecting vessels deep within the skull. The largest and most clinically important of these are the *cavernous sinuses,* located lateral to the body of the sphenoid bone. The clinical significance of the cavernous sinuses is due to the fact that they receive venous blood from the face, as well as from other areas, and are in a vulnerable position when an infection spreads along these channels. The cavernous sinuses provide the means whereby a relatively benign extracranial infection can gain access to the meninges and the brain. The inaccessibility of such infections made them particularly pernicious before the days of antibiotics.

The location of the cavernous sinus is lateral to the body of the _____ bone.

ANSWER   sphenoid

QUESTION
43

    The clinical significance of the cavernous sinuses stems from the fact that they may channel _____ to the brain and meninges together with the venous drainage received from parts of the _____.

ANSWER   infection . . . face

QUESTION
44

    A benign infection in an extracranial area becomes serious when it spreads to the brain and meninges by way of the _____ sinus.

ANSWER   cavernous

ITEM
20

THE CAVERNOUS AND SPHENOPARIETAL SINUSES: LOCATION

    Figure 10–7 shows the position of the cavernous sinus, lateral to the body of the sphenoid bone. It extends posteriorly from the superior orbital fissure to the petrous bone. This area, formed by a dilatation of the space between the fibrous and the meningeal durae, is unique in that it encloses not only venous blood but also several structures to be discussed in Items 21 and 22.

    In Figure 10–7, also notice the location of the *sphenoparietal sinus*, which extends along the crest of the lesser wing of the sphenoid bone. Blood from the sphenoparietal sinus is received into the cavernous sinus.

QUESTION
45

Blood from the _____ sinus drains into the cavernous sinus.

ANSWER   sphenoparietal

QUESTION
46

    The cavernous sinus is formed by a dilatation of the space between _____ _____ and _____ durae.

ANSWER   fibrous . . . meningeal

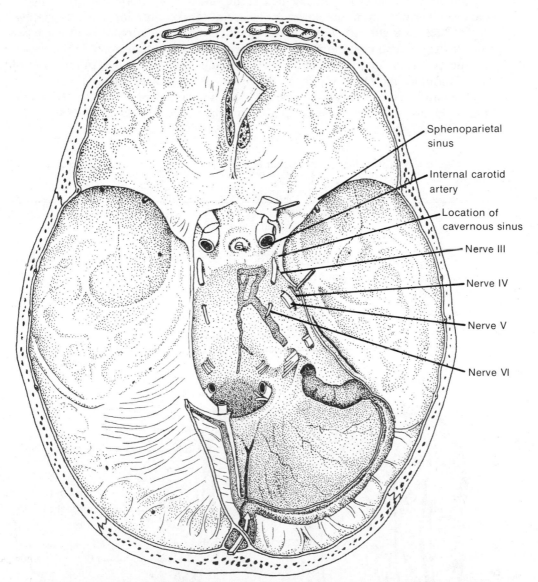

Figure 10-7.   Horizontal section showing locations of the cavernous sinus and the sphenoparietal sinus, and structures within the cavernous sinus. (Redrawn from Wolf-Heidegger: Atlas of Systematic Human Anatomy. Vol. III. Basel, S. Karger AG.)

ITEM
21

THE INTERNAL CAROTID ARTERY WITHIN THE CAVERNOUS SINUS

A frontal section of the cavernous sinus, Figure 10–8, shows the internal carotid artery within the venous blood of the sinus. This artery is enclosed by the cavernous sinus from the foramen lacerum to the anterior clinoid process. Refer back to Figure 10–7 and notice the cut ends of the internal carotid arteries where they extend posteriorly and superiorly from the anterior clinoid processes. At this point, the internal carotid arteries branch and become part of the cerebral arterial circle, the blood supply to the brain. To the lower left of Figure 10–8, notice how the cavernous sinus lies between the two layers of dura mater. At the top of Figure 10–8 can be seen the diaphragma sellae, the dural covering of the hypophysis (pituitary gland).

QUESTION
47

Enclosed within the cavernous sinus is the _____ _____ artery.

ANSWER

internal carotid

QUESTION
48

The portion of the internal carotid artery contained within the cavernous sinus extends from the foramen _____ to the anterior _____ process.

ANSWER

lacerum . . . clinoid

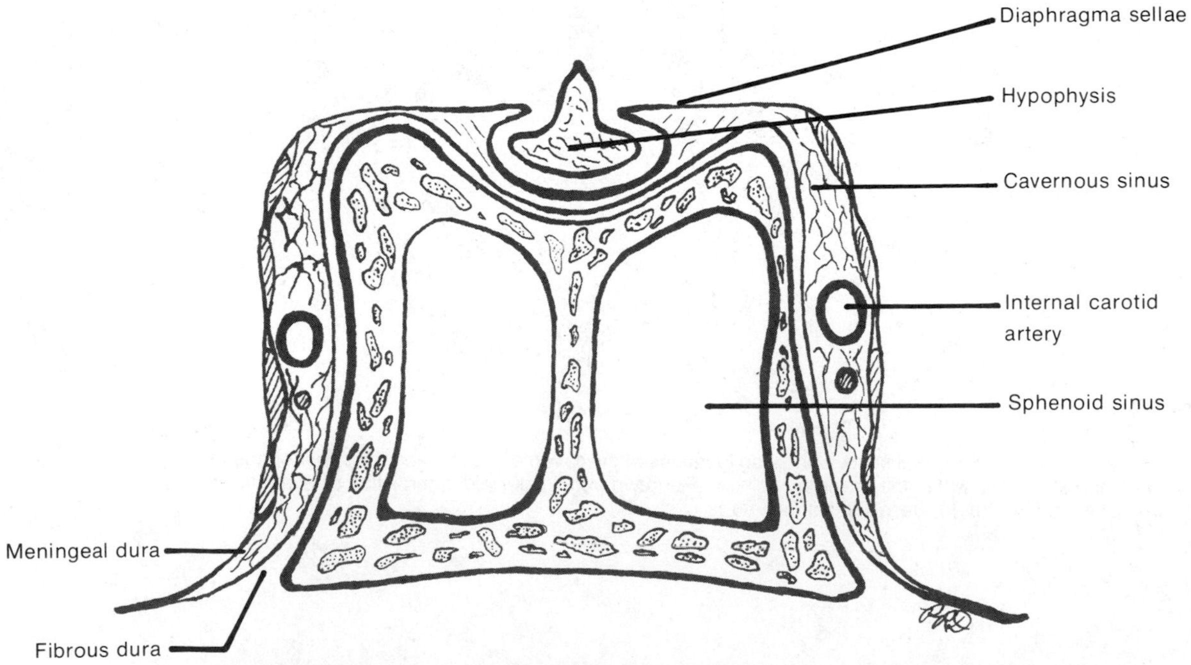

Diaphragma sellae

Hypophysis

Cavernous sinus

Internal carotid artery

Sphenoid sinus

Meningeal dura

Fibrous dura

Figure 10-8. Frontal section through the cavernous sinus. (Redrawn from Woodburne: Essentials of Human Anatomy. 4th Ed. New York, Oxford University Press.)

THE CRANIAL NERVES WITHIN THE CAVERNOUS SINUS

ITEM 22

Several cranial nerves contained within the cavernous sinus can be seen in Figure 10–9. The abducens nerve (VI), seen on the left, occupies a position below the internal carotid artery. Also contained in the lateral wall of the cavernous sinus are the oculomotor (III) and trochlear (IV) nerves, as well as the ophthalmic and maxillary divisions of the trigeminal nerve (V), all of which can be seen on the right of the illustration. Look back to Figure 10–7 and note the positions of these nerves in the horizontal section. Although it does not appear in Figure 10–9, the trigeminal ganglion is located just posterolateral to the cavernous sinus.

Structures contained within the cavernous sinus, surrounded by venous blood, include

QUESTION 49

1. _____ _____ arteries
2. _____ nerves
3. _____ nerves
4. _____ nerves
5. _____ division of the trigeminal nerve
6. _____ division of the trigeminal nerve

---

1. internal carotid
2. oculomotor
3. trochlear
4. abducens
5. ophthalmic
6. maxillary

ANSWER

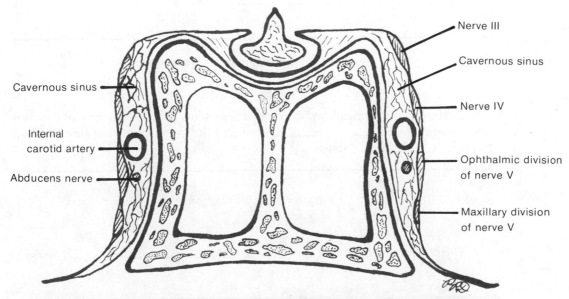

Figure 10-9. Frontal section showing cranial nerves contained within the cavernous sinus. (Redrawn from Woodburne: Essentials of Human Anatomy. 4th Ed. New York, Oxford University Press.)

QUESTION
50

Posterolateral to the cavernous sinus is the site of the _____ ganglion.

ANSWER

trigeminal

ITEM 23   THE CAVERNOUS SINUS AND RELATED SINUSES

The ophthalmic veins empty into the cavernous sinuses from the front. Ophthalmic veins are continuous with the angular veins of the face, which, in turn, are continuous with various extracranial veins from above and below. These veins provide open channels for the spread of infection from the face into the cavernous sinus. Thromboses in the cavernous sinus can lead to compression of the associated cranial nerves.

The cavernous sinus communicates posteriorly with the superior petrosal sinus, leading to the transverse sinus, and with the inferior petrosal sinus, leading to the sigmoid sinus. The cavernous sinus also communicates with the pterygoid plexus of veins by way of emissary veins through the foramen ovale. The pterygoid plexus is in the infratemporal fossa.

QUESTION
51

Connecting veins between the face and the cavernous sinus include the _____ veins, the _____ veins, and the _____ plexus of veins.

ANSWER

angular . . . ophthalmic . . . pterygoid

QUESTION
52

Posterior communications of the cavernous sinus include the superior petrosal sinus leading to the _____ sinus and the inferior petrosal sinus leading to the _____ sinus.

ANSWER

transverse . . . sigmoid

QUESTION
53

The pterygoid plexus of veins is located in the _____ fossa.

ANSWER

infratemporal

As a review of the locations of the dural sinuses, label the accompanying diagram. Using the Word Bank, write in the numbered spaces the names of the corresponding numbered structures in the diagram.

QUESTION
54

Word Bank

cavernous sinus	sigmoid sinus
confluens of sinuses	sphenoparietal sinus
inferior petrosal sinus	superior petrosal sinus
inferior sagittal sinus	superior sagittal sinus
internal carotid artery	straight sinus
occipital sinus	transverse sinus

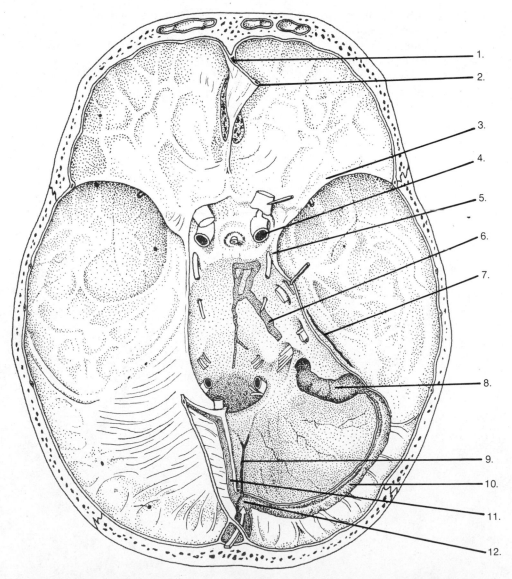

1.
2.
3.
4.
5.
6.
7.
8.
9.
10.
11.
12.

(Redrawn from Wolf-Heidegger: Atlas of Systematic Human Anatomy. Vol. III. Basel, S. Karger AG.)

Labels

1. _____ sinus
2. _____ sinus
3. _____ sinus
4. _____ artery
5. _____ sinus
6. _____ sinus
7. _____ sinus
8. _____ sinus
9. _____ sinus
10. _____ sinus
11. _____ sinus
12. _____ of _____

ANSWER

1. superior sagittal
2. inferior sagittal
3. sphenoparietal
4. internal carotid
5. cavernous
6. inferior petrosal
7. superior petrosal
8. sigmoid
9. occipital
10. transverse
11. straight
12. confluens . . . sinuses

SUMMARY OF UNIT TEN

THE MENINGES

Meninges are connective tissue coverings enclosing the brain and spinal cord. The meninges include the dura mater, the arachnoid, and the pia mater. The outer fibrous layer of dura mater adheres closely to bone. The inner meningeal layer of dura extends into the brain as a double partition enclosing venous channels. The fold of meningeal dura between the cerebral hemispheres is called the falx cerebri; that between the cerebellar hemispheres, the falx cerebelli; that between the cerebrum and the cerebellum, the tentorium cerebelli. The meningeal covering over the hypophysis, or pituitary gland, is termed the diaphragma sellae.

The middle layer of meninges, the arachnoid, is a delicate meshwork of trabeculae which encloses cerebrospinal fluid. The arachnoid membrane follows the meningeal folds into major fissures of the brain, but bridges over sulci without dipping into them. The pia mater, the innermost layer of meninges, closely adheres to brain tissue and dips into all convolutions of the brain, carrying blood vessels deep into the sulci.

Meningeal arteries extend between bone and the fibrous layer of dura. Rupture of one of these vessels causes the dura to separate from bone, forming an extradural hematoma. Injury which results in rupture of a vessel beneath the dura is termed a subdural hematoma. Hemorrhage of one of the arteries enclosed within subarachnoid space causes bleeding into the cerebrospinal fluid, known as a subarachnoid hemorrhage.

CIRCULATION OF THE CEREBROSPINAL FLUID

Cerebrospinal fluid is elaborated from blood by choroid plexuses, a series of semipermeable membranes extending into the cavities of the lateral, third, and fourth ventricles. Cerebrospinal fluid extends through the two lateral ventricles, the interventricular foramina, the third ventricle, the cerebral aqueduct, the fourth ventricle and its medial and lateral recesses, and through subarachnoid space surrounding the brain and spinal cord. At the arachnoid granulations along the superior sagittal sinus in the upper midline, cerebrospinal fluid passes through a membranous partition to join venous blood.

THE VENOUS DURAL SINUSES

The venous dural sinuses are channels of collection enclosed within partitions between the two layers of dura mater. Enclosed within folds of the falx cerebri are three unpaired midline sinuses: the superior sagittal sinus, the inferior sagittal sinus, and the straight sinus. The superior sagittal sinus occupies the triangular space between the meningeal folds and the fibrous layer; the inferior sagittal sinus, the lower fold of the meningeal layer; the straight sinus, the line of junction between the falx cerebri and the tentorium cerebelli. The transverse sinuses are paired sinuses which occupy a position in the posterior attached border of the tentorium cerebelli. At the internal occipital protuberance is the confluens of sinuses, a dilatation where the two transverse sinuses joing with the superior sagittal, straight, and occipital sinuses.

The superior sagittal sinus receives blood from cerebral, diploic, meningeal, and emissary veins along its route; the inferior sagittal sinus, from veins on the medial surface of the brain; the straight sinus, from the great cerebral vein which drains deep regions of brain tissue. At its posterior limit, the straight sinus also receives blood from the occipital sinus, which extends into the midline from below.

Blood drains from the confluens of sinuses laterally through the transverse sinuses to enter the larger sigmoid sinuses, which are channels occupying a position posterior to the petrous bone in the posterior cranial fossa. The superior and inferior petrosal sinuses also drain into the sigmoid sinuses. Receiving blood from the lower cerebrum, the cerebellum, local emissary veins, and adjacent sinuses, the sigmoid sinuses themselves terminate in the internal jugular vein. Sinuses draining blood from more anterior regions of the base of the brain include the sphenoparietal sinus and the cavernous sinus, the former draining into the latter. The cavernous sinus extends from the anterior clinoid processes along the sides of the base of the sphenoid bone to the posterior clinoid processes. Structures within the cavernous sinus include the internal carotid artery; the oculomotor, trochlear, and abducens nerves; and the ophthalmic and maxillary divisions of the trigeminal nerve. The cavernous sinus receives blood from ophthalmic veins, which are continuations of the angular veins of the face, and from the pterygoid plexus of veins in the infratemporal fossa. It is through these channels that extracranial infections can gain intracranial access to the brain and meninges. Thromboses in the cavernous sinus can lead to compression of the enclosed cranial nerves.

QUESTION
55

The meninges are connective tissue coverings of the _____ and the _____ _____.

ANSWER

brain . . . spinal cord

QUESTION
56

The three layers of meninges are _____ mater, _____, and _____ mater.

ANSWER

dura . . . arachnoid . . . pia

QUESTION
57

The outer layer of dura adheres to _____, while the inner layer of dura forms folds between the cerebral and cerebellar _____ as well as between the cerebrum and cerebellum.

ANSWER

bone . . . hemispheres

QUESTION
58

The fold of dura between cerebral hemispheres is called the _____ cerebri, that between cerebellar hemispheres is called the _____ cerebelli, and that between cerebrum and cerebellum is called the _____ cerebelli.

ANSWER

falx . . . falx . . . tentorium

The diaphragma sallae is a covering of the _____.

QUESTION
59

hypophysis (pituitary gland)

ANSWER

Cerebrospinal fluid is enclosed within the *dura mater/arachnoid/pia mater* (circle one).

QUESTION
60

arachnoid

ANSWER

While the arachnoid bridges over sulci without dipping into them, the _____ dips into sulci.

QUESTION
61

pia mater

ANSWER

Rupture of a meningeal artery between the fibrous dura and bone is called an _____ hematoma; rupture of a vessel underneath the fibrous dura is called a _____ hematoma.

QUESTION
62

extradural . . . subdural

ANSWER

Cerebrospinal fluid is elaborated by the _____ plexuses and circulates through _____ and _____ space.

QUESTION
63

choroid . . . ventricles . . . subarachnoid

ANSWER

The venous channels between layers of dura are called _____ sinuses.

QUESTION
64

venous dural

ANSWER

The superior sagittal, inferior sagittal, and straight sinuses are enclosed within folds of the falx _____.

QUESTION
65

cerebri

ANSWER

The sinuses located in the tentorium cerebelli are the paired _____ sinuses.

QUESTION
66

ANSWER

transverse

QUESTION
67

The juncture of unpaired sinuses with the transverse sinuses is called the
_____ of sinuses.

ANSWER

confluens

QUESTION
68

The drainage of blood from deep regions of brain tissue flows into the (circle
one)
A. superior sagittal sinus
B. inferior sagittal sinus
C. straight sinus

ANSWER

The correct answer is C. The straight sinus receives blood from the great
cerebral vein, which drains deep brain regions, as well as from the occipital sinus.

QUESTION
69

Transverse sinuses drain into the _____ sinuses.

ANSWER

sigmoid

QUESTION
70

The sphenoparietal sinus drains into the _____ sinus.

ANSWER

cavernous

QUESTION
71

Structures located within the cavernous sinus include the
1. _____ _____ artery
2. _____ nerve
3. _____ nerve
4. _____ nerve
5. _____ division of the trigeminal nerve
6. _____ division of the trigeminal nerve

ANSWER

1. internal carotid   4. abducens
2. oculomotor   5. ophthalmic
3. trochlear   6. maxillary

QUESTION
72

Veins through which extracranial infection can pass into the cavernous sinus
include the _____ veins and the _____ plexus of veins.

ANSWER

ophthalmic . . . pterygoid

Unit Eleven □ BLOOD SUPPLY TO THE HEAD

ORIGIN OF THE BLOOD SUPPLY TO THE HEAD

ITEM 1

The blood supply to the head falls into two main categories: (1) supply to the brain, and (2) supply to extracranial structures of the head. Blood to the brain is received from the *internal carotid arteries* and the *vertebral arteries*. Extracranial structures of the head are mainly supplied by branches of the *external carotid arteries*.

The internal carotid and vertebral arteries supply the (circle one) *brain/extracranial structures*.

QUESTION 1

---

brain

ANSWER

Most extracranial structures of the head receive their blood supply from the (circle one) *internal/external* carotid artery.

QUESTION 2

External. Associate *ex*tracranial with *external* carotid artery and *in*tracranial (within the brain) with *internal* carotid artery and you will have no difficulty in remembering the distinction.

ANSWER

BRANCHES OF THE AORTA

ITEM 2

Examine Figure 11–1 and trace the course of the principal branches of the aorta which supply the head. The *ascending aorta* gives off, on the right, the *brachiocephalic trunk,* which bifurcates to form the *right common carotid* artery and the *right subclavian* artery. The *arch of the aorta* directly gives off the *left common carotid* and *left subclavian* arteries. The *right* and *left vertebral*

429

arteries arise as the first branches off the right and left subclavian arteries, respectively. The vertebral arteries ascend through transverse foramina in cervical vertebrae to enter the foramen magnum.

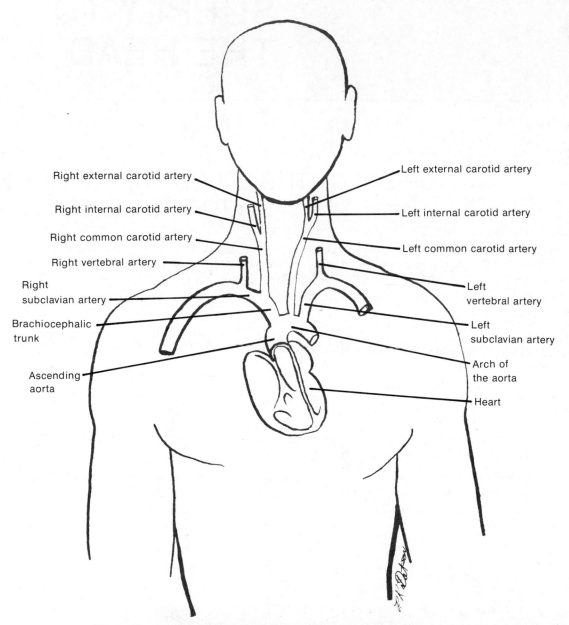

Figure 11–1. Origin of the carotid and vertebral arteries. (Modified from Jacob and Francone: Structure and Function in Man. 3rd Ed. Philadelphia, W. B. Saunders Co.)

QUESTION
3

The brachiocephalic trunk is given off the *right/left* (circle one) part of the ascending aorta.

ANSWER   right

The left common carotid and left subclavian arteries arise from the _____ of the aorta.

arch

The right common carotid artery and the right subclavian artery are formed from a bifurcation of the _____ trunk.

brachiocephalic

The vertebral arteries are branches of the _____ arteries.

subclavian

The vertebral arteries pass through transverse foramina to enter the foramen _____.

magnum

Using the Word Bank, fill in the names of the numbered structures on the diagram, page 432, in the corresponding numbered labels that follow.

Word Bank
ascending aorta
arch of the aorta
brachiocephalic trunk
left common carotid artery
right common carotid artery
left external carotid artery
right external carotid artery
left internal carotid artery
right internal carotid artery
left subclavian artery
right subclavian artery
left vertebral artery
right vertebral artery

Labels
1. _____
2. _____
3. _____
4. _____
5. _____
6. _____
7. _____

8. _____
9. _____
10. _____
11. _____
12. _____
13. _____

ANSWER   Check your labels with those on Figure 11–1.

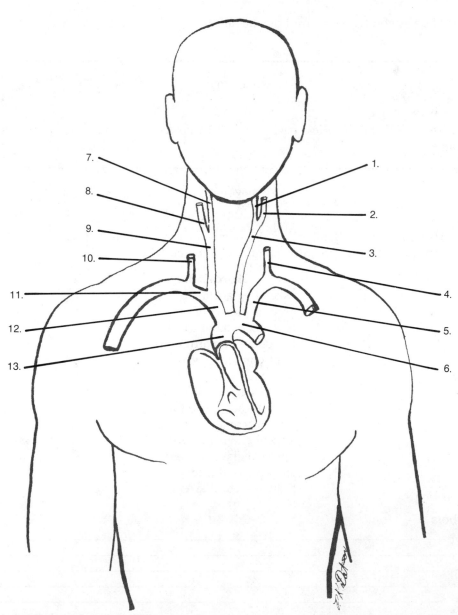

(Modified from Jacob and Francone: Structure and Function in Man. 3rd Ed. Philadelphia, W. B. Saunders Co.)

THE COMMON CAROTID ARTERIES   ITEM 3

Figure 11–2 shows the course of the right common carotid artery. The common carotid ascends in the neck from the level of the sternoclavicular joint to the superior border of the thyroid cartilage, where it bifurcates into internal and external carotid arteries. No branches are given off the common carotid artery in the neck.

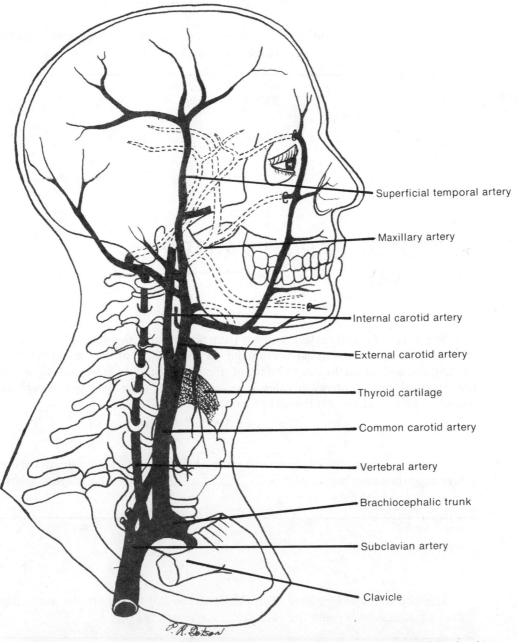

— Superficial temporal artery

— Maxillary artery

—Internal carotid artery

—External carotid artery

—Thyroid cartilage

—Common carotid artery

—Vertebral artery

—Brachiocephalic trunk

—Subclavian artery

— Clavicle

Figure 11–2. Course of the right common carotid artery. (Redrawn and modified from Jacob and Francone: Structure and Function in Man. 3rd Ed. Philadelphia, W. B. Saunders Co.)

Also in Figure 11–2 observe the vertebral artery, which, together with the internal carotid artery, supplies the brain.

QUESTION
9

The common carotid arteries begin at the _____ joint and extend to the upper level of the _____ cartilage.

ANSWER

sternoclavicular . . . thyroid

QUESTION
10

The common carotid artery divides into internal and external carotid arteries at the level of the *sternoclavicular joint/thyroid cartilage* (circle one).

ANSWER

thyroid cartilage

ITEM 4   EXTERNAL CAROTID ARTERY: PATHWAY

The external carotid artery ascends from a point near the upper border of the thyroid cartilage, running posteromedial to the ramus of the mandible, and passing through, or on the deep surface of, the parotid gland. At the parotid gland, the external carotid artery divides into its terminal branches, the *superficial temporal* and *maxillary* arteries, shown in Figure 11–2.

QUESTION
11

The external carotid artery runs from the bifurcation of the common carotid artery near the upper border of the _____ cartilage upward through the _____ gland.

ANSWER

thyroid . . . parotid

QUESTION
12

The two terminal branches of the external carotid artery are the superficial _____ artery and the _____ artery.

ANSWER

temporal . . . maxillary

THE EXTERNAL CAROTID ARTERY: MAIN BRANCHES

ITEM 5

In its course, the external carotid artery gives off eight main branches, which are illustrated in Figure 11–3. Four of these branches, the *superior thyroid,* the *lingual,* the *ascending pharyngeal,* and the *facial* arteries, arise in the carotid triangle of the neck, just above the point of bifurcation.

The two posterior branches of the external carotid are the *occipital* artery,

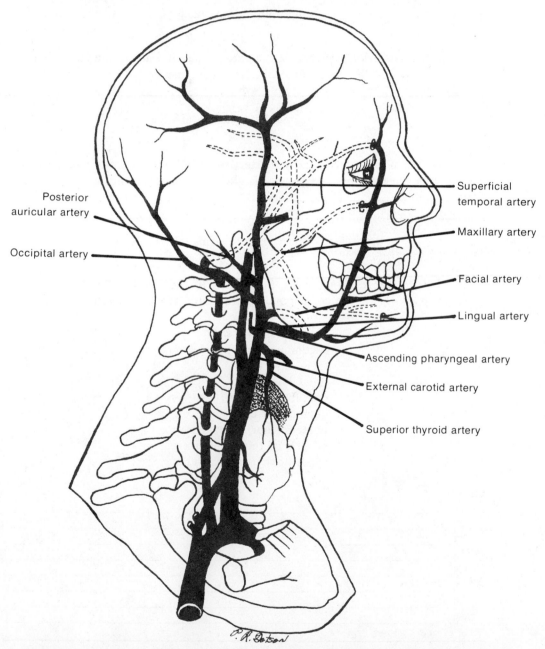

Figure 11–3. Main branches of the external carotid artery. (Redrawn and modified from Jacob and Francone: Structure and Function in Man. 3rd Ed. Philadelphia, W. B. Saunders Co.)

which arises at the level of the hyoid bone, and the *posterior auricular* artery, which arises below the ear.

The terminal branches of the external carotid artery are the *maxillary* and *superficial temporal* arteries mentioned in Item 4. These branches are given off deep to the neck of the mandible.

QUESTION
13

The two terminal branches of the external carotid artery are the superficial _____ artery and the _____ artery.

ANSWER

temporal . . . maxillary

QUESTION
14

The two posterior branches of the external carotid artery are the _____ _____ artery and the posterior _____ artery.

ANSWER

occipital . . . auricular

QUESTION
15

Branches of the external carotid artery given off in the carotid triangle of the neck include the superior _____ branch, the ascending _____ branch, and the _____ and _____ branches.

ANSWER

thyroid . . . pharyngeal . . . lingual . . . facial

QUESTION
16

Using the Word Bank, write the names of the numbered arteries on the diagram, page 437, in the corresponding numbered labels that follow.

Word Bank
ascending pharyngeal artery
facial artery
lingual artery
maxillary artery
occipital artery
posterior auricular artery
superficial temporal artery
superior thyroid artery

Labels

1. _____
2. _____
3. _____
4. _____
5. _____
6. _____
7. _____
8. _____

ANSWER

Check your labels with those in Figure 11–3.

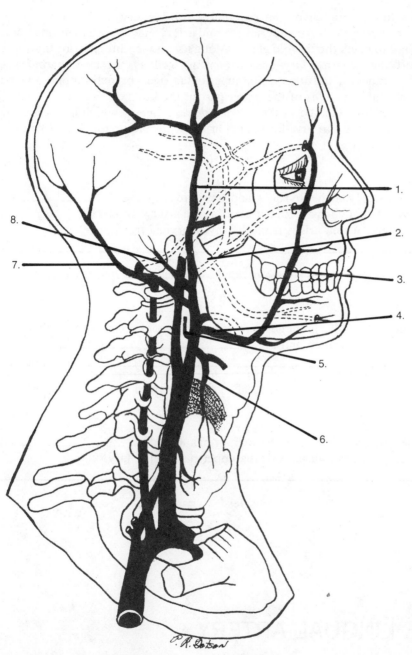

1.

2.

3.

4.

5.

6.

7.

8.

(Redrawn and modified from Jacob and Francone: Structure and Function in Man. 3rd Ed. Philadelphia, W. B. Saunders Co.)

ITEM 6 — THE SUPERIOR THYROID ARTERY

The lowest branch of the external carotid artery is the superior thyroid artery. In Figure 11–4 the superior thyroid artery may be seen curving anteriorly downward to reach the thyroid gland. Along its course, the superior thyroid artery gives off the *superior laryngeal artery* as well as the *cricothyroid branch,* muscular branches, and others. The superior laryngeal branch supplies the mucous membranes and muscles of the upper part of the larynx.

Figure 11–4 also shows the *inferior thyroid artery,* which is not a branch of the external carotid artery, but which arises from the *thyrocervical* trunk of the subclavian artery.

QUESTION 17

Blood supply to the thyroid gland is provided by the _____ thyroid artery, which branches off the external carotid artery, and by the _____ thyroid artery, which arises from the thyrocervical trunk.

ANSWER

superior . . . inferior

QUESTION 18

Besides muscular branches, the superior thyroid artery gives off the superior _____ branch and the _____ branch.

ANSWER

laryngeal . . . cricothyroid

QUESTION 19

The superior laryngeal branch brings blood to _____ and to _____ membranes of the upper part of the larynx.

ANSWER

muscles . . . mucous

ITEM 7 — THE LINGUAL ARTERY

The *lingual artery* arises from the external carotid artery at the level of the hyoid bone. Locate this branch on Figure 11–5. The lingual artery runs forward and upward deep to the suprahyoid muscles and the submandibular gland, giving off branches to muscles during its approach to the tongue.

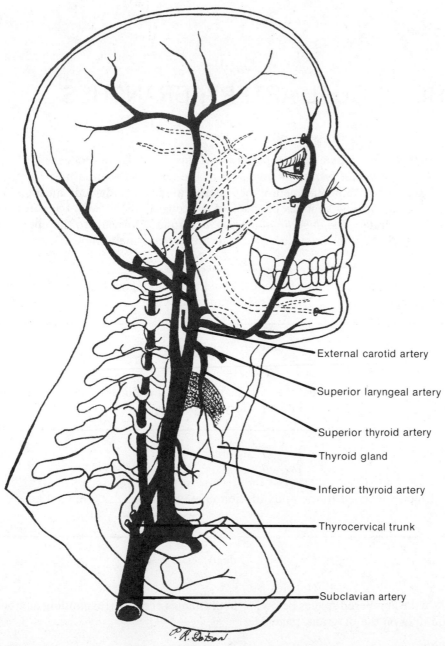

External carotid artery

Superior laryngeal artery

Superior thyroid artery

Thyroid gland

Inferior thyroid artery

Thyrocervical trunk

Subclavian artery

Figure 11–4. The superior and inferior thyroid arteries. (Redrawn and modified from Jacob and Francone: Structure and Function in Man. 3rd Ed. Philadelphia, W. B. Saunders Co.)

QUESTION
20

In its forward course to the tongue, the lingual artery travels deep to the _____ gland and to the _____ muscles.

ANSWER

submandibular . . . suprahyoid

ITEM
8

THE LINGUAL ARTERY: BRANCHES

In Figure 11–5, examine the pathways of the three main branches of the lingual artery. A *sublingual branch* is given off at the floor of the mouth to supply the sublingual gland, mucous membranes of the area, and adjacent muscles. The *dorsal lingual branch* supplies the back of the tongue, the tonsils, the soft palate, and the epiglottis. The *deep lingual branch* continues forward to the apex of the tongue along the inferior surface, deep to the mucous membrane.

QUESTION
21

Besides supplying the sublingual gland, the sublingual branch of the lingual artery supplies _____ membranes and _____ of the area.

ANSWER

mucous . . . muscles

QUESTION
22

The back of the tongue, the soft palate, and the epiglottis receive blood supply from the _____ lingual artery.

ANSWER

dorsal

QUESTION
23

Blood is carried to the apex of the tongue by the _____ lingual artery.

ANSWER

deep

QUESTION
24

In the numbered spaces below, fill in the names of the corresponding numbered structures on the diagram, page 442.

Labels

1. _____ artery
2. _____ artery
3. _____ artery
4. _____ artery

ANSWER

Check your labels with those in Figure 11–5.

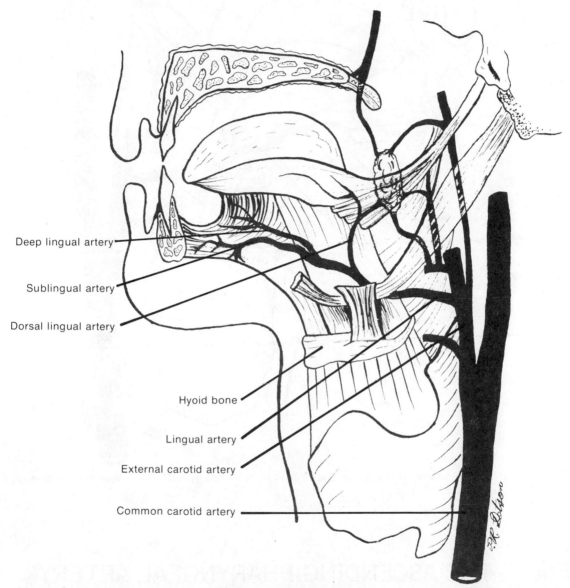

Deep lingual artery

Sublingual artery

Dorsal lingual artery

Hyoid bone

Lingual artery

External carotid artery

Common carotid artery

Figure 11–5.   Branches of the lingual artery. (Redrawn from Woodburne: Essentials of Human Anatomy. 4th Ed. New York, Oxford University Press.)

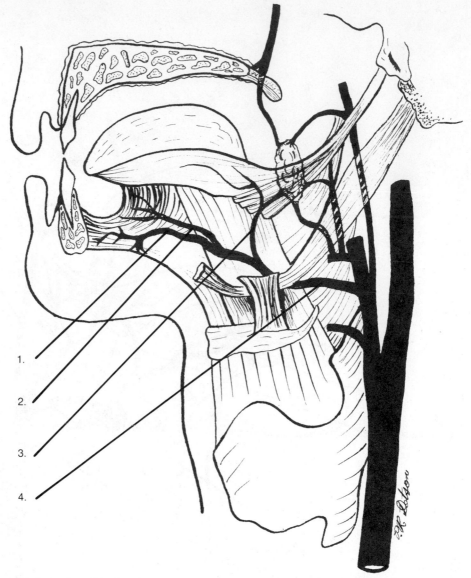

1.

2.

3.

4.

(Redrawn from Woodburne: Essentials of Human Anatomy. 4th Ed. New York, Oxford University Press.)

ITEM 9   THE ASCENDING PHARYNGEAL ARTERY

Examine Figure 11–6 and note the *ascending pharyngeal* artery arising from the medial side of the external carotid artery near its origin. It ascends superiorly to the lateral wall of the superior pharyngeal constrictor muscle. The ascending pharyngeal artery supplies the muscular wall of the pharynx and the deep muscles of the vertebral column. A *palatine branch*, given off above the superior pharyngeal constrictor muscle, goes to the soft palate and the palatine tonsil.

The point of origin of the ascending pharyngeal artery is the medial side of the _____ _____ artery.

external carotid

Structures supplied by the ascending pharyngeal artery include deep muscles of the _____ column and the muscular wall of the _____.

vertebral . . . pharynx

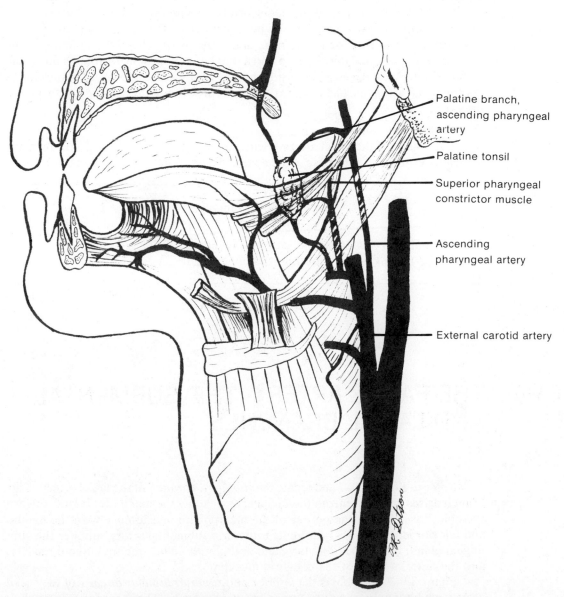

Palatine branch, ascending pharyngeal artery

Palatine tonsil

Superior pharyngeal constrictor muscle

Ascending pharyngeal artery

External carotid artery

Figure 11–6. The ascending pharyngeal artery and its palatine branch. (Redrawn from Woodburne: Essentials of Human Anatomy. 4th Ed. New York, Oxford University Press.)

QUESTION
27

The palatine branch of the ascending pharyngeal artery supplies the _____ palate and the _____ tonsil.

ANSWER

soft . . . palatine

ITEM 10

THE FACIAL ARTERY: PATHWAY

The *facial artery* branches off the external carotid below the angle of the mandible. Notice the course and branches of the facial artery shown in Figure 11–7. Arching forward and upward, the facial artery curves over the lower border of the mandible and follows a tortuous oblique route across the face, terminating as the *angular artery* at the base of the nose and eyes. As it crosses the mandible, the facial artery is covered only by skin and a thin layer of muscle, so that its pulse can be felt. Sometimes, it can be felt inside the oral cavity in the upper part of the cheek. As the facial artery ascends, it runs more deeply among the muscles of facial expression.

QUESTION
28

The course of the facial artery begins below the _____ of the mandible and terminates at the base of the nose and eyes as the _____ artery.

ANSWER

angle . . . angular

QUESTION
29

The pulse of the facial artery can be palpated as it crosses the _____ and can be felt inside the mouth in the upper _____.

ANSWER

mandible . . . cheek

ITEM 11

THE FACIAL ARTERY: THE SUBMENTAL AND LABIAL BRANCHES

Refer to Figure 11–7 and locate the *submental branch* of the facial artery. This branch arises anteriorly from the facial artery below the mandible. It runs toward the chin, turning over the border of the mandible to anastomose with the mental and inferior labial arteries. Along its route, the submental artery supplies the sublingual gland, the submandibular gland and lymph nodes, the mylohyoid muscle, and the anterior belly of the digastric muscle.

Figure 11–7 also shows the *inferior* and *superior labial branches* of the facial artery, which supply lower and upper lips, respectively. These branches run below and above the mouth, deep to the orbicularis oris muscle.

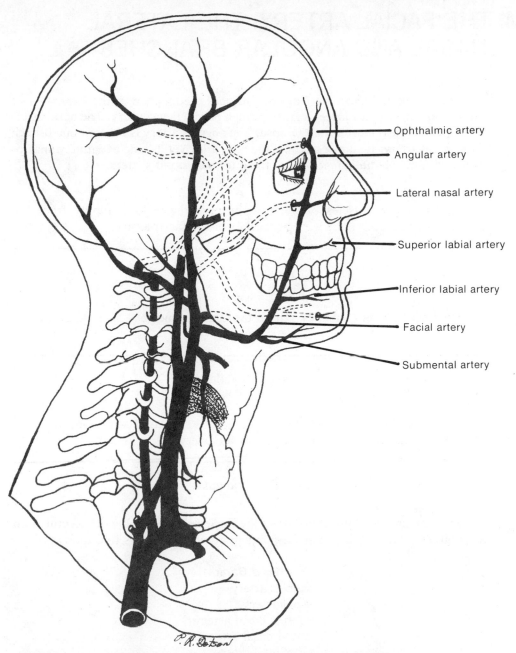

Figure 11–7. Course and main branches of the facial artery. (Redrawn and modified from Jacob and Francone: Structure and Function in Man. 3rd Ed. Philadelphia, W. B. Saunders Co.)

Muscles supplied by the submental artery include the _____ muscle and the anterior belly of the _____ muscle.

QUESTION
30

---

mylohyoid . . . digastric

ANSWER

Both inferior and superior labial branches of the facial artery run deep to the _____ _____ muscle.

QUESTION
31

---

orbicularis oris

ANSWER

ITEM   THE FACIAL ARTERY: THE LATERAL
12   NASAL AND ANGULAR BRANCHES

Look back to Figure 11–7 again, and note the location of the *lateral nasal arteries* and the *angular artery* as they branch off the facial artery. The nasal arteries supply skin and muscles of the nose. The angular artery is the terminal branch of the facial artery. It supplies skin of the nose and eyelids, and eventually anastomoses with the *ophthalmic artery* of the internal carotid system.

QUESTION
32

The skin and muscles of the nose receive their blood supply from the _____ _____ branches of the facial artery.

---

lateral nasal

QUESTION
33

The angular artery supplies skin of the _____ and the _____.

ANSWER

nose . . . eyelids

QUESTION
34

The ophthalmic branch of the _____ carotid artery anastomoses with the _____ branch of the facial artery.

ANSWER

internal . . . angular

QUESTION
35

Drawing on the Word Bank, write the names of the numbered structures on the diagram, page 447, in the corresponding numbered spaces that follow.

Word Bank
angular artery
facial artery
inferior labial artery
lateral nasal arteries
submental artery
superior labial artery

Labels
1. _____
2. _____
3. _____
4. _____
5. _____
6. _____

ANSWER

Check your labels with Figure 11–7.

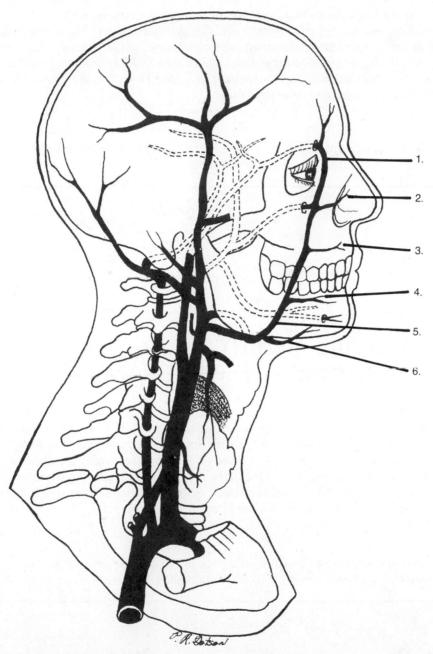

1.

2.

3.

4.

5.

6.

(Redrawn and modified from Jacob and Francone: Structure and Function in Man. 3rd Ed. Philadelphia, W. B. Saunders Co.)

ITEM
13

THE FACIAL ARTERY: BRANCHES
IN THE NECK

Figure 11–8 shows two branches of the facial artery which do not reach the face, the *ascending palatine branch* and the *tonsillar branch*. The ascending palatine artery supplies muscles and mucous membranes of the pharynx. The tonsillar artery is the main supply to the palatine tonsil. The facial artery also gives off other branches in the neck which do not appear in Figure 11–8, notably the submandibular, sublingual, and muscular branches.

QUESTION
36

The ascending palatine artery supplies mucous membranes and muscles of the _____; the tonsillar artery supplies the _____ tonsil.

ANSWER

pharynx . . . palatine

ITEM
14

THE FACIAL ARTERY:
ANASTOMOSES OF THE BRANCHES

Branches of the facial artery on opposite sides of the face anastomose (connect) freely with each other as well as with branches of the deeper maxillary artery. Consequently, when a branch is severed or ligated, establishing a collateral blood supply is usually not a problem. One of the more important anastomoses, that of the angular artery with the ophthalmic artery, was mentioned in Item 12. It connects the external carotid system with the internal carotid system.

QUESTION
37

The functional and clinical significance of the anastomoses of the facial arteries is that an alternate pathway is readily established if an artery is _____.

ANSWER

cut (or ligated)

QUESTION
38

The angular artery of the _____ carotid system anastomoses with the ophthalmic artery of the _____ carotid system.

ANSWER

external . . . internal

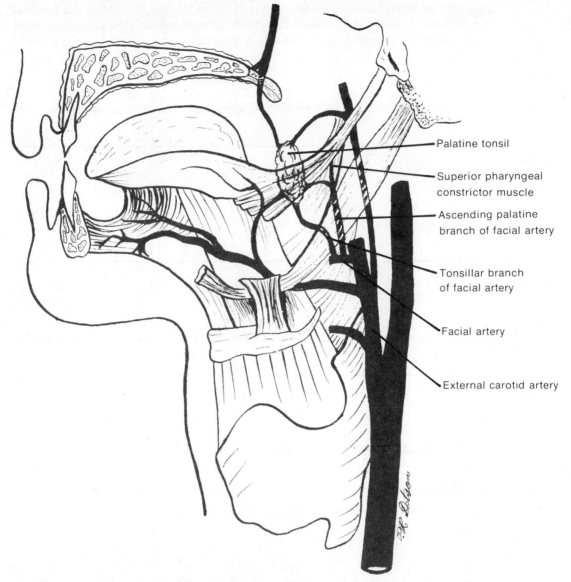

Figure 11 –8. Ascending palatine and tonsillar branches of the facial artery. (Redrawn from Woodburne: Essentials of Human Anatomy. 4th Ed. New York, Oxford University Press.)

THE FACIAL VEIN   ITEM 15

The *facial vein* is the companion vein to the facial artery. Although arterial supply to the forehead does not come from the facial artery, the *supratrochlear* and *supraorbital veins* which drain the forehead form the beginning of the facial vein. Medial to the eye, the supratrochlear and supraorbital veins join to form the *angular vein*. At the side of the nose, the angular vein becomes the facial vein proper, continuing downward into the neck to terminate by joining the internal jugular vein. In its downward pathway, the facial vein parallels the ascending facial artery, and its contributing branches correspond to the branches of the facial artery.

QUESTION
39

The supratrochlear and supraorbital veins carry the venous drainage of the
_____.

ANSWER

forehead

QUESTION
40

The vein medial to the eye is called the _____ vein.

ANSWER

angular

QUESTION
41

The site where the angular vein becomes the facial vein proper is the side of the _____.

ANSWER

nose

QUESTION
42

The termination of the facial vein is in the _____ _____ vein.

ANSWER

internal jugular

ITEM
16
THE OCCIPITAL AND POSTERIOR AURICULAR ARTERIES

The *occipital artery* and the *posterior auricular artery* arise posteriorly from the external carotid artery, as can be seen in Figure 11–9. The occipital artery arises slightly superior to the facial artery, and runs obliquely superiorly and posteriorly to supply the sternocleidomastoid muscle, the deep muscles of the neck, and the posterior part of the scalp.

The posterior auricular artery arises in the retromandibular fossa and ascends behind the ear. It supplies the tympanic cavity, the outer ear, and the adjacent scalp.

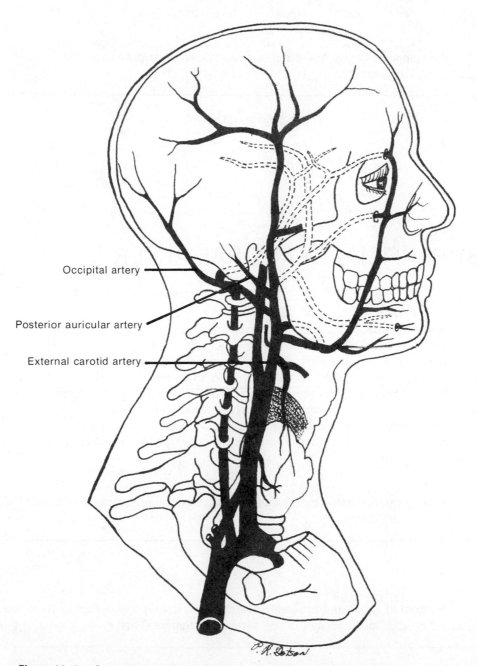

Occipital artery

Posterior auricular artery

External carotid artery

Figure 11–9. Occipital and posterior auricular arteries. (Redrawn and modified from Jacob and Francone: Structure and Function in Man. 3rd Ed. Philadelphia, W. B. Saunders Co.)

QUESTION
43

The occipital artery supplies the posterior part of the _____, deep muscles of the _____, and the _____ muscle.

ANSWER

scalp . . . neck . . . sternocleidomastoid

QUESTION
44

The tympanic cavity and outer ear receive blood supply from the _____ _____ artery.

ANSWER

posterior auricular

ITEM 17   SUPERFICIAL TEMPORAL ARTERY

The two terminal branches of the external carotid artery, shown in Figure 11–10, are the *superficial temporal artery* and the *maxillary artery*. The superficial temporal artery ascends through the parotid gland immediately in front of the ear. Its pulse can be felt as it crosses the posterior border of the zygomatic arch. The superficial temporal artery gives off, at the upper level of the parotid gland, the *transverse facial artery,* which runs anteriorly forward to supply the parotid gland and the masseter muscle. The superficial temporal artery also sends branches to the external ear, the temporomandibular joint, and the scalp above the ear.

QUESTION
45

Running anterior to the ear, the superficial temporal artery passes through the _____ gland.

ANSWER

parotid

QUESTION
46

The parotid gland and masseter muscle derive their blood supply from the _____ facial branch of the superficial temporal artery.

ANSWER

transverse

QUESTION
47

The temporomandibular joint receives its blood supply from the _____ _____ _____ artery.

ANSWER

superficial temporal

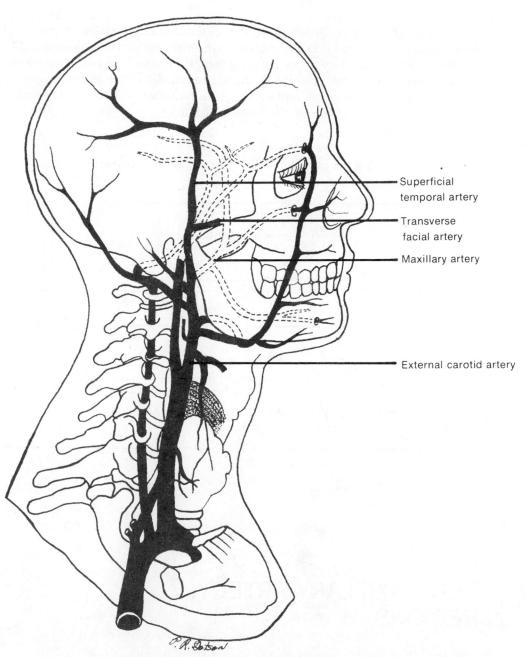

Superficial
temporal artery

Transverse
facial artery

Maxillary artery

External carotid artery

Figure 11–10. Terminal branches of the external carotid artery. (Redrawn and modified from Jacob and Francone: Structure and Function in Man. 3rd Ed. Philadelphia, W. B. Saunders Co.)

ITEM 18
THE MAXILLARY ARTERY: PATHWAY

The maxillary artery arises from the external carotid artery at the level of the neck of the mandible. Running between the mandible and the sphenomandibular ligament, the maxillary artery continues anteriorly and superiorly through the infratemporal fossa. After crossing the infratemporal fossa, the artery enters the pterygopalatine fossa, where it forms its terminal branches. The terminal branches emerge onto the face through the infraorbital foramen.

QUESTION 48

Prior to entering the pterygopalatine fossa, the maxillary artery crosses the _____ fossa.

ANSWER

infratemporal

QUESTION 49

The maxillary artery forms its terminal branches in the (circle one) *infratemporal/pterygopalatine* fossa.

ANSWER

pterygopalatine

QUESTION 50

The maxillary artery emerges onto the face through the (circle one) *infraorbital foramen/pterygopalatine fissure*.

ANSWER

infraorbital foramen

ITEM 19
THE MAXILLARY ARTERY: REGIONS

The numerous branches of the maxillary artery supply parts of the ear, the maxillary teeth and jaws, the muscles of mastication, the palate, the dura mater, and part of the nasal cavity. The extensive maxillary branches can be learned more easily if they are assigned arbitrarily to three specific regions: the mandibular, the pterygoid, and the pterygopalatine. Figure 11–11 shows the position of each of

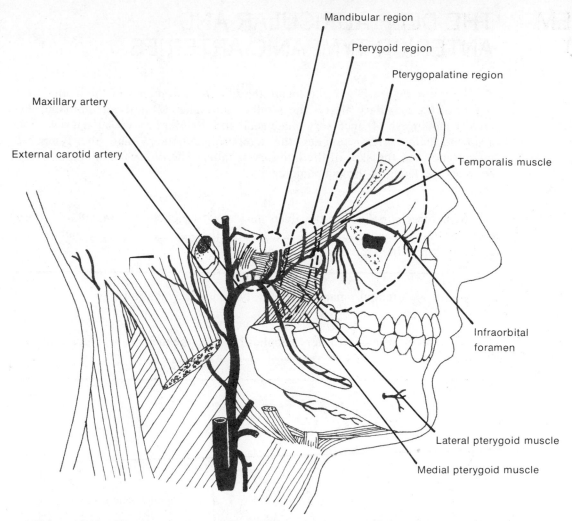

Figure 11-11. The three regions of the maxillary artery. (Redrawn from Romanes (Ed.): Cunningham's Textbook of Anatomy. 10th Ed. New York, Oxford University Press.)

these three areas. The mandibular part of the maxillary artery is behind the neck of the mandible; the pterygoid part, in the infratemporal fossa; the pterygopalatine part, in the pterygopalatine fossa.

The three parts of the maxillary artery are
1. the _____ area behind the neck of the _____
2. the _____ area in the _____ fossa
3. the _____ area in the _____ fossa

QUESTION
51

1. mandibular . . . mandible
2. pterygoid . . . infratemporal
3. pterygopalatine . . . pterygopalatine

ANSWER

ITEM 20

THE DEEP AURICULAR AND ANTERIOR TYMPANIC ARTERIES

Examine Figure 11–12 and locate the five main branches of the mandibular region of the maxillary artery: the (1) deep auricular, (2) anterior tympanic, (3) middle meningeal, (4) accessory meningeal, and (5) inferior alveolar arteries. The *deep auricular artery* supplies the temporomandibular joint, the tympanic membrane, and the skin of the auditory meatus. The *anterior tympanic artery* supplies the lining of the tympanic cavity.

QUESTION
52

Structures supplied by the deep auricular branch of the maxillary artery include the _____ joint, the _____ membrane, and the skin of the _____ meatus.

ANSWER

temporomandibular . . . tympanic . . . auditory

QUESTION
53

The anterior tympanic artery supplies blood to the membrane which lines the tympanic _____.

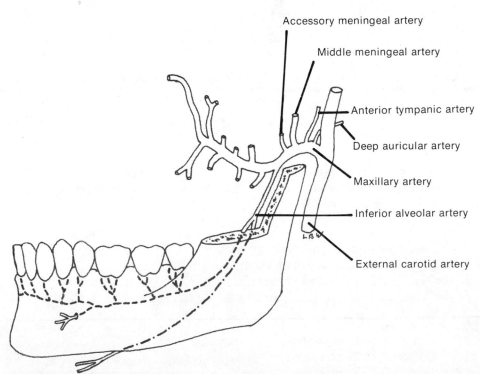

Figure 11–12.   Main branches of the mandibular area of the maxillary artery, seen from the left side, with a portion of the mandible removed.

cavity   *ANSWER*

Using the Word Bank, write the names of the numbered structures on the   QUESTION
accompanying diagram in the corresponding numbered spaces that follow.   **54**

Word Bank

accessory meningeal artery
anterior tympanic artery
deep auricular artery
inferior alveolar artery
maxillary artery
middle meningeal artery

Labels

1. _____
2. _____
3. _____
4. _____
5. _____
6. _____

Check your labels with Figure 11–12.   *ANSWER*

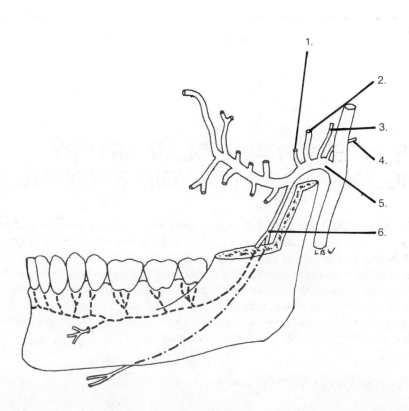

ITEM 21

THE MIDDLE AND ACCESSORY MENINGEAL ARTERIES

Return to Figure 11–12 and locate the middle and the accessory meningeal arteries. The *middle meningeal artery* runs lateral to the sphenomandibular ligament between two roots of the auriculotemporal nerve. It passes through the foramen spinosum along with the meningeal branch of the mandibular nerve. Inside the cranial cavity, the middle meningeal artery branches extensively, forming grooves in the undersurface of the dura mater, which it supplies, and in the adjacent bone. It also sends branches to the tympanic cavity.

The *accessory meningeal artery* travels through the foramen ovale to supply the trigeminal ganglion and adjacent dura.

QUESTION
55

The middle meningeal artery supplies the _____ _____ of most of the cranial cavity, whereas the accessory meningeal artery supplies dura mater adjacent to the _____ ganglion itself.

ANSWER

dura mater . . . trigeminal

QUESTION
56

The middle meningeal artery enters the cranium through the foramen _____; the accessory meningeal artery, through the foramen _____.

ANSWER

spinosum . . . ovale

ITEM 22

THE INFERIOR ALVEOLAR ARTERY: LINGUAL AND MYLOHYOID BRANCHES

In the mandibular region of the maxillary artery are three main branches of the *inferior alveolar artery:* the *mylohyoid, mental,* and *incisive arteries.* On Figure 11–13, follow the course of the inferior alveolar artery as it descends, in company with the inferior alveolar nerve, to the mandibular fossa where it enters bone.

Near its origin, the inferior alveolar artery gives off a *lingual branch* (not shown in the drawing) which runs with the lingual nerve to the tongue. A second branch is the mylohyoid branch, which travels medial to the mandible with the mylohyoid nerve to supply the mylohyoid muscle.

QUESTION
57

The lingual and mylohyoid arteries travel with _____ of the same names.

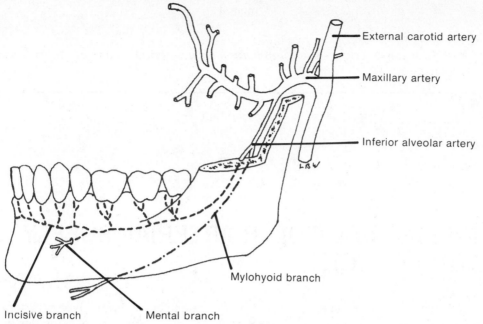

External carotid artery

Maxillary artery

Inferior alveolar artery

Mylohyoid branch

Incisive branch   Mental branch

Figure 11–13.   Branches of the inferior alveolar artery. Intraosseous portions are indicated by dotted lines.

nerves   *ANSWER*

The lingual artery supplies the _____; the mylohyoid artery   QUESTION
supplies the mylohyoid _____.   **58**

tongue . . . muscle   *ANSWER*

THE INFERIOR ALVEOLAR ARTERY: ITEM
MENTAL AND INCISIVE BRANCHES 23

Look at Figure 11–13 again, and locate the mental and incisive branches of the inferior alveolar artery. At the mental foramen, the *mental branch* leaves the main trunk to supply skin of the chin and mucous membranes of the lower lip. Beyond the mental foramen, the continuation of the inferior alveolar artery within the mandible is the *incisive artery*. The incisive branch on one side, together with the incisive branch of the other side, forms a continuous branch to the anterior mandibular teeth.

Skin of the chin and mucous membrane of the lower lip receive blood supply   QUESTION
from the _____ branch of the inferior alveolar artery.   **59**

ANSWER   mental

QUESTION   The incisive artery is a *continuation/branch* (circle one) of the inferior
60   alveolar artery.

ANSWER   continuation

ITEM 24   INFERIOR ALVEOLAR ARTERIAL SUPPLY TO THE TEETH

Running in the mandibular canal within bone, the inferior alveolar artery gives off branches to each of the lower teeth, as does the accompanying nerve. Branches are also given off to the alveolar process and to marrow spaces of bone. Two types of vessels extend upward from the inferior alveolar artery to the teeth and adjacent structures: *dental arteries* and *alveolar arteries*.

Dental arteries enter the teeth through apical foramina, ascend the root canals, and supply dental pulp and a small area of the periodontal ligament. Alveolar arteries ascend through canals in septa at the roots of the teeth. Branches of the alveolar arteries supply the periodontal ligament and the buccal and lingual gingiva.

QUESTION   The inferior alveolar artery runs within bone in the _____ canal.
61

ANSWER   mandibular

QUESTION   The two types of arteries which extend upward to the teeth from the
62   inferior alveolar artery are _____ arteries and _____ arteries.

ANSWER   dental . . . alveolar

QUESTION   Arteries which ascend through canals in septa at the roots of the teeth are the
63   _____ arteries; those which ascend through apical foramina and through
the root canals are _____ arteries.

ANSWER   alveolar . . . dental

THE MAXILLARY ARTERY: BRANCHES OF THE PTERYGOID AREA

ITEM 25

The second region of the maxillary artery is the pterygoid area. Branches of the maxillary artery in this area are shown in Figure 11–14. The pterygoid portion runs through the infratemporal fossa, either lateral or medial to the lateral pterygoid muscle. Each of the six branches of this region travels with a branch of the mandibular nerve of the same name: (1) masseteric, (2) posterior deep temporal, (3) anterior deep temporal, (4) lateral pterygoid, (5) medial pterygoid, or (6) buccal.

The pterygoid portion of the maxillary artery occupies the *pterygopalatine/infratemporal* (circle one) fossa.

QUESTION **64**

infratemporal

ANSWER

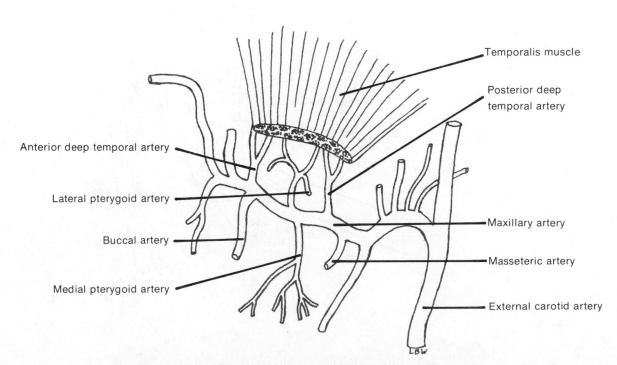

Figure 11–14. Branches of the pterygoid region of the maxillary artery.

Labels: Temporalis muscle; Posterior deep temporal artery; Maxillary artery; Masseteric artery; External carotid artery; Anterior deep temporal artery; Lateral pterygoid artery; Buccal artery; Medial pterygoid artery.

QUESTION
65

Using the Word Bank, write the names of the numbered arteries on the accompanying diagram in the corresponding numbered blanks.

Word Bank

anterior deep temporal artery
buccal artery
lateral pterygoid artery
masseteric artery
medial pterygoid artery
posterior deep temporal artery

ANSWER

Labels

1. _____
2. _____
3. _____
4. _____
5. _____
6. _____

Check your labels with Figure 11–14.

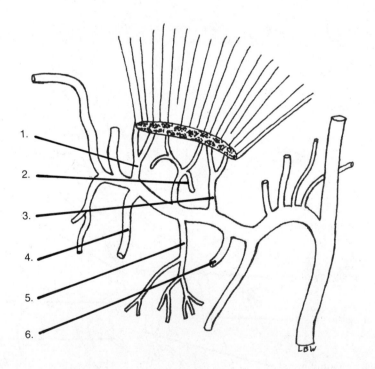

THE MASSETERIC AND DEEP TEMPORAL ARTERIES

ITEM 26

Look back to Figure 11–14 and notice the location of the *masseteric artery*. This branch of the maxillary artery passes laterally through the mandibular notch to reach the masseter muscle which it supplies. The *posterior* and *anterior deep temporal arteries*, and an occasional *middle deep temporal artery*, arch over the infratemporal crest to supply the temporalis muscle. The masseteric and deep temporal arteries travel with nerves having the same names.

The masseteric artery distributes with the _____ nerve to the masseter muscle.

QUESTION 66

---

masseteric

ANSWER

The temporalis muscle receives its blood supply from the anterior and posterior _____ _____ arteries.

QUESTION 67

---

deep temporal

ANSWER

THE PTERYGOID REGION: PTERYGOID AND BUCCAL BRANCHES

ITEM 27

A variable number of *pterygoid branches* supply blood to the medial and lateral pterygoid muscles. Two such branches appear in Figure 11–14. Also shown is the *buccal artery*, which travels with the buccal branch of the mandibular nerve to supply the buccinator muscle as well as skin and mucous membrane of the cheek.

Pterygoid branches of the _____ artery supply the medial and lateral pterygoid muscles.

QUESTION 68

---

maxillary

ANSWER

Skin and mucous membrane of the cheek receive their blood supply from the _____ artery.

QUESTION 69

---

buccal

ANSWER

The buccal artery supplies the _____ muscle.

QUESTION 70

---

buccinator

ANSWER

ITEM 28

THE MAXILLARY ARTERY: THE PTERYGOPALATINE REGION

The third part of the maxillary artery, the pterygopalatine region, contains branches which supply the maxillae, maxillary teeth, nasal cavities, and palate. The maxillary artery terminates on the infraorbital region of the cheek. All branches of the maxillary artery in the pterygopalatine area distribute with branches of the maxillary division of the trigeminal nerve (V).

The six principal branches of the pterygopalatine area appear in Figure 11–15: (1) posterior superior alveolar, (2) infraorbital, (3) descending palatine, (4) artery of the pterygoid canal, (5) pharyngeal, and (6) sphenopalatine branches. Locate each of these branches on the drawing.

QUESTION 71

The maxillary artery exits onto the face at the _____ foramen and terminates in the _____ region of the cheek.

ANSWER

infraorbital . . . infraorbital

QUESTION 72

Branches of the maxillary artery in the pterygopalatine area travel with branches of the _____ division of the _____ nerve.

ANSWER

maxillary . . . trigeminal

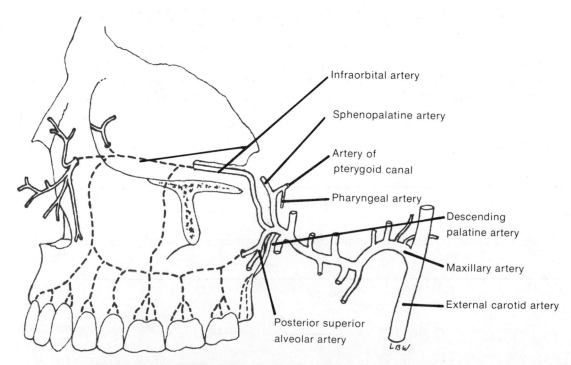

Figure 11–15.   Main branches of the pterygopalatine region of the maxillary artery, seen from the left side. Intraosseous portions are indicated by dotted lines.

The mandibular teeth receive blood from vessels which branch off the maxillary artery in the _____ area; the maxillary teeth, from vessels which branch off in the _____ area.

---

mandibular . . . pterygopalatine

Drawing on the Word Bank, write the names of the numbered arteries on the accompanying diagram in the corresponding numbered labels.

Word Bank

artery of pterygoid canal
descending palatine artery
infraorbital artery
pharyngeal artery
posterior superior alveolar artery
pharyngeal artery

Labels

1. _____
2. _____
3. _____
4. _____
5. _____
6. _____

Check your labels with Figure 11–15.

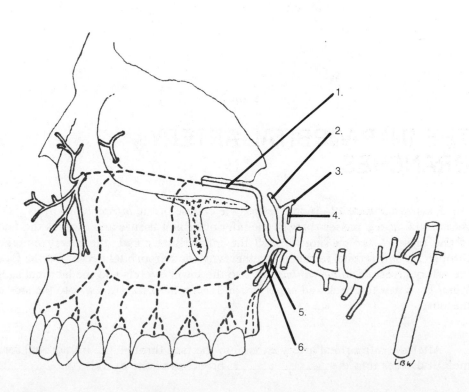

LBW

ITEM 29

THE POSTERIOR SUPERIOR ALVEOLAR ARTERY

Re-examine Figure 11–15 and take special note of the course of the *posterior superior alveolar artery*. This artery arises where the maxillary artery enters the pterygopalatine fossa. It descends the posterior surface of the maxilla with the posterior superior alveolar nerve. Branches enter the maxilla at the posterior superior alveolar canals to supply the upper molar teeth. Other branches continue downward to supply the alveolar process and the mucous membranes adjacent to the molar and premolar teeth.

The general arrangement of the blood supply to the maxillary teeth is the same as that described for the mandibular teeth in Item 24. Dental branches enter the apical foramina to supply dental pulp; alveolar branches traverse the alveolar canals to supply the periodontal ligaments and adjacent gingiva.

QUESTION 75

Besides supplying upper molar teeth, the posterior superior alveolar artery supplies the _____ process and adjacent _____ membranes.

ANSWER

alveolar . . . mucous

QUESTION 76

Dental arteries from the posterior superior alveolar artery supply the _____ _____; alveolar arteries supply the _____ ligament and _____.

ANSWER

dental pulp . . . periodontal . . . gingiva

ITEM 30

THE INFRAORBITAL ARTERY: BRANCHES

Examine Figure 11–16 and follow the course of the *infraorbital artery*. The infraorbital artery passes through the inferior orbital fissure and crosses the floor of the orbit. After passing through the infraorbital canal, the artery emerges through the infraorbital foramen together with the infraorbital nerve. On the face, the artery gives off *palpebral branches* to the lower eyelids and the lacrimal sacs, *labial branches* to cheek and upper lip, and *external nasal branches* to the side of the nose.

QUESTION 77

After the infraorbital artery exits onto the face through the infraorbital foramen, it divides into the _____ branches to the eyelids, the _____

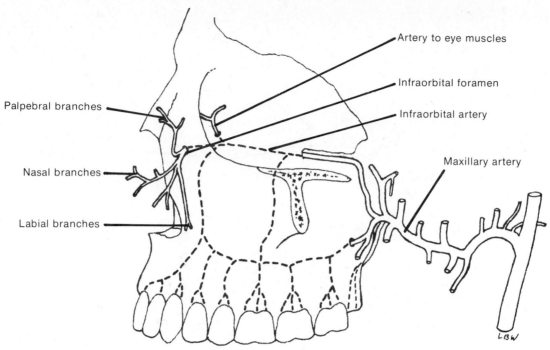

Figure 11–16. Palpebral, nasal, and labial branches of the infraorbital artery.

branches to the side of the nose, and the _____ branches to cheek and upper lip.

---

palpebral . . . nasal . . . labial

ANSWER

The infraorbital artery enters the infraorbital canal through the _____ _____ fissure and exits through the _____ foramen.

QUESTION 78

---

inferior orbital . . . infraorbital

ANSWER

THE ANTERIOR AND MIDDLE SUPERIOR ALVEOLAR ARTERIES

ITEM 31

Figure 11–17 shows the *anterior, middle,* and *posterior* superior alveolar arteries as dotted lines. Notice that the anterior and middle branches are offshoots of the infraorbital artery, given off within the infraorbital canal. The posterior artery, on the other hand, branches directly off the maxillary artery. These three branches anastomose with each other, as is apparent in Figure 11–17.

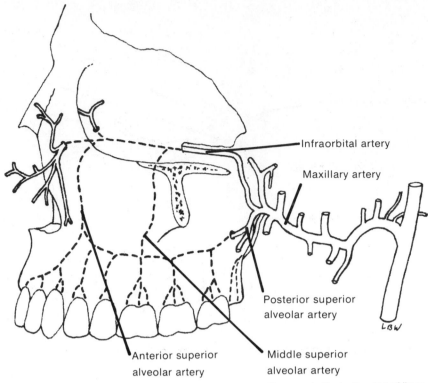

Figure 11–17.   The superior alveolar arteries. Intraosseous portions are indicated by dotted lines.

QUESTION
79

Circle the letters before the superior alveolar branches which arise from the infraorbital artery.
  A. anterior branch
  B. posterior branch
  C. middle branch

ANSWER

You should have circled A and C. The anterior superior alveolar artery, and the middle superior alveolar when present, are given off the infraorbital artery within the infraorbital canal. The posterior superior alveolar artery arises directly from the maxillary artery.

ITEM
32

THE DESCENDING PALATINE ARTERY: BRANCHES

The descending palatine artery and its branches are shown in Figure 11–18. The *descending palatine branch* runs inferiorly in the greater palatine canal and, in company with the greater palatine nerve, emerges through the greater palatine foramen as the *greater palatine artery*. It turns forward in a groove just medial to the alveolar process and runs to the incisive canal. The greater palatine branch supplies gingiva, palatine glands, and the roof of the mouth.

A *lesser palatine branch* is given off in the palatine canal, and emerges at the lesser palatine foramen to supply the soft palate and the palatine tonsil.

The descending palatine artery gives off two branches: the _____ palatine artery and the _____ palatine artery.

QUESTION
80

greater . . . lesser (in either order)

ANSWER

The soft palate is supplied with blood by the _____ palatine artery; the roof of the mouth is supplied by the _____ palatine artery.

QUESTION
81

lesser . . . greater

ANSWER

The palatine glands are supplied with blood by the _____ palatine artery; the palatine tonsil is supplied by the _____ palatine artery.

QUESTION
82

greater . . . lesser

ANSWER

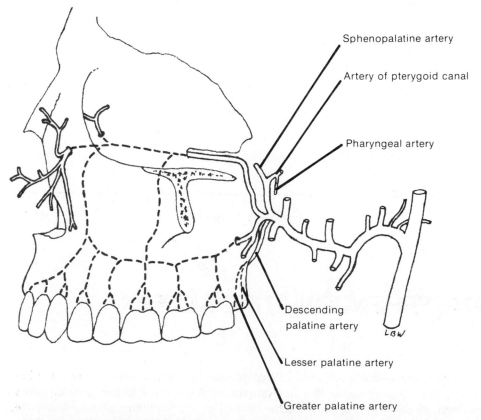

Figure 11–18. Palatine, pharyngeal, and sphenopalatine branches of the maxillary artery, and the artery of the pterygoid canal.

QUESTION
83
Gingiva is supplied by the *greater/lesser* (circle one) palatine artery.

ANSWER   greater

ITEM 33   ARTERY OF THE PTERYGOID CANAL AND THE PHARYNGEAL ARTERY

Locate the position of the artery of the pterygoid canal and the pharyngeal artery on Figure 11–18. The *artery of the pterygoid canal* runs posteriorly in a canal at the base of the pterygoid plates to supply the tympanic cavity, auditory tube, and upper area of the pharynx. Its course follows that of the nerve of the pterygoid canal.

The *pharyngeal artery* passes posteriorly to supply the auditory tube, sphenoid sinus, and upper pharynx.

QUESTION
84
Circle the letters before the structures which receive blood supply from both the pharyngeal artery and the artery of the pterygoid canal.
A. auditory tube
B. upper pharynx
C. sphenoid sinus
D. tympanic cavity

ANSWER   The letters which should have been circled are A and B.

QUESTION
85
The sphenoid sinus is supplied by the (circle one) *pharyngeal artery/artery of the pterygoid canal.*

ANSWER   pharyngeal artery

ITEM 34   THE SPHENOPALATINE ARTERY

The *sphenopalatine branch* of the maxillary artery is also shown in Figure 11–18. This branch leaves the pterygopalatine fossa through the sphenopalatine foramen, along with the nasopalatine branch of the maxillary nerve. The artery gives off the *posterior lateral nasal branches,* which supply mucosa of the lateral nasal wall and adjacent sinuses.

A *septal branch* of the sphenopalatine artery supplies the nasal septum. The septal branch crosses the roof of the sinus and runs anteriorly and inferiorly down the septal wall to the incisive foramen, where it anastomoses with terminal branches of the greater palatine artery.

The sphenopalatine artery travels with the _____ nerve.

QUESTION
86

nasopalatine

ANSWER

Branches of the sphenopalatine artery include the posterior _____ nasal branches and the _____ branch.

QUESTION
87

lateral . . . septal

ANSWER

The greater palatine artery terminates by anastomosing with (circle one) *lateral nasal/septal* branches of the sphenopalatine artery.

QUESTION
88

septal

ANSWER

BLOOD SUPPLY TO THE BRAIN   ITEM 35

Thus far this unit has dealt with the arterial supply to extracranial structures. The remaining items in this unit will deal with the blood supply to the brain. As you trace the route of the internal carotid arteries to the interior of the skull, it would be extremely helpful to have a skull at hand.

Blood supply to intracranial structures is derived from branches of two *internal carotid arteries* and two *vertebral arteries*. The internal carotid arteries originate at the bifurcation of the common carotid arteries below the angle of the mandible. Entering the carotid canal in the petrous part of the temporal bone, the internal carotid arteries extend anteromedially through the canal to ascend above the foramen lacerum. Internal carotid arteries extend anteriorly within the cavernous sinus, then at the lesser wing of the sphenoid they turn abruptly up and back between the anterior and middle clinoid processes to reach the brain.

Blood reaches the brain by way of the _____ _____ arteries and the _____ arteries.

QUESTION
89

internal carotid . . . vertebral

ANSWER

QUESTION
90

The carotid canal runs anteromedially through the petrous part of the _____ bone.

ANSWER

temporal

QUESTION
91

From the foramen lacerum, the internal carotid artery runs anteriorly through the _____ sinus.

ANSWER

cavernous

QUESTION
92

The internal carotid arteries reach the brain by turning upward and backward behind the anterior _____ process.

ANSWER

clinoid

ITEM 36
THE OPHTHALMIC AND ANTERIOR CHOROID ARTERIES

The internal carotid artery gives off no branches in the neck. All of its branches are within the cranial cavity.

The *ophthalmic artery* is given off the internal carotid artery at its point of emergence from the cavernous sinus. The *anterior choroid artery* arises just before the internal carotid divides into its terminal branches.

QUESTION
93

The first two branches of the internal carotid artery are the _____ artery and the anterior _____ artery.

ANSWER

ophthalmic . . . choroid

QUESTION
94

The ophthalmic artery arises at the site where the internal carotid artery emerges from the _____ sinus.

ANSWER

cavernous

THE ANTERIOR AND MIDDLE CEREBRAL ARTERIES

ITEM
37

As it reaches the inferior surface of the brain lateral to the optic chiasma, the internal carotid artery divides into *anterior* and *middle cerebral arteries*. Locate these branches on Figure 11–19. Anterior cerebral arteries course medially forward in the longitudinal cerebral fissure, contributing to the blood supply for the frontal lobes of the brain. Middle cerebral arteries extend laterally between the temporal and parietal lobes to the lateral sulcus, giving off branches to both temporal and parietal lobes along their course.

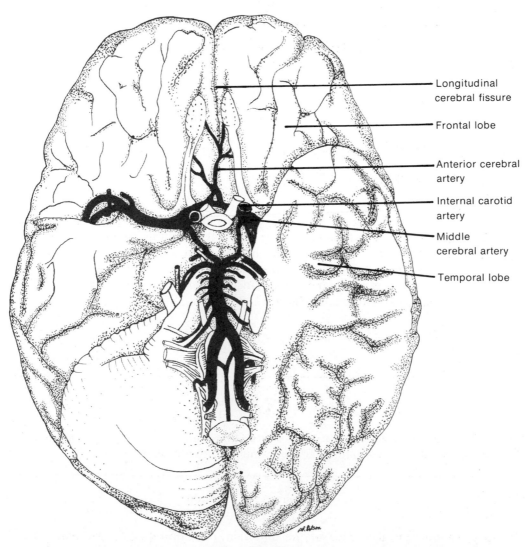

Figure 11–19. Blood supply to the brain, ventral aspect, showing anterior and middle cerebral arteries. (Redrawn from Wolf-Heidegger: Atlas of Systematic Human Anatomy. Vol. III. Basel, S. Karger AG.)

QUESTION
95

Terminal branches of the internal carotid artery are the anterior and middle _____ arteries.

ANSWER

cerebral

QUESTION
96

The frontal lobes of the brain are supplied by the _____ cerebral arteries.

ANSWER

anterior

QUESTION
97

The middle cerebral arteries supply lateral parts of the _____ and _____ lobes of the brain.

ANSWER

parietal . . . temporal (in either order)

ITEM 38   THE VERTEBRAL ARTERIES AND THE BASILAR ARTERY

Vertebral arteries branch off the subclavian artery and ascend in the neck through the transverse foramina of the cervical vertebrae. Superior to the first cervical vertebra, the vertebral arteries penetrate the atlanto-occipital membrane and enter the cranial vault in the subarachnoid space of the foramen magnum. The two vertebral arteries join to form a single *basilar artery* on the ventral surface of the pons, as can be seen in Figure 11–20.

QUESTION
98

Vertebral arteries are branches of the _____ artery.

ANSWER

subclavian

QUESTION
99

In the neck, vertebral arteries course through _____ foramina of the cervical vertebrae and enter the cranium at the foramen _____.

ANSWER

transverse . . . magnum

QUESTION
100

At the ventral surface of the midbrain, vertebral arteries terminate as a single vessel called the _____ artery.

ANSWER

basilar

THE VERTEBRAL ARTERIES: BRANCHES

ITEM 39

On Figure 11–20, locate the *anterior spinal artery* which courses medially downward from the lower part of the vertebral arteries to supply the spinal cord. *Posterior inferior cerebellar arteries* are given off laterally from the vertebral arteries to supply part of the cerebellum. Additional branches off the vertebral arteries supply the medulla.

Branches from vertebral arteries include _____ arteries, posterior inferior _____ arteries, and branches to the _____.

----

spinal . . . cerebellar . . . medulla

BRANCHES OF THE BASILAR ARTERY

ITEM 40

In Figure 11–20, notice the branches of the basilar artery as it runs forward on the lower surface of the pons. The *anterior inferior cerebellar arteries* are given off at the level of the abducens, facial, and vestibulocochlear nerves, between the pons and the medulla. *Labyrinthine branches* of the basilar artery follow the vestibulocochlear and facial nerves into the internal acoustic meatus. In addition, several small branches of the basilar artery supply the ventral and lateral surfaces of the pons.

Branches of the basilar artery given off at the level of the abducens, facial, and vestibulocochlear nerves are the (circle one)
 A. anterior inferior cerebellar arteries
 B. posterior inferior cerebellar arteries

The correct answer is A. If you look back to Figure 11–20, you will notice that the anterior inferior cerebellar arteries branch off the basilar artery, while the posterior inferior cerebellar arteries branch off the vertebral arteries before the latter join to form the basilar artery.

Labyrinthine arteries follow the course of the vestibulocochlear and facial nerves into the internal _____ meatus.

----

acoustic

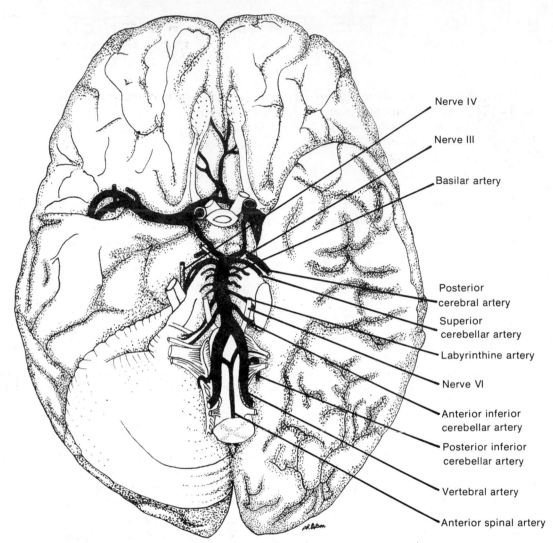

Figure 11–20.   Blood supply to the brain, ventral aspect, showing vertebral artery and branches of the basilar artery. (Redrawn from Wolf-Heidegger: Atlas of Systematic Human Anatomy. Vol. III. Basel, S. Karger AG.)

ITEM 41   THE SUPERIOR CEREBELLAR AND POSTERIOR CEREBRAL ARTERIES

Look again at Figure 11–20, and take note of the *superior cerebellar arteries,* which are given off the basilar artery just before it ends at the upper level of the pons. At this point, the superior cerebellar arteries are in close proximity to the oculomotor and trochlear nerves near the junction of the pons and the midbrain. Extending laterally around the pons, superior cerebellar arteries supply adjacent regions of the brain stem and the upper cerebellum.

Finally, in Figure 11–20, note the *posterior cerebral arteries,* which are the terminal branches of the basilar artery.

Branches of the basilar artery given off at the level of the oculomotor and trochlear nerves are the superior _____ arteries.

QUESTION
104

cerebellar

ANSWER

Posterior cerebral arteries are the terminal branches of the _____ artery.

QUESTION
105

basilar

ANSWER

Drawing on the Word Bank, write the names of the numbered arteries on the diagram, page 478, in the corresponding numbered blank labels that follow.

QUESTION
106

Word Bank
anterior cerebral artery
anterior inferior cerebellar artery
basilar artery
internal carotid artery
middle cerebral artery
posterior cerebral artery
posterior inferior cerebellar artery
spinal arteries
superior cerebellar arteries
vertebral arteries

Labels
1. _____
2. _____
3. _____
4. _____
5. _____
6. _____
7. _____
8. _____
9. _____
10. _____

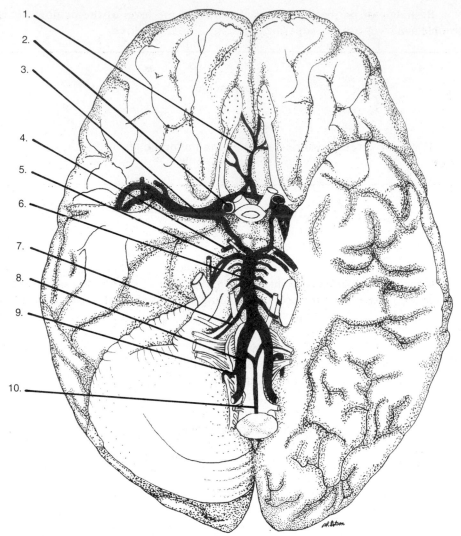

(Redrawn from Wolf-Heidegger: Atlas of Systematic Human Anatomy. Vol. III. Basel, S. Karger AG.)

ANSWER

1. anterior cerebral artery
2. internal carotid artery
3. middle cerebral artery
4. posterior cerebral artery
5. superior cerebellar artery

6. basilar artery
7. anterior inferior cerebellar artery
8. vertebral artery
9. posterior inferior cerebellar artery
10. spinal artery

ITEM 42   THE CEREBRAL ARTERIAL CIRCLE

Items 35 to 37 traced the route of the internal carotid arteries to their termination in the brain as anterior and middle cerebral arteries. Items 38 to 41 traced the continuation of the vertebral arteries as a single basilar artery terminating as the posterior cerebral arteries. The *cerebral arterial circle* is a continuous network of vessels connecting the internal carotid arteries with the basilar artery at the base of the brain near the sella turcica. Observe the relationships of these vessels as depicted in Figure 11–21. Notice particularly the *anterior* and *posterior communicating arteries*.

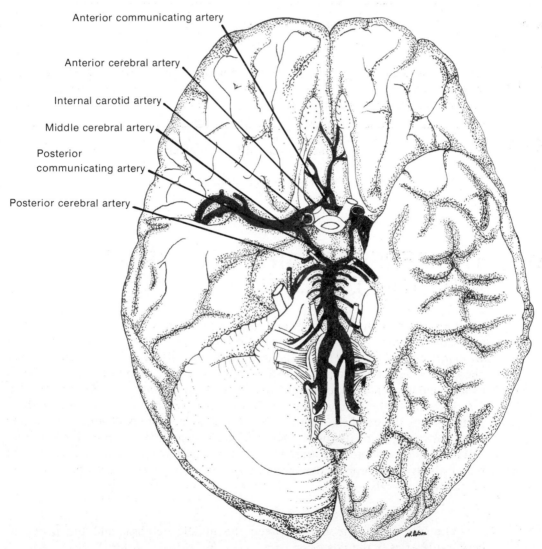

Anterior communicating artery

Anterior cerebral artery

Internal carotid artery

Middle cerebral artery

Posterior communicating artery

Posterior cerebral artery

Figure 11–21.   The brain, ventral aspect, showing the cerebral arterial circle. (Redrawn from Wolf-Heidegger: Atlas of Systematic Human Anatomy. Vol. III. Basel, S. Karger AG.)

The circular formation of arteries at the base of the brain is called the
_____ _____ circle.

cerebral arterial

The internal carotid arteries terminate in the brain in a bifurcation into
_____ and _____ cerebral arteries; the basilar artery terminates as the _____ cerebral arteries.

anterior . . . middle . . . posterior

The anterior part of the cerebral arterial circle is formed from terminal
branches of the _____ _____ arteries; the posterior part,
from terminal branches of the _____ artery.

internal carotid . . . basilar

ITEM 43   THE CEREBRAL ARTERIAL CIRCLE: ANASTOMOSES

Observe how the posterior cerebral arteries from the basilar artery connect
with continuations of the internal carotid artery by a *posterior communicating
branch,* shown in Figure 11–21. If either the carotid artery or the vertebral artery
becomes occluded over a period of time, the posterior communicating artery will
usually enlarge enough to supply the area. A single *anterior communicating
artery* connects the two anterior cerebral arteries as they enter the longitudinal
fissure. Thus the cerebral arterial circle forms a continuous channel connecting
posterior cerebral, posterior communicating, internal carotid, anterior cerebral,
and anterior communicating arteries. Anastomoses allow for some equalization of
blood supply to the brain under conditions of fluctuating pressure in one or another
of the input vessels.

The vascular connection between the middle cerebral and the posterior
cerebral arteries is the posterior _____ artery.

communicating

The single anterior communicating artery connects the two _____
_____ arteries.

Anastomoses (connections) of the network of vessels in the cerebral arterial circle permit equalization of fluctuating _____ _____.   QUESTION
112

---

blood pressure   *ANSWER*

In the space below, sketch the cerebral arterial circle and label its branches. Refer back to Figure 11–21 as necessary.   QUESTION
113

THE CEREBRAL ARTERIAL CIRCLE: THE MEDIAL ASPECT

ITEM 44

Figure 11–21 illustrated the cerebral arterial circle from the ventral aspect. Now examine Figure 11–22, which shows the arteries of the arterial circle on the medial aspect of the right cerebral hemisphere and on the lateral surface of the left cerebellar hemisphere. Notice the right internal carotid artery and the anterior cerebral artery which branches from it. Locate the anterior communicating artery as it branches off the right anterior cerebral artery. In the lower part of the illustration, the left vertebral artery can be seen as it ascends to fuse into the basilar artery. Finally, note the left posterior cerebral artery and the left posterior communicating artery.

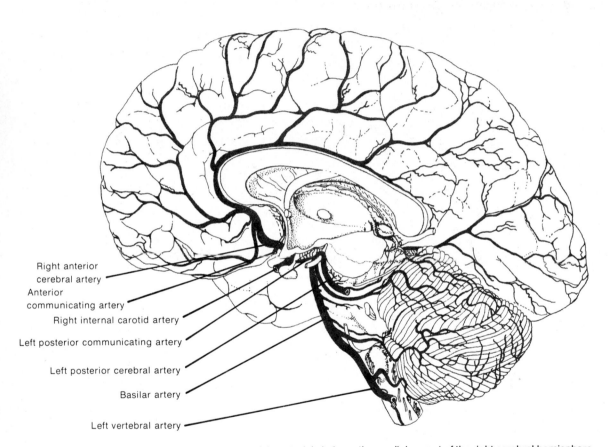

Right anterior
cerebral artery
Anterior
communicating artery
Right internal carotid artery
Left posterior communicating artery
Left posterior cerebral artery
Basilar artery
Left vertebral artery

Figure 11–22. Arteries of the arterial circle on the medial aspect of the right cerebral hemisphere and on the lateral surface of the left cerebellar hemisphere. (Redrawn from Wolf-Heidegger: Atlas of Systematic Human Anatomy. Vol. III. Basel, S. Karger AG.)

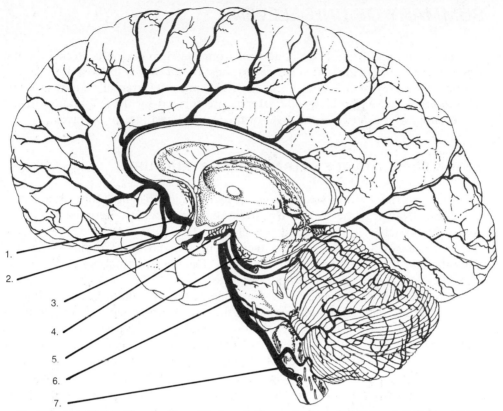

(Redrawn from Wolf-Heidegger: Atlas of Systematic Human Anatomy. Vol. III. Basel, S. Karger AG.)

In the numbered spaces below write the names of the corresponding numbered arteries shown in the accompanying diagram.

QUESTION
114

Labels

1. _____
2. _____
3. _____
4. _____
5. _____
6. _____
7. _____

1. anterior cerebral artery
2. anterior communicating artery
3. internal carotid artery
4. posterior communicating artery
5. posterior cerebral artery
6. basilar artery
7. vertebral artery

ANSWER

SUMMARY OF UNIT ELEVEN

Blood supply to the brain is derived from the right and left internal carotid arteries and the right and left vertebral arteries; blood supply to most of the extra-cranial structures of the head, from the right and left external carotid arteries. The internal and external carotid arteries are formed by the bifurcation of the common carotid arteries at the level of the thyroid cartilage in the neck.

BLOOD SUPPLY TO THE EXTRACRANIAL STRUCTURES

The external carotid artery gives off eight main branches: four branches in the carotid triangle of the neck, two posterior branches, and two terminal branches. The four branches in the carotid triangle are the superior thyroid, the lingual, the ascending pharyngeal, and the facial. The two posterior branches are the occipital and the posterior auricular arteries. The two terminal branches are the maxillary and the superficial temporal arteries.

The facial artery begins below the angle of the mandible, travels obliquely across the face, and terminates medial to the eye. In the neck, several branches arise which do not reach the face: (1) the ascending palatine, supplying muscles and mucous membranes of the pharynx; (2) the tonsillar, which is the main artery to the tonsils; and (3) the submental, supplying the chin, mylohyoid muscle, and anterior belly of the digastric muscle. In the face, the facial artery gives off inferior and superior labial branches below and above the mouth, and lateral nasal branches to skin and muscle of the nose. The termination of the facial artery is the angular artery, supplying skin of the nose and the eyelids.

The superficial temporal artery, one of the two terminal branches of the external carotid, ascends through the parotid gland and supplies the external ear, scalp, and temporomandibular joint. It gives off the transverse facial artery which supplies the parotid gland and the masseter muscle.

The final terminal branch of the external carotid artery is the maxillary. Its extensive branchings supply parts of the ear, the maxillary teeth and jaws, the muscles of mastication, the palate, the dura mater, and part of the nasal cavity. The maxillary artery is usually categorized as three regions: the mandibular, the pterygoid, and the pterygopalatine. The mandibular part, occupying the area behind the neck of the mandible, includes (1) the deep auricular artery to the temporomandibular joint, tympanic membrane, and skin of the meatus; (2) the anterior tympanic artery to the membrane lining the tympanic cavity; (3) the middle meningeal artery to the dura mater; (4) the accessory meningeal artery to the trigeminal ganglion and adjacent dura; and (5) the inferior alveolar artery supplying the lower molar teeth, peridontal ligaments, and gingiva. The branches of the inferior alveolar artery are the lingual branch to mucous membranes of the mouth, the mylohyoid branch to the mylohyoid muscle, the mental branch to skin of the chin, and the incisive branch, which is actually a continuation of the artery beyond the mental foramen.

The pterygoid part of the maxillary artery, occupying the infratemporal fossa, includes the masseteric branch to the masseter muscle, posterior and anterior deep temporal branches to the temporalis muscle, pterygoid branches to medial and lateral pterygoid muscles, and the buccal branch to mucous membranes of the mouth and skin of the cheek.

The pterygopalatine region of the maxillary artery, occupying the pterygo-palatine fossa, gives off the posterior superior alveolar artery, which supplies the upper molar teeth, the alveolar process, and the mucous membranes near the molar and premolar teeth. A second branch of the pterygopalatine portion is the infraorbital artery from which the anterior superior alveolar branches go to the upper canine and incisor teeth and the maxillary sinus. As the infraorbital artery surfaces onto the face, it divides into palpebral branches to the lower eyelid, labial branches to the cheek and upper lip, and nasal branches to the side of the nose. A third branch of the pterygopalatine region is the descending palatine artery, which divides into greater and lesser palatine arteries. The greater palatine artery supplies palatine gingiva, palatine glands, and the roof of the mouth; the lesser palatine, the soft palate and palatine tonsil. Fourth and fifth branches of the pterygopalatine part, the artery of the pterygoid canal and the pharyngeal artery, supply the tympanic cavity, upper pharynx, auditory tube, and sphenoid sinus. The final branch of the third part of the maxillary artery is the sphenopalatine artery. This branch courses with the nasopalatine nerve and gives off branches to the mucosa of the lateral nasal wall and to the nasal septum.

BLOOD SUPPLY TO THE INTRACRANIAL STRUCTURES

The blood supply to the brain derives from two internal carotid arteries and two vertebral arteries. Internal carotid arteries enter the carotid canal at the base of the skull, run anteriorly and medially through the canal, and emerge into the middle cranial fossa at the foramen lacerum. At this point the internal carotid arteries enter the cavernous sinus, turn anteriorly and superiorly, and emerge between the anterior and middle clinoid processes to reach the brain. Ophthalmic arteries and the anterior choroid arteries are given off just anterior to the cavernous sinus. Internal carotid arteries bifurcate into anterior and middle cerebral arteries. Anterior cerebral arteries supply the medial anterior regions of the brain; the middle cerebral arteries, the outermost parts of the parietal and temporal lobes.

Vertebral arteries branch off the subclavian artery and ascend in the neck through transverse foramina of the cervical vertebrae. They penetrate the atlanto-occipital membrane to enter the cranium at the foramen magnum. Branches of the vertebral arteries include spinal arteries, the posterior inferior cerebellar arteries, and branches to the medulla. Vertebral arteries join to form a single basilar artery on the ventral midline of the pons. The basilar artery gives off the anterior inferior and the superior cerebellar arteries, labyrinthine arteries, and branches to the pons. The basilar artery terminates by bifurcating into two posterior cerebral arteries.

Branches of the internal carotid artery which approach the brain from the front communicate with branches from the basilar artery which approach from behind. This communicating network of arteries forms the cerebral arterial circle, an arrangement which allows for equalization of blood supply to the brain under conditions of fluctuating pressure in one or the other of the input vessels. In the circle, a single anterior communicating artery connects the two anterior cerebral arteries; two posterior communicating arteries connect the posterior cerebral arteries with the middle cerebral arteries. If either a carotid or a vertebral artery becomes occluded over a period of time, communicating channels will usually enlarge sufficiently to supply distal vessels within the circle.

Blood supply to the brain is supplied by the _____ carotid arteries and the _____ arteries.

QUESTION
115

ANSWER

internal . . . vertebral

QUESTION
116

Most of the extracranial structures of the head are supplied by the _____
_____ artery.

ANSWER

external carotid

QUESTION
117

Four branches given off the external carotid artery in the carotid triangle of
the neck include the superior _____, the ascending _____,
the _____, and the _____ arteries.

ANSWER

thyroid . . . pharyngeal . . . lingual . . . facial

QUESTION
118

Branches of the facial artery in the neck which do not reach the face itself
include the ascending _____ artery to the pharynx and the _____
artery to the tonsils.

ANSWER

palatine . . . tonsillar

QUESTION
119

Three branches of the facial artery supplying the face itself include the superior
and inferior _____ arteries above and below the mouth, the lateral
_____ arteries to the skin and muscle of the nose, and the _____
artery to eyelids and part of skin of the nose.

ANSWER

labial . . . nasal . . . angular

QUESTION
120

The terminal branch of the external carotid artery which supplies the temporomandibular joint is the superficial _____ artery.

ANSWER

temporal

QUESTION
121

The transverse facial artery, which supplies the parotid gland, is a branch of
the (circle one) *facial artery/superficial temporal artery*.

ANSWER

superficial temporal artery

QUESTION
122

The extensive branchings of the maxillary artery are conveniently grouped
into three regions:
1. the _____ part, located behind the neck of the _____
2. the _____ part, occupying the _____ fossa
3. the _____ part, occupying the _____ fossa

---

1. mandibular . . . mandible
2. pterygoid . . . infratemporal
3. pterygopalatine . . . pterygopalatine

The deep auricular artery and the anterior tympanic artery, which supply structures in the tympanic area, are branches of the *mandibular/pterygoid/pterygopalatine* (circle one) area of the maxillary artery.

mandibular

Two branches of the mandibular part of the maxillary artery which supply dura mater are the middle and accessory _____ arteries.

meningeal

The posterior inferior alveolar artery supplies mandibular _____ teeth.

molar

Four branches of the posterior inferior alveolar artery are (1) the _____ branch supplying mucous membranes of the floor of the mouth, (2) the _____ branch supplying skin of the chin, (3) the _____ branch supplying the mylohyoid muscle, and (4) the _____ branch, which is the continuation of the posterior inferior alveolar artery beyond the mental foramen.

lingual . . . mental . . . mylohyoid . . . incisive

The masseter, deep temporal, pterygoid, and buccal arteries branch off the maxillary artery in the _____ region occupying the infratemporal fossa.

pterygoid

The posterior inferior alveolar artery branches off the maxillary artery in the _____ area; the posterior superior alveolar artery branches off in the _____ area.

mandibular . . . pterygopalatine

The *anterior/posterior* (circle one) superior alveolar artery is a branch of the infraorbital artery.

ANSWER

anterior

QUESTION
130

The terminal branches of the infraorbital artery on the face are the _____ branches to the region of the eye, the _____ branches to the region of the upper lip, and the _____ branches to the side of the nose.

ANSWER

palpebral . . . labial . . . nasal

QUESTION
131

The anterior and middle superior alveolar arteries supply _____ and _____ teeth.

ANSWER

canine . . . incisor (in either order)

QUESTION
132

The soft palate and the palatine tonsil are supplied by the _____ palatine artery; the roof of the mouth and the palatine gland, by the _____ palatine artery.

ANSWER

lesser . . . greater

QUESTION
133

The ascending palatine artery is a branch of the _____ artery; the descending palatine artery is a branch of the _____ artery.

ANSWER

facial . . . maxillary

QUESTION
134

The artery of the pterygoid canal and the pharyngeal artery supply the _____ tube and the upper _____ .

ANSWER

auditory . . . pharynx

QUESTION
135

The lateral nasal wall and the nasal septum receive blood supply from the _____ artery.

ANSWER

sphenopalatine

QUESTION
136

The anterior and anterior medial regions of the brain receive blood supply from branches of the _____ _____ arteries; the cerebellum, medulla, pons, and posterior cerebrum are supplied by extensions of the _____ arteries.

ANSWER

internal carotid . . . vertebral

The ophthalmic artery is a branch of the *internal/external* (circle one) carotid artery.

---

internal

The juncture of the two vertebral arteries in the pons is called the _____ _____ artery.

---

basilar

The cerebral arterial circle is formed from communicating branches of the _____ _____ arteries anteriorly and branches of the _____ arteries posteriorly.

---

internal carotid . . . vertebral

Unit Twelve □ LYMPHATICS OF THE HEAD AND NECK

ITEM 1   THE LYMPHATIC SYSTEM

The lymphatic system is a network of vessels and lymph nodes which are located in most major tissues of the body with the exception of the central nervous system. The lymphatic channels return fluid from tissue spaces into venous blood. Lymph nodes produce *lymphocytes* and filter toxic products from tissue fluid to prevent entry into general circulation.

QUESTION 1

The major function of lymphatic channels is the return of _____ from interstitial space to _____ blood.

_____

ANSWER

fluids . . . venous

QUESTION 2

Lymph nodes filter _____ substances from tissue fluid.

_____

ANSWER

toxic

QUESTION 3

The principal body tissue in which lymphatic channels are not found is that of the _____ _____ system.

_____

ANSWER

central nervous

THE COMPOSITION OF LYMPH   ITEM 2

The tissue fluid collected in lymphatic vessels is called *lymph*. Lymph is a colorless liquid similar in composition to plasma, rich in protein and particulate matter. Lymph is the principal fluid medium for the transport of assimilable fats collected from the intestines. Large numbers of white cells in the lymph, mostly lymphocytes, detoxify bacteria. Lymph also transports infectious substances, and sometimes cancer cells, from one part of the body to another.

The three predominant substances transported in lymph are (1) _____, (2) _____, and (3) toxic substances associated with _____.   QUESTION 4

protein . . . fat . . . infection (tumors)   *ANSWER*

The predominant white cells found in the lymph are called _____.   QUESTION 5

lymphocytes   *ANSWER*

THE LYMPHATIC CHANNELS   ITEM 3

There are three types of lymphatic channels: capillaries, vessels, and ducts. The *lymphatic capillaries* are blind ended endothelial tubes, without valves, which collect fluid from tissue spaces. In a manner similar to the converging of veins, capillaries converge into the larger *lymphatic vessels*. The lymphatic vessels are larger and thicker than the capillaries and, unlike the capillaries, have valves. The vessels eventually converge into one of two *lymphatic ducts,* which empty into the venous circulation.

The function of lymphatic capillaries is to collect fluid from _____ _____.   QUESTION 6

tissue spaces   *ANSWER*

The lymphatic ducts are the two terminal channels through which lymph enters the _____.   QUESTION 7

ANSWER   veins (venous circulation)

QUESTION   Lymphatic vessels are channels into which the smaller lymphatic
8   _____ converge, and through which lymph flows into the two
lymphatic _____.

ANSWER   capillaries . . . ducts

ITEM 4   THE LYMPHATIC DUCTS

Examine Figure 12–1 and notice the dashed line which separates the upper
right quadrant of the body from the other three quadrants. Lymphatic vessels of
the upper right quadrant converge eventually into the *right lymphatic duct,* which
joins the venous system at the junction of the right subclavian and right internal
jugular veins. Lymphatic vessels of the remaining three quadrants of the body
converge into the *thoracic* (left lymphatic) *duct,* which joins the venous system
at the junction of the left subclavian and left internal jugular veins. Lymph from the
right side of the head and neck drains through the *right jugular trunk* directly
into the venous system, as illustrated in Figure 12–1. Lymph from the left side
of the head and neck drains through the *left jugular trunk* into the thoracic duct.

QUESTION   The thoracic duct enters the venous circulation at the junction of the (circle
9   one)
    A. right subclavian and right internal jugular veins
    B. left subclavian and left internal jugular veins

ANSWER   The correct answer is B. The thoracic duct receives lymph from the left side
of the body above the diaphragm and from all of the body below the diaphragm;
it enters the venous circulation at the point where left subclavian and left internal
jugular veins unite.

QUESTION   The right lymphatic duct drains *one quadrant/three quadrants* (circle one) of
10   the body.

ANSWER   one quadrant

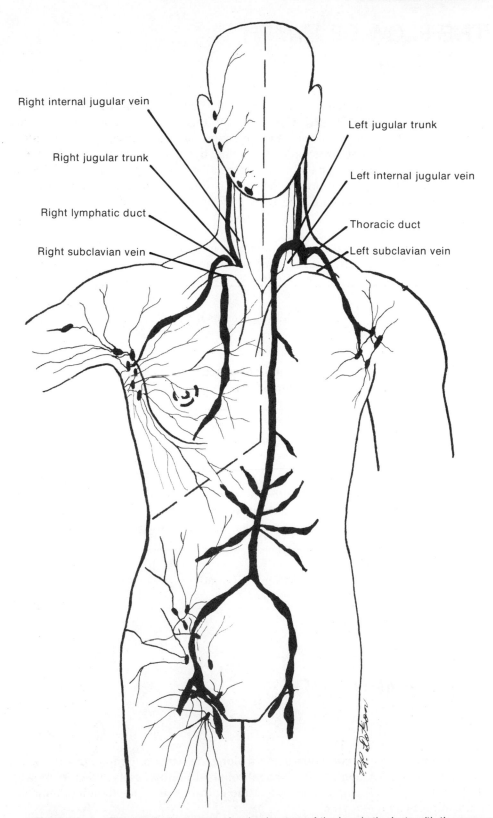

Right internal jugular vein

Right jugular trunk

Right lymphatic duct

Right subclavian vein

Left jugular trunk

Left internal jugular vein

Thoracic duct

Left subclavian vein

Figure 12–1. The lymphatic system, showing juncture of the lymphatic ducts with the venous circulation. (Modified from Jacob and Francone: Structure and Function in Man. 3rd Ed. Philadelphia, W. B. Saunders Co.)

ITEM 5

THE FLOW OF LYMPH

The lymphatic system has no contractile apparatus for the propulsion of lymph through the channels. Consequently the flow of lymph depends on compression of vessels by means of muscle contraction and pressure differential. Pressures are such that direction of flow is always from tissue spaces to venous blood. Valves of the lymphatic vessels further ensure this oneway flow. Vital substances, mainly plasma protein, as well as infectious material and malignant tumors, can spread through the body by way of the lymphatic system.

QUESTION 11

Movement of fluid through lymphatic capillaries into lymphatic vessels is accomplished by _____ contraction and _____ differences.

ANSWER

muscle . . . pressure

QUESTION 12

The oneway flow of lymph from tissue space to veins is ensured in part by the _____ with which lymphatic vessels are equipped.

ANSWER

valves

QUESTION 13

A disadvantage connected with the lymphatic system of returning plasma protein to the blood is the fact that the lymphatic mechanism also allows the spread of _____ and _____ cells through the body.

ANSWER

infection . . . tumor

ITEM 6

THE LYMPH NODES

Located in a fairly consistent pattern along the paths of lymphatic vessels are the *lymph nodes*. Lymph enters a node through afferent vessels and exits by way of efferent vessels. Lymph nodes effect the entrapment of bacteria and their detoxification by *lymphocytes*.

Lymph from a particular region drains into *regional* (or *primary*) *nodes*. Regional nodes, in turn, drain into *central* (or *secondary*) *nodes*. Consequently a pathologic process from an obscure area will, in many cases, manifest itself first in the regional nodes. For this reason, knowledge of the location and drainage area of these nodes is clinically important. However, it also must be recognized that a wide variation of lymph node distribution may occur among individuals.

The major function of lymph nodes is to trap _____ so that they can be detoxified by _____.

QUESTION
14

bacteria . . . lymphocytes

ANSWER

Primary nodes are *regional/central* (circle one); secondary nodes are *regional/central* (circle one).

QUESTION
15

regional . . . central

ANSWER

The clinical value of knowing the area drained by each of the various lymph nodes is that this knowledge enables one to trace a pathologic condition from the region in which it appears to the more obscure site where it _____.

QUESTION
16

originates

ANSWER

SUPERFICIAL AND DEEP LYMPH NODES OF THE HEAD AND NECK

ITEM 7

Groups of superficial lymph nodes are distributed in the head, and both deep and superficial nodes are found in the neck. The superficial nodes of the head and neck are associated with arteries, veins, or muscle fascia; the deep cervical network is associated with connective tissue surrounding veins.

Lymph nodes of the head are (circle one)
A. all superficial
B. all deep
C. both superficial and deep

QUESTION
17

The correct answer is A.

ANSWER

QUESTION
18

The lymph nodes of the neck are (circle one)
A. all superficial
B. all deep
C. both superficial and deep

ANSWER

The correct answer is C. Some of the cervical nodes are superficial; others are deep.

QUESTION
19

Superficial nodes are associated with (circle one)
A. connective tissue surrounding veins
B. veins, arteries, and muscle fascia

ANSWER

The correct answer is B.

QUESTION
20

Deep lymphatic nodes of the neck are associated with (circle one)
A. veins, arteries, and muscle fascia
B. connective tissue surrounding veins

ANSWER

The correct answer is B.

ITEM 8   LYMPHATICS OF THE HEAD: THE OCCIPITAL LYMPH NODES

Figure 12–2 shows the sites of five groups of superficial nodes of the head: (1) occipital, (2) retroauricular, (3) anterior auricular, (4) superficial parotid, and (5) facial. The first group of nodes, called the *occipital,* is associated with the occipital artery at the posterior base of the skull. These nodes drain the occipital part of the scalp and upper neck and empty into deep cervical nodes. In the illustration, notice the relationship of the occipital nodes to the superior deep cervical nodes.

QUESTION
21

The occipital nodes are arranged along the occipital _____ and drain into deep _____ nodes.

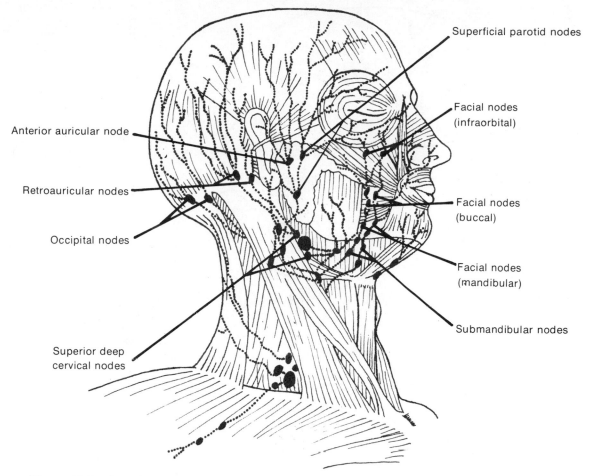

Anterior auricular node

Retroauricular nodes

Occipital nodes

Superior deep
cervical nodes

Superficial parotid nodes

Facial nodes
(infraorbital)

Facial nodes
(buccal)

Facial nodes
(mandibular)

Submandibular nodes

Figure 12–2. Superficial lymphatic nodes of the head. (Redrawn from Goss, C. M., Ed: Gray's Anatomy of the Human Body. 29th Ed. Philadelphia, Lea & Febiger.)

artery . . . cervical

ANSWER

Using the Word Bank, write the names of the corresponding numbered structures in the accompanying diagram into the blank labels.

QUESTION
22

Word Bank
anterior auricular node
facial nodes
occipital node
retroauricular node
superficial parotid node

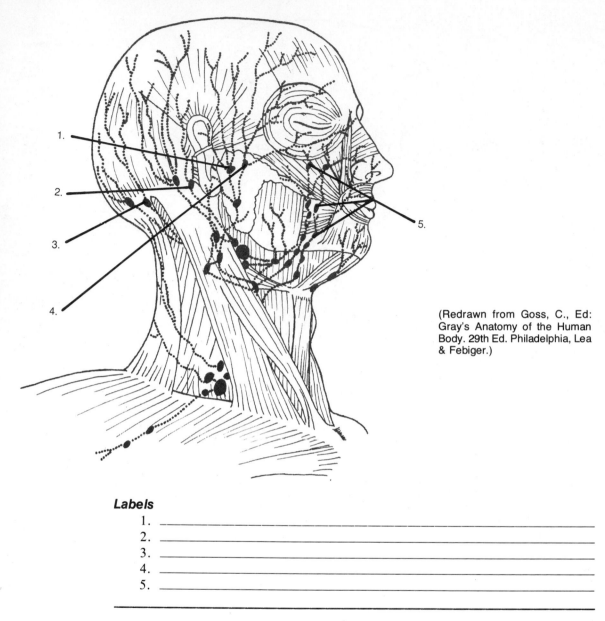

(Redrawn from Goss, C., Ed: Gray's Anatomy of the Human Body. 29th Ed. Philadelphia, Lea & Febiger.)

Labels

1. _____
2. _____
3. _____
4. _____
5. _____

ANSWER   Check your labels with Figure 12–2.

ITEM 9   RETROAURICULAR, ANTERIOR AURICULAR, AND SUPERFICIAL PAROTID NODES

Refer to Figure 12–2 and note the locations of the *retroauricular, anterior auricular,* and *superficial parotid* nodes. The retroauricular and anterior auricular nodes drain the external ear and the lateral surface of the scalp. Efferent channels from retroauricular nodes drain into superior deep cervical nodes and into accessory nodes; efferent channels from anterior auricular nodes drain into superior deep cervical nodes and into superficial parotid nodes. The superficial parotid nodes drain the external ear and adjacent regions of the scalp, their efferent vessels going to the superior deep cervical nodes.

Areas drained by the retroauricular, anterior auricular, and superficial parotid nodes include the external _____ and adjacent regions of the _____.

QUESTION
23

---

ear . . . scalp

ANSWER

The superior deep cervical nodes receive drainage from (circle one)
A. anterior auricular nodes
B. occipital nodes
C. retroauricular nodes
D. superficial parotid nodes
E. all four of the above

QUESTION
24

The correct answer is E.

ANSWER

Accessory nodes receive some of the drainage from (circle one) *anterior auricular/retroauricular* nodes.

QUESTION
25

---

retroauricular

ANSWER

The superficial parotid nodes receive some of the drainage from (circle one) *anterior auricular/retroauricular* nodes.

QUESTION
26

---

anterior auricular

ANSWER

Efferent vessels from superficial parotid nodes drain into superior _____ _____ nodes.

QUESTION
27

---

deep cervical

ANSWER

THE FACIAL NODES   ITEM 10

Small lymph nodes scattered along the facial artery are classified into three groups of *facial nodes*. Nodes below the orbit are called *infraorbital* nodes; nodes at the angles of the mouth, *buccal nodes;* nodes over the mandible, *mandibular nodes*. Locate these three groups of facial nodes on Figure 12–2.

Afferent channels of the facial nodes arise in the skin and mucous membranes of the face; efferent channels extend to the submandibular nodes. Take note of the relationship of the facial nodes to the submandibular nodes as shown on Figure 12–2.

QUESTION
28

The facial nodes below the eye are called _____ nodes; those on the lower jaw are called _____ nodes; those at the angle of the mouth are called _____ nodes.

ANSWER

infraorbital . . . mandibular . . . buccal

QUESTION
29

The facial nodes drain into the _____ nodes.

ANSWER

submandibular

ITEM 11   SUPERFICIAL NODES OF THE NECK: THE SUBMENTAL GROUP

Figure 12–3 shows four groups of superficial lymph nodes of the neck, the (1) *submental,* (2) *submandibular,* (3) *external jugular,* and (4) *anterior jugular* groups. The submental nodes lie on the mylohyoid muscle at the midline between the symphysis of the mandible and the hyoid bone. They receive lymphatic vessels from the chin, lower lip, cheeks, from the incisor teeth and adjacent membranes, and from the tip of the tongue. Efferent vessels extend to the submandibular nodes and to the jugulodigastric group at the upper part of the deep cervical channels.

QUESTION
30

Submental lymph nodes are located on the _____ muscle.

ANSWER

mylohyoid

QUESTION
31

The submental lymph nodes are situated between the symphysis of the _____ and the _____ bone.

ANSWER

mandible . . . hyoid

QUESTION
32

Areas drained by the submental nodes include, in addition to the cheeks, chin, and lower lip, the mandibular _____ teeth and the tip of the _____.

ANSWER

incisor . . . tongue

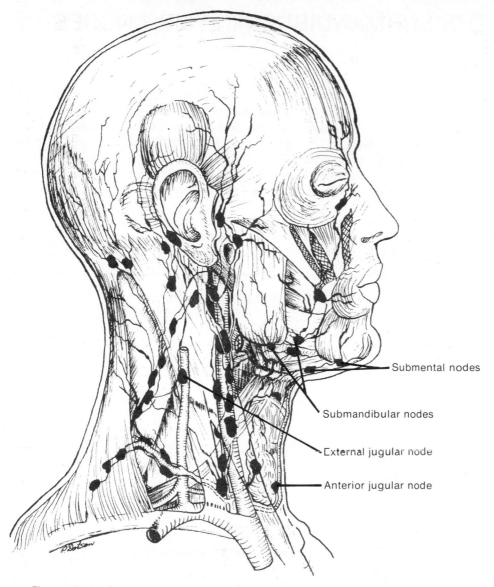

Submental nodes

Submandibular nodes

External jugular node

Anterior jugular node

Figure 12-3. Superficial lymph nodes of the neck. (Redrawn from Woodburne: Essentials of Human Anatomy. 4th Ed. New York, Oxford University Press.)

Submental nodes drain into _____ nodes and into _____ nodes.

QUESTION **33**

submandibular . . . jugulodigastric (in either order)

ANSWER

The four groups of superficial lymph nodes of the neck are the _____ nodes, the _____ nodes, the _____ jugular nodes, and the _____ jugular nodes.

QUESTION **34**

submental . . . submandibular . . . external . . . anterior

ANSWER

ITEM 12

THE SUBMANDIBULAR LYMPH NODES

Look at Figure 12–3 and find the submandibular lymph nodes, which lie along the inferior border of the ramus of the mandible at the submandibular gland. These nodes receive afferent channels from the chin, lips, nose, cheeks, and gingivae; from the anterior region of the hard palate; and from the anterior region of the tongue. Sublingual and submandibular salivary glands also drain into the submandibular lymph nodes. From the submandibular group, efferent vessels extend to the superior deep cervical nodes and to other deep nodes of the neck.

QUESTION 35

Efferent channels from the chin, cheeks, and tongue extend to (circle one) *submental/submandibular/both submental and submandibular* lymph nodes.

ANSWER

both submental and submandibular

QUESTION 36

The anterior region of the _____ palate drains into the submandibular nodes.

ANSWER

hard

QUESTION 37

The salivary glands drained by the submandibular nodes are the _____ and _____ glands.

ANSWER

submandibular . . . sublingual (in either order)

QUESTION 38

The submandibular nodes send efferent vessels to the *superior/inferior* (circle one) deep cervical group.

ANSWER

superior

ITEM 13

THE EXTERNAL AND ANTERIOR JUGULAR NODES

Re-examine Figure 12–3 and find the *external jugular* and the *anterior jugular nodes*. External jugular nodes, lying along the external jugular vein over the sternocleidomastoid muscle, drain the lower part of the ear and the region of the parotid gland. They empty into the superior deep cervical nodes.

Anterior jugular nodes, accompanying the anterior jugular vein, lie just deep to the superficial cervical fascia in the lower levels of the neck. They drain the infrahyoid region of the neck and empty into the inferior deep cervical nodes.

The external jugular nodes drain into the *superior/inferior* (circle one) deep cervical nodes; the anterior jugular nodes, into the *superior/inferior* (circle one) deep cervical nodes.

QUESTION
39

superior . . . inferior

ANSWER

The areas drained by the external jugular nodes are those of the lower part of the ear and the _____ region.

QUESTION
40

parotid

ANSWER

Anterior jugular nodes receive lymphatic vessels from the _____ area of the neck.

QUESTION
41

infrahyoid

ANSWER

THE SUPERIOR AND INFERIOR DEEP CERVICAL NODES: LOCATION

ITEM 14

Figure 12–4 shows the landmarks defining the location of the *superior* and the *inferior deep cervical nodes*. Deep cervical nodes are divided for convenience into superior and inferior subgroups, depending upon whether they lie above or below the point where the omohyoid muscle crosses the internal jugular vein. The deep cervical nodes, the most extensive group of lymph nodes in the neck, are arranged along the internal jugular vein.

The arbitrary line of demarcation between the superior and inferior deep cervical nodes is the crossing of the _____ _____ vein and the _____ muscle.

QUESTION
42

internal jugular . . . omohyoid

ANSWER

The location of the deep cervical nodes is along the route of the _____ _____ vein.

QUESTION
43

internal jugular

ANSWER

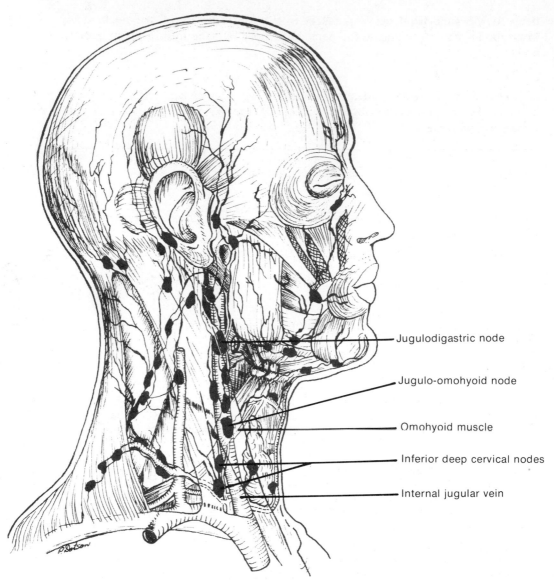

Figure 12–4. The deep cervical lymph nodes. (Redrawn from Woodburne: Essentials of Human Anatomy. 4th Ed. New York, Oxford University Press.)

ITEM 15 THE SUPERIOR DEEP CERVICAL NODES

The most prominent of the superior deep cervical nodes is the *jugulodigastric node,* which lies at the point where the digastric muscle crosses the internal jugular vein. Locate this node in Figure 12–4. The jugulodigastric node drains the tongue and the palatine tonsil. The *jugulo-omohyoid node,* also seen in Figure 12–4, derives its name from its position at the crossing of the internal jugular vein and the omohyoid muscle. The jugulo-omohyoid node receives afferent vessels from the tip of the tongue and from the submental region.

The jugulodigastric node derives its name from its position at the crossing of the internal _____ vein and the _____ muscle.

jugular . . . digastric

The jugulo-omohyoid node derives its name from its position at the crossing of the _____ muscle and the internal _____ vein.

omohyoid . . . jugular

The tip of the tongue and the submental area drain into the _____ _____ node; the tongue and the palatine tonsil drain into the _____ _____ node.

jugulo-omohyoid . . . jugulodigastric

THE RETROPHARYNGEAL AND DEEP PAROTID NODES

ITEM 16

Marginal members of the superior deep cervical series, lying at the upper end of the chain, include the *retropharyngeal nodes* and the *deep parotid nodes*. The retropharyngeal nodes drain the pharynx and palate, as well as the nose and the paranasal sinuses. The deep parotid nodes drain the external acoustic meatus, the auditory tube, and the tympanic cavity, in addition to draining the parotid gland.

The retropharyngeal nodes drain the pharynx and the _____, as well as the nose and the _____ sinuses.

palate . . . paranasal

Areas drained by the deep parotid nodes include, in addition to the parotid gland, structures associated with the _____.

ear

The superior deep cervical nodes include the _____ node, the _____ node, the _____ nodes, and the _____ _____ nodes.

ANSWER   jugulodigastric . . . jugulo-omohyoid . . . retropharyngeal . . . deep parotid

QUESTION
50

The retropharyngeal and deep parotid nodes lie near the *upper/lower* (circle one) margin of the superior deep cervical chain.

ANSWER   upper

ITEM 17   THE INFERIOR DEEP CERVICAL NODES

The *inferior deep cervical nodes,* shown in Figure 12–4, are a continuation of the superior group below the omohyoid muscle. Like the superior deep cervical group, the inferior deep cervical nodes follow the internal jugular vein. Lymphatic efferent channels from the superior nodes drain either into the inferior nodes or directly into one of the two jugular trunks. As was explained in Item 4, the left jugular trunk is a short vessel emptying into the thoracic duct; the right jugular trunk drains directly into the venous system.

QUESTION
51

Efferent lymphatic channels from the superior deep cervical nodes may take either of two routes to the venous system; they may feed into the _____ _____ _____ nodes, or directly into the _____ trunks.

ANSWER   inferior deep cervical . . . jugular

QUESTION
52

Lymph from the left jugular trunk reaches the venous system via the _____ duct; that from the right jugular trunk empties directly into the _____ circulation.

ANSWER   thoracic . . . venous

ITEM 18   THE ACCESSORY NODES

The inferior nodes, discussed in Item 17, are continuations of the superior deep cervical nodes. Additional deep nodes of the neck are the *accessory nodes,* the *transverse cervical nodes,* and the *juxtavisceral nodes.* Examine Figure 12–5 and locate these three groups.

The accessory nodes, which are associated with the accessory nerve, are a

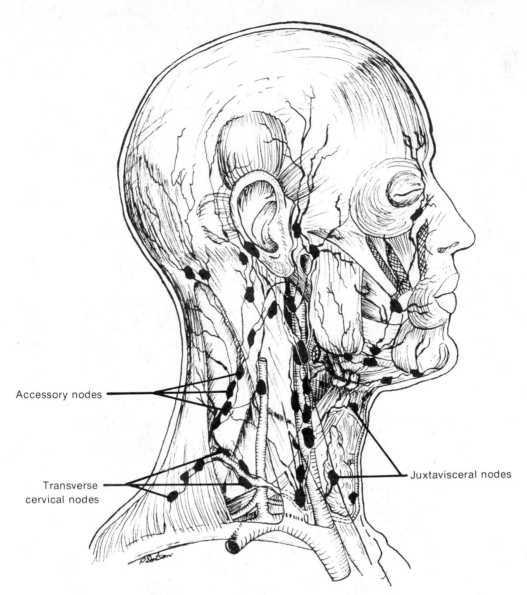

Accessory nodes

Transverse
cervical nodes

Juxtavisceral nodes

Figure 12-5. Accessory, transverse cervical, and juxtavisceral lymph nodes. (Redrawn from Woodburne: Essentials of Human Anatomy. 4th Ed. New York, Oxford University Press.)

posterior extension of the deep cervical chain. They receive the occipital and retroauricular groups, and drain downward to join the transverse cervical chain.

The superior deep cervical chain continues inferiorly and posteriorly as the _____ nodes.

QUESTION
53

accessory

ANSWER

Lymph drains into the accessory nodes from the _____ and _____ nodes.

QUESTION
54

ANSWER   occipital . . . retropharyngeal (in either order)

QUESTION
55   Efferent vessels from the accessory nodes drain into the _____ cervical nodes.

ANSWER   transverse

ITEM 19   THE TRANSVERSE CERVICAL NODES

Note the location of the transverse cervical nodes, shown in Figure 12–5. As explained in the previous Item, this chain of nodes receives efferent vessels from the accessory nodes. The transverse cervical nodes may empty into one of the jugular trunks, into the thoracic or the right lymphatic duct, or directly into the venous system.

QUESTION
56   Lymph flowing in efferent channels from the transverse cervical nodes reaches the venous circulation through four routes: through a _____ trunk, through the _____ duct, through the _____ lymphatic duct, or directly into the _____ system.

ANSWER   jugular . . . thoracic . . . right . . . venous

ITEM 20   THE JUXTAVISCERAL LYMPH NODES

Locate the *juxtavisceral lymph nodes* in Figure 12–5. These nodes are adjacent to the structures which they drain: the larynx, the trachea, the esophagus, and the thyroid gland. Juxtavisceral nodes drain into the superior and inferior deep cervical chains.

QUESTION
57   Efferent vessels of the juxtavisceral nodes extend to the _____ and _____ deep cervical nodes.

ANSWER   superior . . . inferior (in either order)

The thyroid gland, larynx, esophagus, and trachea are drained by (circle one) *transverse cervical/juxtavisceral* nodes.

QUESTION
58

juxtavisceral

ANSWER

LYMPHATIC DRAINAGE OF STRUCTURES ADJACENT TO THE TEETH
ITEM 21

Certain components of the lymphatic system and the structures they drain have immediate relevance to dental studies. These components and their areas of drainage are summarized in this and the next two Items.

The soft palate, most of the hard palate, the base of the tongue, and most of the sublingual region drain along the retromandibular vein into the superior deep cervical nodes.

The anterior region of the hard palate and the base of the tongue drain into the submandibular nodes. Vessels which drain the labial and buccal gingivae also extend to the submandibular nodes, as well as to the submental nodes.

Lymph from the region of the mandibular incisors drains into the submental nodes. Lymph from the lingual portion of the upper jaw courses posteriorly to the superior deep cervical group.

The soft palate, the upper jaw, and the sublingual region are drained by the _____ deep cervical nodes.

QUESTION
59

superior

ANSWER

The hard palate and the base of the tongue drain into two groups of nodes, the _____ deep cervical nodes and the _____ nodes.

QUESTION
60

superior . . . submandibular

ANSWER

Buccal and labial gingivae drain into the _____ and _____ nodes.

QUESTION
61

submental . . . submandibular (in either order)

ANSWER

QUESTION
62

The mandibular incisor teeth drain into the (circle one)
A. submandibular nodes
B. submental nodes

ANSWER

The correct answer is B. The mandibular incisor teeth, the lower lip, and the chin drain into the submental nodes. Efferent vessels from the submental nodes extend in turn to the submandibular nodes.

ITEM 22   LYMPHATIC DRAINAGE OF THE TEETH AND THE PERIODONTAL MEMBRANE

Except for those of the lower incisors, which drain into the submental nodes, most of the vessels of the teeth drain into the submandibular nodes. A few lymphatic vessels from the maxillary region may reach the superior deep cervical nodes directly.

Lymphatics draining the pulp and periodontal membrane of the incisors and canines extend anteriorly to reach the submental nodes; drainage from the molars extends posteriorly into the submandibular nodes. Lymphatics from the premolar region may drain in either direction.

QUESTION
63

Lymphatic drainage of the lower incisor teeth is effected by the _____ nodes; that of most of the other teeth, by the _____ nodes.

ANSWER

submental . . . submandibular

QUESTION
64

The submandibular nodes drain pulp and periodontal membrane of the _____ teeth; the submental nodes, pulp and periodontal membrane of the _____ and _____ teeth.

ANSWER

molar . . . incisor . . . canine

QUESTION
65

Lymphatic drainage from the premolar teeth may go either posteriorly to the _____ nodes or anteriorly to the _____ nodes.

ANSWER

submandibular . . . submental

LYMPHATIC DRAINAGE OF THE MAXILLARY REGION

Dental lymphatics from the maxillary region take two routes. The channels from the anterior region of the maxillary teeth and periodontal structures drain into the infraorbital channels, then into the facial group of nodes. Lymphatic channels from the posterior maxillary region follow the retromandibular vein and drain into submandibular nodes.

Facial lymph nodes drain the *anterior/posterior* (circle one) region of the maxillary teeth and periodontal structures; submandibular nodes drain the *anterior/posterior* (circle one) maxillary region.

QUESTION
66

---

anterior . . . posterior

ANSWER

SUMMARY OF UNIT TWELVE

The lymphatic capillaries absorb interstitial fluid. Lymphatic vessels transport lymph through a series of regional and central nodes in which it is detoxified by lymphocytes. Lymph is delivered into two terminal lymphatic ducts which join the venous system at the junction of the subclavian and jugular veins. The right lymphatic duct drains the upper right quadrant of the body into the venous system; the thoracic (left lymphatic) duct drains the other three quadrants.

The lymph itself is rich in plasmalike protein. It transports assimilable fats, but it may also transport various noxious substances. Pressure and muscular activity, in combination with the valves in the lymphatic vessels, effect a oneway flow of lymph from tissue space to the venous circulation.

Superficial lymph nodes are found in the head; the neck contains both superficial and deep nodes. Superficial nodes of the head include the occipital, retroauricular, anterior auricular, superficial parotid, and facial groups. Superficial lymph nodes of the neck include the submental, submandibular, external jugular, and anterior jugular nodes.

The deep nodes of the neck can be divided conveniently into superior deep and inferior deep cervical nodes, according to their position above or below the crossing of the omohyoid muscle and the internal jugular vein. The superior deep cervical nodes include the retropharyngeal, the deep parotid, the jugulodigastric, and the jugulo-omohyoid. The inferior deep cervical nodes include continuations of the superior nodes in addition to the accessory, transverse cervical, and juxtavisceral groups.

Lymph nodes of particular significance in dentistry are, (1) the superior deep cervical, (2) the submandibular, (3) the submental, (4) the retromandibular, and (5) the facial.

The superior deep cervical nodes drain parts of the soft palate, most of the hard palate, the base of the tongue, the sublingual region, and the upper jaws. The submandibular nodes drain parts of the hard palate and the base of the tongue, the pulp and periodontal membrane of the molar teeth, and vessels of most other teeth with the exception of the lower incisors. The submental nodes drain the region of the mandibular incisor teeth, the buccal and labial gingivae, and the pulp and periodontal membrane of the canine teeth. The facial nodes drain the anterior maxillary region; the submandibular nodes drain the posterior maxillary region.

QUESTION
67

The channels of the lymphatic system include (1) lymphatic _____, which collect fluid from tissue space, (2) lymphatic _____, which transport lymph, and (3) lymphatic _____, which deliver lymph into the venous circulation.

ANSWER

capillaries . . . vessels . . . ducts

QUESTION
68

The thoracic duct is the *right/left* (circle one) terminal lymphatic channel and drains *one quadrant/three quadrants* (circle one) of the body.

ANSWER

left . . . three quadrants

The principal kinds of substance carried through the lymphatic channels are (1) _____, (2) _____, and (3) _____ substances.

QUESTION 69

proteins . . . fats . . . toxic

ANSWER

The oneway flow of lymph is from _____ space to the _____ circulation.

QUESTION 70

tissue (interstitial) . . . venous

ANSWER

Factors effecting the oneway flow of lymph are _____ action and pressure plus the _____ with which lymphatic vessels are equipped.

QUESTION 71

muscular . . . valves

ANSWER

The occipital, retroauricular, anterior auricular, and facial nodes are *superficial/deep* (circle one) nodes of the *head/neck* (circle one).

QUESTION 72

superficial . . . head

ANSWER

The principal superficial nodes of the neck are the _____ nodes, the _____ nodes, the exterior _____ nodes, and the anterior _____ nodes.

QUESTION 73

submental . . . submandibular . . . jugular . . . jugular

ANSWER

The retropharyngeal, deep parotid, jugulodigastric, and jugulo-omohyoid nodes are *superior/inferior* (circle one) deep cervical nodes.

QUESTION 74

superior

ANSWER

Inferior deep cervical nodes are continuations of the _____ ____ _____ nodes.

QUESTION 75

superior deep cervical

ANSWER

The accessory, transverse cervical, and juxtavisceral nodes are *superficial/deep* (circle one) nodes of the neck.

QUESTION 76

deep

ANSWER

QUESTION
77

Four groups of lymph nodes which are of special significance in dentistry are the

1. _____ nodes
2. _____ nodes
3. _____ nodes
4. _____ deep cervical nodes

ANSWER

1. submental 2. submandibular 3. facial 4. superior

QUESTION
78

The soft palate, upper jaws, and sublingual region are drained by _____ _____ _____ nodes.

ANSWER

superior deep cervical

QUESTION
79

The hard palate and the base of the tongue drain into the superior deep cervical nodes as well as into the _____ nodes.

ANSWER

submandibular

QUESTION
80

The mandibular incisor teeth drain into the _____ nodes; most of the other teeth, into the _____ nodes.

ANSWER

submental . . . submandibular

QUESTION
81

The submandibular nodes drain pulp and periodontal membrane of the _____ teeth; the submental nodes, pulp and periodontal membrane of the mandibular _____ and _____ teeth.

ANSWER

molar . . . canine . . . incisor

QUESTION
82

The anterior maxillary region drains into the _____ nodes; the posterior maxillary region, into the _____ nodes.

ANSWER

facial . . . submandibular

PART THREE

□

REGIONS

Unit Thirteen □ TEMPORAL AND INFRA-TEMPORAL FOSSAE

REGIONAL STUDY OF THE HEAD AND NECK

The first 12 units of this program explained various structures of the head and neck in terms of systems: skeletal, muscular, nervous, and vascular. Units Thirteen through Sixteen will discuss structures on the basis of regions. All of the structures of a particular area of the head and neck will be dealt with simultaneously, with emphasis on surface landmarks, on bony landmarks, and, above all, on the relationships among various structures within a given region.

In this and the next three units, the discussion of each area will point out which structures are superficial, which deep; which are lateral, which medial; which are superior, which inferior. Positional visualization of this sort is an essential skill in clinical anatomy.

The regions studied in the present unit are the *temporal fossa* and the *infratemporal fossa*. While studying these structures, use a skull to help you to understand relationships and identify bony landmarks.

A systematic approach to anatomy deals with a single system throughout a number of _____ of the body; a regional approach studies a number of _____ within a single area.

QUESTION 1

---

areas (regions) . . . structures (systems)

ANSWER

A regional study calls special attention to _____ and gives particular emphasis to _____ of structures to one another.

QUESTION 2

---

landmarks . . . relationships

ANSWER

517

ITEM 2   THE TEMPORAL FOSSA AND ITS BOUNDARIES

The *temporal fossa* is a depression on the lateral side of the skull, above the zygomatic arch. The temporalis muscle and its nerves and vessels lie within this fossa, whose boundaries are shown in Figure 13–1.

The superior and posterior limits of the temporal fossa are demarcated by temporal lines. The superficial inferior border is the zygomatic arch; the deep inferior border is the infratemporal crest of the sphenoid bone. The anterior boundary is formed by the frontal process of the zygoma and the zygomatic process of the frontal bone.

Locate these landmarks on Figure 13–1.

QUESTION 3

The temporal fossa is occupied by the _____ muscle and its _____ and _____.

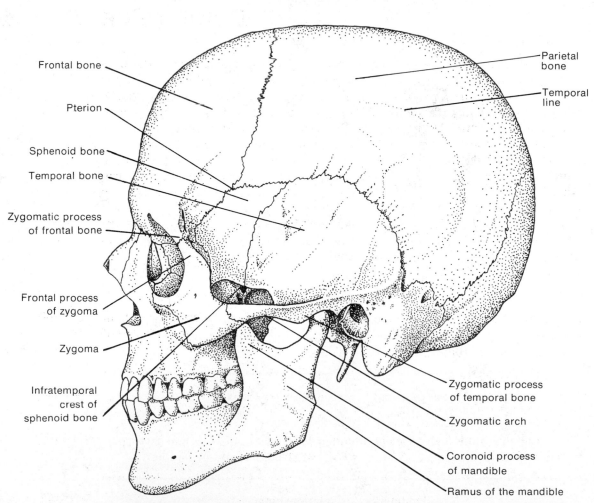

Figure 13–1. Boundaries of the temporal fossa, lateral aspect. (Redrawn from Wolf-Heidegger: Atlas of Systematic Human Anatomy. Vol. I. Basel, S. Karger AG.)

ANSWER

temporalis . . . nerves . . . arteries

The temporal lines form the _____ and _____ bound- QUESTION
4
aries of the temporal fossa.

ANSWER

superior . . . posterior (in either order)

The temporal fossa is bounded anteriorly by the _____ and QUESTION
5
_____ bones.

ANSWER

frontal . . . zygomatic (in either order)

The superficial inferior boundary of the temporal fossa is the _____ QUESTION
6
arch; the deep inferior boundary, the infratemporal crest of the _____
bone.

ANSWER

zygomatic . . . sphenoid

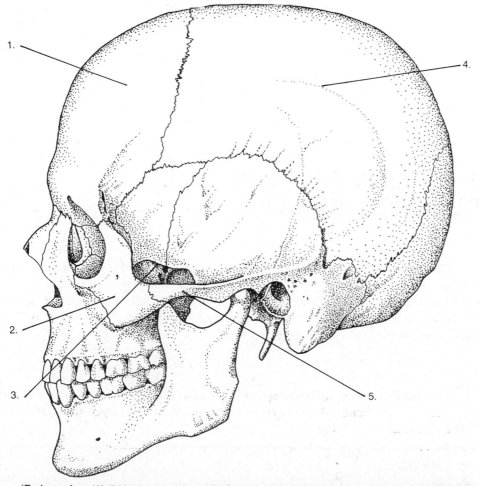

(Redrawn from Wolf-Heidegger: Atlas of Systematic Human Anatomy. Vol. I. Basel, S. Karger AG.)

QUESTION 7

Using the Word Bank, write the names of the numbered structures in the diagram, page 519, in the corresponding blank labels.

Word Bank

frontal bone
infratemporal crest of the sphenoid bone
temporal line
zygomatic arch
zygomatic bone

Labels

1. _____
2. _____
3. _____
4. _____
5. _____

ANSWER   Check your labels with Figure 13–1.

ITEM 3   THE TEMPORAL FOSSA: THE SUPERIOR BORDER

The temporal lines, which are the upper border of the temporal fossa, form an almost complete circle. Look at Figure 13–1 again and notice that the temporal lines begin at the *zygomatic process of the frontal bone* anteriorly, and arch over the temporal and parietal bones to become continuous with the posterior part of the *zygomatic process of the temporal bone*.

QUESTION 8

The anterior origin of the temporal lines is at the zygomatic process of the _____ bone; the posterior termination, at the zygomatic process of the _____ bone.

ANSWER   frontal . . . temporal

THE TEMPORAL FOSSA: THE ANTERIOR BORDER

ITEM 4

Details of the anterior border of the temporal fossa can be seen in Figure 13–1. The anterior border is formed by the posterior surface of the *zygomatic process of the frontal bone* and the *frontal process of the zygoma*. Not shown in Figure 13–1 is the *inferior orbital fissure*, through which the temporal fossa communicates anteriorly with the orbit. This fissure transmits the infraorbital nerve and artery.

The anterior border of the temporal fossa is constituted by the _____ process of the zygoma and the _____ process of the frontal bone.

QUESTION 9

---

frontal . . . zygomatic

ANSWER

The infraorbital nerve and artery enter the orbit through the _____ _____ fissure.

QUESTION 10

---

inferior orbital

ANSWER

The temporal fossa and the orbit communicate via the _____ _____ fissure.

QUESTION 11

---

inferior orbital

ANSWER

THE TEMPORAL FOSSA: THE MEDIAL WALL

ITEM 5

The medial wall, or floor, of the temporal fossa is formed by portions of the frontal and parietal bones, a portion of the greater wing of the sphenoid bone, and squamous portions of the temporal bone. Refer to Figure 13–1 and locate the bones of the floor of the temporal fossa. The point at which these four bones most nearly approach each other is called the *pterion*. The pterion lies over the anterior branch of the middle meningeal artery, which grooves the inner surface of the skull. The lower limit of the medial wall of the temporal fossa is the infratemporal crest of the greater wing of the sphenoid bone.

The four bones forming the floor of the temporal fossa are the _____ bone, the _____ bone, the _____ bone, and the _____ bone.

QUESTION 12

ANSWER   frontal . . . parietal . . . temporal . . . sphenoid (in any order)

QUESTION
13

The point where the four bones forming the medial wall of the temporal fossa converge is the _____ .

ANSWER   pterion

QUESTION
14

The infratemporal crest of the sphenoid bone is the lower limit of the _____ of the temporal fossa.

ANSWER   floor (medial wall)

QUESTION
15

The anterior branch of the middle meningeal artery is situated just under the _____ .

ANSWER   pterion

ITEM 6   THE INFRATEMPORAL FOSSA

The *infratemporal fossa* is the cavity below and medial to the zygomatic arch. This fossa contains most of the muscles of mastication, as well as blood vessels and nerves which reach the mouth. The infratemporal fossa is continuous with the temporal fossa above, the space between the two fossae being filled by the temporalis muscle and the deep temporal nerves and vessels.

QUESTION
16

The structures occupying the infratemporal fossa include vessels and nerves to the _____ , as well as muscles of _____ .

ANSWER   mouth . . . mastication

QUESTION
17

The interval between the points of communication of the temporal and infratemporal fossae is occupied by deep _____ nerves and vessels and by the _____ muscle.

ANSWER   temporal . . . temporalis

THE INFRATEMPORAL FOSSA: BOUNDARIES   ITEM 7

Figure 13–2 shows the boundaries of the infratemporal fossa from the inferior aspect. The medial roof is formed by the *infratemporal crest of the greater wing of the sphenoid bone*. The medial limit is the *lateral pterygoid plate*. The relationship of the infratemporal fossa to the mandible can be seen in Figure 13–1. The anterior border is the *infratemporal surface of the maxilla;* the posterior border, the posterior edge of the mandible. The lateral boundaries are the ramus and the coronoid process of the mandible.

The infratemporal crest of the greater wing of the sphenoid bone is the medial _____ of the infratemporal fossa; the medial limit of this fossa is the lateral _____ plate.

QUESTION 18

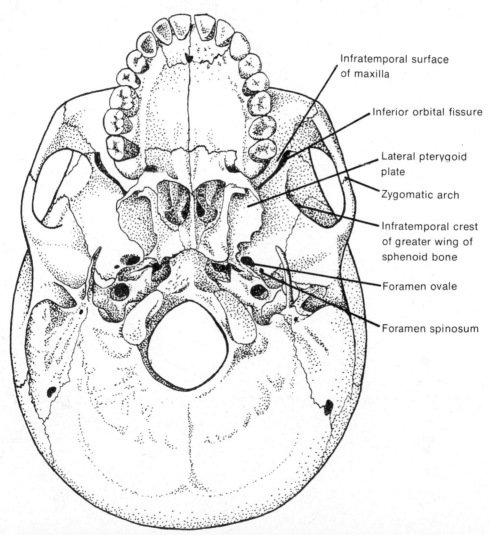

Infratemporal surface of maxilla

Inferior orbital fissure

Lateral pterygoid plate

Zygomatic arch

Infratemporal crest of greater wing of sphenoid bone

Foramen ovale

Foramen spinosum

Figure 13–2.   Infratemporal fossa, seen from below with mandible removed. (Redrawn from Wolf-Heidegger: Atlas of Systematic Human Anatomy. Vol. I. Basel, S. Karger AG.)

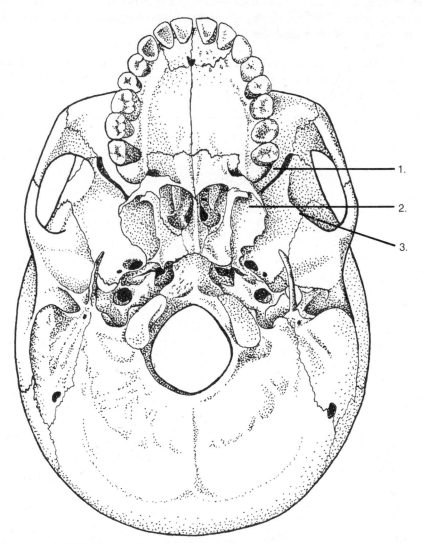

1.

2.

3.

(Redrawn from Wolf-Heidegger: Atlas of Systematic Human Anatomy. Vol. I. Basel, S. Karger AG.)

roof . . . pterygoid

The ramus of the mandible forms part of the _____ border of the infratemporal fossa.

---

lateral

The anterior boundary of the infratemporal fossa is the infratemporal surface of the _____ ; the posterior limit is the posterior border of the _____ .

---

maxilla . . . mandible

Using the Word Bank, write the names of the numbered structures on the diagram, page 524, in the corresponding blank labels.

Word Bank

infratemporal crest of the sphenoid bone
infratemporal surface of the maxilla
lateral pterygoid plate

Labels

1. _____
2. _____
3. _____

Check your labels with Figure 13–2.

FORAMEN OVALE, FORAMEN SPINOSUM, AND ALVEOLAR CANAL   ITEM 8

The *foramen ovale* and the *foramen spinosum* can be seen opening onto the roof of the infratemporal fossa in Figure 13–2. The *alveolar canal,* which is not shown in this Figure, opens on the anterior wall of the infratemporal fossa.

The foramen ovale transmits the mandibular division of the trigeminal (fifth cranial) nerve and the accessory meningeal artery, the foramen spinosum, the middle meningeal artery and the meningeal branch of the mandibular nerve. The alveolar canal transmits the posterior superior alevolar artery and nerve to the upper molar teeth.

A meningeal nerve and artery pass through the foramen _____ ,
while the mandibular division of the trigeminal nerve passes through the foramen
_____ .

ANSWER
spinosum . . . ovale

QUESTION
23
The _____ _____ alveolar nerve and artery pass through
the alveolar canal en route to the upper _____ teeth.

ANSWER
posterior superior . . . molar

ITEM 9   THE INFERIOR ORBITAL FISSURE

The anterior part of the infratemporal fossa communicates with the orbit
through the *inferior orbital fissure*. This fissure is a cleft between the posterior
superior surface of the maxilla and the greater wing of the sphenoid bone. Look
back to Figure 13–2 and locate it.
The inferior orbital fissure transmits the infraorbital artery and nerve, the
zygomatic nerve, and orbital branches from the pterygopalatine ganglion. It also
transmits veins which connect orbital veins with a plexus lateral to the pterygoid
muscles, called the *pterygoid venous plexus*.

QUESTION
24
The inferior orbital fissure connects the _____/_____ fossa with
the _____.

ANSWER
infratemporal . . . orbit

QUESTION
25
The nerves which pass through the inferior orbital fissure include the
_____ nerve, the _____ nerve, and _____
branches from the pterygopalatine ganglion.

ANSWER
infraorbital . . . zygomatic . . . orbital

Blood vessels passing through the inferior orbital fissure include the infra-orbital artery as well as connecting veins which join orbital veins with the _____ plexus.

pterygoid venous

The inferior orbital fissure is an opening between the superior surface of the _____ and the _____ _____ of the sphenoid bone.

maxilla . . . greater wing

THE PTERYGOMAXILLARY FISSURE ITEM 10

The *pterygomaxillary fissure* is an opening between the upper infratemporal surface of the maxilla and the base of the lateral pterygoid plate. The inferior orbital fissure is continuous posteriorly and inferiorly with it. The pterygomaxillary fissure forms the route of the maxillary artery from the infratemporal fossa to the pterygopalatine fossa, where the terminal branches of the maxillary artery are given off.

The pterygomaxillary fissure is continuous with the posterior and inferior parts of the _____ _____ fissure.

inferior orbital

The pterygomaxillary fissure is a cleft between the base of the lateral _____ plate and the upper infratemporal surface of the _____.

pterygoid . . . maxilla

The maxillary artery goes through the pterygomaxillary fissure as this artery passes from the _____ fossa to the _____ fossa.

infratemporal . . . pterygopalatine

ITEM 11   THE PTERYGOPALATINE FOSSA

The *pterygopalatine fossa* is bounded by the pterygoid plates of the sphenoid bone, the maxilla, and the palatine bone. The bony structures related to this fossa can be seen in Figure 13–3. The pterygopalatine fossa contains the maxillary artery with its terminal branches, the maxillary division of the trigeminal (fifth cranial) nerve, and the pterygopalatine ganglion.

The pterygomaxillary fissure in the lateral wall of the pterygopalatine fossa allows entry of the maxillary artery. The foramen rotundum permits entry of the maxillary nerve.

QUESTION 31

Structures occupying the pterygopalatine fossa include the _____ artery, the _____ ganglion, and the _____ division of the trigeminal nerve.

ANSWER

maxillary . . . pterygopalatine . . . maxillary

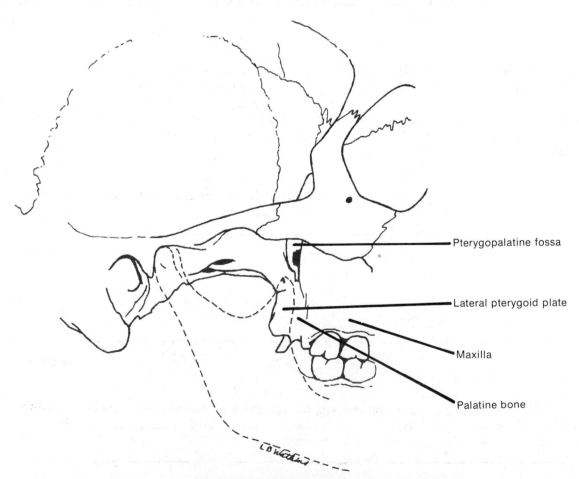

Figure 13–3.   The pterygopalatine fossa, lateral aspect.

The bony landmarks which enclose the pterygopalatine fossa are the pterygoid plates of the _____ bone, the _____ bone, and the _____.

---

sphenoid . . . palatine . . . maxilla

The maxillary nerve enters the pterygopalatine fossa through the foramen _____; the maxillary artery, through the _____ fissure.

---

rotundum . . . pterygopalatine

THE PTERYGOPALATINE FOSSA: THE OPENINGS

Besides the pterygomaxillary fissure and foramen rotundum, there are three other important openings of the pterygopalatine fossa: (1) the palatine canals, (2) the sphenopalatine foramen, and (3) the pterygoid canal.

The *palatine canals* are openings in the inferior surface of the pterygopalatine fossa which transmit the greater and lesser palatine nerves and arteries to the roof of the mouth.

On the medial surface of the fossa, the *sphenopalatine foramen* communicates with the nasal cavity and transmits the sphenopalatine artery and the nasopalatine nerve.

The *pterygoid canal,* situated on the posterior and inferior surface of the fossa, transmits the nerve and artery of the pterygoid canal through the base of the pterygoid plates.

The palatine canals open from the _____ surface of the pterygo-palatine fossa; the pterygoid canal opens on the _____ surface; the sphenopalatine foramen opens on the _____ surface.

---

inferior . . . posterior . . . medial

The greater and lesser _____ nerves and arteries pass through the palatine canals to the roof of the mouth.

---

palatine

QUESTION
36
Through the sphenopalatine foramen, the _____ nerve and the _____ artery enter the nasal cavity.

_____

ANSWER
nasopalatine . . . sphenopalatine

QUESTION
37
The pterygoid canal transmits the nerve and artery of the pterygoid canal through the base of the _____ _____.

_____

ANSWER
pterygoid plates

ITEM 13   THE TEMPORAL AND INFRATEMPORAL FOSSAE: THE SUPERFICIAL CONTENTS

It is important to be able to visualize the structures of the temporal and infratemporal fossae in terms of the relationship of superficial to deep. In trying to picture these soft tissues, you will find it extremely helpful to refer frequently to a skull.

The most superficial structures in the temporal and infratemporal region are the temporalis muscle and the ramus of the mandible, as can be seen in Figure 13–4. The temporalis muscle attaches above to the temporal line and splits below to attach to the lateral and medial edges of the upper rim of the zygoma. Small blood vessels occupy the space thus formed on the upper edge of the zygomatic arch. The temporalis muscle inserts on the anterior border of the ramus of the mandible.

QUESTION
38
The point of attachment of the temporalis muscle superiorly is the _____ _____.

_____

ANSWER
temporal line

QUESTION
39
The lower point of attachment of the temporalis muscle is at the medial and lateral edges of the upper rim of the _____.

_____

ANSWER
zygoma

QUESTION
40
The space between the lower points of attachment of the temporalis muscle is occupied by _____ _____.

_____

ANSWER
blood vessels

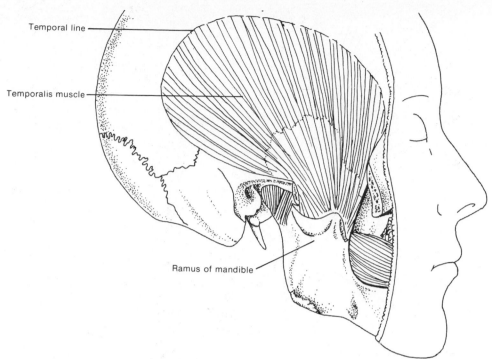

Figure 13–4. Temporalis muscle in the temporal and infratemporal fossae, seen with zygomatic arch and masseter muscle removed. (Redrawn from Wolf-Heidegger: Atlas of Systematic Human Anatomy. Vol. I. Basel, S. Karger AG.)

THE TEMPORAL AND INFRATEMPORAL FOSSAE: THE DEEP CONTENTS

ITEM 14

Deep to the temporalis muscle and deep to the zygomatic arch and the ramus of the mandible are the *lateral* and *medial pterygoid muscles.* Locate these muscles on Figure 13–5. Various nerves occupy the space between the muscles and the superficial structures.

The *lateral pterygoid muscle,* as was explained earlier, extends from the lateral surface of the lateral pterygoid plate and the greater wing of the sphenoid, to the condyle of the mandible and the articular disk.

The *medial pterygoid muscle* extends from the medial surface of the lateral pterygoid plate to the lower medial surface of the ramus of the mandible. Anterior to the medial pterygoid muscle, Figure 13–5 shows the *buccinator muscle.*

The lateral and medial pterygoid muscles are situated in the temporal fossa deep to the _____ muscle and to the _____ arch.

QUESTION
41

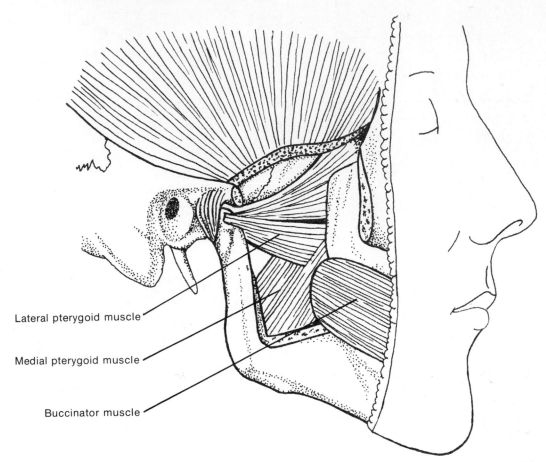

Figure 13–5. Lateral pterygoid, medial pterygoid, and buccinator muscles in the region of the temporal and infratemporal fossae. (Redrawn from Wolf-Heidegger: Atlas of Systematic Human Anatomy. Vol. I. Basel, S. Karger AG.)

Lateral pterygoid muscle

Medial pterygoid muscle

Buccinator muscle

ANSWER   temporalis . . . zygomatic

QUESTION
42

The span of the lateral pterygoid muscle is from the lateral surface of the lateral _____ _____ and the greater wing of the _____ bone, to the _____ of the mandible.

ANSWER   pterygoid plate . . . sphenoid . . . condyle

QUESTION
43

The span of the medial pterygoid muscle is from the medial surface of the lateral _____ _____ to the _____ of the mandible.

ANSWER   pterygoid plate . . . ramus

THE TEMPORAL AND INFRATEMPORAL FOSSAE: STRUCTURES IN ADJACENT AREAS

ITEM 15

Figure 13–6 shows several structures which are not actually within the temporal and infratemporal fossae, but which appropriately are mentioned in a regional treatment of this area. First, notice the *external carotid artery* ascending in the area behind the mandible, the retromandibular space. In this area, the external carotid gives off the *maxillary* and *superficial temporal arteries*. The *transverse facial* and the *zygomatico-orbital arteries* can be seen branching off the superficial temporal artery.

Also seen in Figure 13–6 are the *parotid duct* entering the buccinator muscle, the lateral and medial pterygoid muscles, the buccal artery and nerve, the masseteric artery and nerve, and the inferior alveolar artery and nerve.

Another important structure of this general region, although also not a part of the infratemporal fossa, is the *masseter muscle*. This muscle overlies the ramus of the mandible. In Figure 13–6, the masseter muscle has been removed to reveal underlying structures.

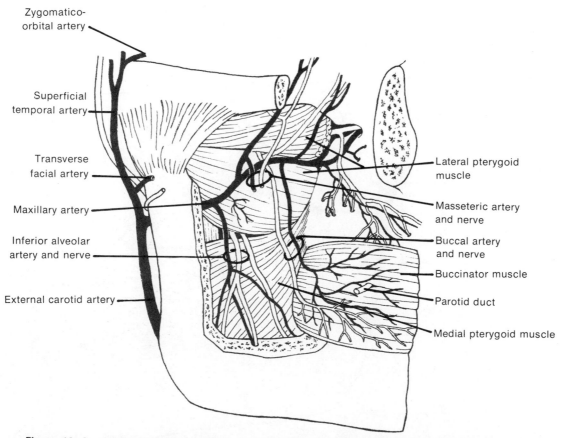

Figure 13–6. Adjacent structures lying outside the temporal and infratemporal fossae, seen with masseter muscle removed. (Redrawn from Woodburne: Essentials of Human Anatomy. 4th Ed. New York, Oxford University Press.)

QUESTION
44

Terminal arteries given off the external carotid in the retromandibular space are the _____ and the _____ _____ arteries.

ANSWER

maxillary . . . superficial temporal

QUESTION
45

Branches of the superficial temporal artery given off in the general vicinity of the temporal region are the _____ _____ artery and the _____ artery.

ANSWER

transverse facial . . . zygomatico-orbital

QUESTION
46

Two important muscles of the face lying adjacent to, but outside, the infratemporal fossa are the _____ and the _____ muscles.

ANSWER

masseter . . . buccinator (in either order)

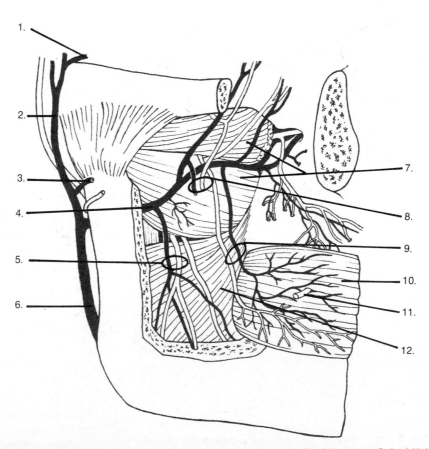

(Redrawn from Woodburne: Essentials of Human Anatomy. 4th Ed. New York, Oxford University Press.)

Using the Word Bank, fill in the numbered blank labels with the names of the corresponding numbered structures in the diagram, page 534.

QUESTION
47

Word Bank

buccal artery and nerve
buccinator muscle
external carotid artery
inferior alveolar artery and nerve
lateral pterygoid muscle
masseteric artery and nerve
maxillary artery
medial pterygoid muscle
parotid duct
superficial temporal artery
transverse facial artery
zygomatico-orbital artery

Labels

1. _____
2. _____
3. _____
4. _____
5. _____
6. _____
7. _____
8. _____
9. _____
10. _____
11. _____
12. _____

Check your labels with Figure 13–6.   *ANSWER*

SUMMARY OF UNIT THIRTEEN

A study of structures of various systems in the particular region of the temporal and infratemporal fossae calls attention to significant anatomical landmarks as well as to the interrelationships of structures in the same area.

THE TEMPORAL FOSSA

The temporal fossa is a depression on the lateral side of the skull, containing the temporalis muscle with its nerves and arteries. Overlying the muscle is the sheath of dense connective tissue called the temporal fascia. The superior and posterior boundaries of the temporal fossa are the temporal lines, which extend in a circle from the zygomatic process of the frontal bone to the zygomatic process of the temporal bone. Anterior limits of the fossa include processes of the frontal and zygomatic bones. The superficial lower border is the zygomatic arch; the deep lower border, the infratemporal crest of the sphenoid bone. The temporal fossa has a floor, or medial wall, formed by parts of the frontal bone, the parietal bone, the greater wing of the sphenoid bone, and the squamous portion of the temporal bone.

THE INFRATEMPORAL FOSSA

The infratemporal fossa, continuous with the temporal fossa above, is the cavity below and medial to the zygomatic arch. The contents of the infratemporal fossa include muscles of mastication, nerves and arteries to the mouth, and deep temporal nerves and vessels. The anterior border of the infratemporal fossa is formed by the infratemporal surface of the maxilla; the posterior border, by the posterior edge of the mandible; the lateral border, by the ramus and coronoid process of the mandible; the medial roof, by the infratemporal crest of the greater wing of the sphenoid bone; and the medial limit, by the lateral pterygoid plate.

Openings in the infratemporal fossa permit passage of nerves and vessels. The foramen ovale transmits the mandibular division of the trigeminal nerve and the accessory meningeal artery through the roof of the fossa. The foramen spinosum, also in the roof, transmits the middle meningeal artery and the meningeal branch of the mandibular nerve. The alveolar canals, opening on the anterior wall of the fossa, admit the posterior superior alveolar artery and the nerve to the upper molar teeth. The infratemporal fossa communicates anteriorly with the orbit via the inferior orbital fissure, through which pass the infraorbital nerve and artery, the zygomatic nerve, and orbital branches from the pterygopalatine ganglion. Continuous with the inferior orbital fissure is the pterygomaxillary fissure, through which the maxillary artery makes its way to the pterygopalatine fossa. The foramen rotundum admits the maxillary division of the trigeminal nerve into the pterygopalatine fossa.

A number of structures not actually within the temporal and infratemporal fossae are situated in this general region of the head. These include the external carotid artery and parts of its terminal branches, the buccinator and masseter muscles, and the nerves and arteries supplying these two muscles.

QUESTION
48

The value of a regional study of anatomy in complementing a systems approach is clarification of the spatial _____ of structures of diverse systems to one another, and the identification of the location of structures by means of anatomical _____.

---

relationships . . . landmarks

The temporal fossa contains the _____ muscle, which is covered by the dense temporal _____.

---

temporalis . . . fascia

The temporal lines constitute the _____ and _____ boundaries of the temporal fossa; processes of the zygomatic and frontal bones, the _____ boundary; the zygomatic arch and the infratemporal crest of the sphenoid, the _____ boundary.

---

superior . . . posterior . . . anterior . . . inferior

The point of convergence of the bones of the floor of the temporal fossa is called the _____.

---

pterion

The medial roof of the infratemporal fossa is the _____ _____ of the greater wing of the sphenoid bone; the anterior border, the infratemporal surface of the _____.

---

infratemporal crest . . . maxilla

The lateral border of the infratemporal fossa is formed by the _____ process and _____ of the mandible.

---

coronoid . . . ramus

The contents of the infratemporal fossa include muscles of _____, nerves and arteries to the _____, in addition to the deep _____ nerves and arteries.

---

mastication . . . mouth . . . temporal

The foramen rotundum admits the _____ division of the trigeminal nerve to the pterygopalatine fossa.

ANSWER   maxillary

QUESTION   The mandibular division of the trigeminal nerve enters the infratemporal fossa
56   through the foramen _____.

ANSWER   ovale

QUESTION   The middle meningeal artery enters the infratemporal fossa through the fora-
57   men _____.

ANSWER   spinosum

QUESTION   Muscles near but not within the temporal and infratemporal fossae are the
58   _____ muscle and the _____ muscle.

ANSWER   masseter . . . buccinator (in either order)

Unit Fourteen □ THE MOUTH AND RELATED STRUCTURES

THE ORAL CAVITY

The oral cavity is bounded anteriorly by the lips, posteriorly by the pharynx, laterally by the cheeks, inferiorly by the muscles of the floor, and superiorly by the palate. The opening from the oral cavity to the exterior is called the *oral fissure*. The arched opening from the oral cavity into the pharynx is called the *fauces*. The teeth and the alveolar processes divide the oral cavity into two regions: the *oral cavity proper,* within the teeth, and the *vestibule,* between the teeth and the cheeks and lips.

The fauces forms the opening of the oral cavity into the _____; the oral fissure, the opening to the _____.

QUESTION 1

---

pharynx . . . exterior

ANSWER

The vestibule is the space between the _____ and the _____ and lips.

QUESTION 2

---

teeth . . . cheeks

ANSWER

The boundaries of the oral cavity are
1. laterally, the _____
2. anteriorly, the _____
3. posteriorly, the _____
4. superiorly, the _____
5. inferiorly, the _____ of the floor

QUESTION 3

ANSWER

1. cheeks	4. palate
2. lips	5. muscles
3. pharynx	

ITEM 2

THE LIPS: THE UPPER LIP

The lips are extremely mobile muscular folds covered by mucous membrane on the inside and by skin on the outside. Structures of the lips include the orbicularis oris muscle, connective tissue, outer skin, inner mucous membrane, labial glands, and associated blood vessels and nerves.

The upper lip is bounded superiorly by the nose and laterally by the *nasolabial sulcus* between the upper lip and cheeks. The furrow extending down the midline, the *philtrum,* ends in a thicker area of the upper lip, the *tubercle.* Locate these markings on Figure 14–1.

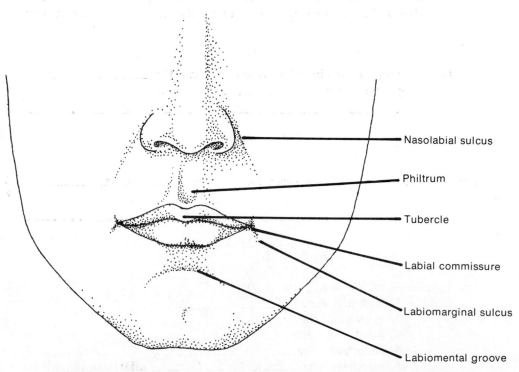

Nasolabial sulcus

Philtrum

Tubercle

Labial commissure

Labiomarginal sulcus

Labiomental groove

Figure 14–1.   Lower part of the face, showing grooves bordering the lips. (Redrawn from Wolf-Heidegger: Atlas of Systematic Human Anatomy. Vol. II. Basel, S. Karger AG.)

The lips are composed of the _____ _____ muscle and connective tissue, covered by an outer _____ and an inner _____ membrane.

orbicularis oris . . . skin . . . mucous

The furrow between cheeks and upper lip is the _____ sulcus.

nasolabial

The philtrum is the groove in the _____ of the upper lip which terminates inferiorly in the thicker _____.

midline . . . tubercle

THE LIPS: THE LOWER LIP   ITEM 3

The lower lip extends down to the *horizontal labiomental groove* which separates it from the chin. A *labiomarginal sulcus,* extending downward from the corner of the mouth toward the mandible, usually develops with age. These two grooves can be seen in Figure 14–1. The fold connecting the upper and lower lips is known as the *labial commissure,* or angle of the mouth.

The labial commissure forms the _____ of the mouth.

angle

The furrow running from the corner of the mouth inferiorly across the mandible is the _____ sulcus; that between the lower lip and the chin, the _____ groove.

labiomarginal . . . labiomental

ITEM 4

THE LIPS: THE RED ZONE

The transition zone between the skin of the lips and the mucous membrane of the oral cavity is the *red zone*. It is characterized by thin nonkeratinized epithelium and dense connective tissue papillae. The fact that the capillaries in the connective tissue papillae are near the surface and covered only by thin epithelium gives this area its typical red coloration. The mucous membrane of the lips is composed of stratified squamous epithelium with numerous labial glands.

QUESTION
9

The red zone of the lips is the area between _____ and _____ membrane of the lips.

ANSWER

skin . . . mucous

QUESTION
10

The red zone derives its particular coloration from the nearness of the _____ to the surface and the thinness of the covering _____.

ANSWER

capillaries . . . epithelium

QUESTION
11

Labial glands are located in the (circle one) *skin/red zone/mucous membrane* of the lips.

ANSWER

mucous membrane

ITEM 5

THE CHEEKS

The cheeks are composed of the horizontally oriented buccinator muscle anteriorly and the vertically oriented masseter muscle posteriorly. Between these two muscles is an area of fat tissue, the *buccal fat pad*. Figure 14–2 shows these two cheek muscles in relation to other muscles of the face and neck. These muscles are bounded by fascia and skin superficially, and by mucous membrane on the oral surface.

QUESTION
12

Two major muscles in the cheek are the vertical _____ muscle posteriorly and the horizontal _____ muscle anteriorly.

ANSWER

masseter . . . buccinator

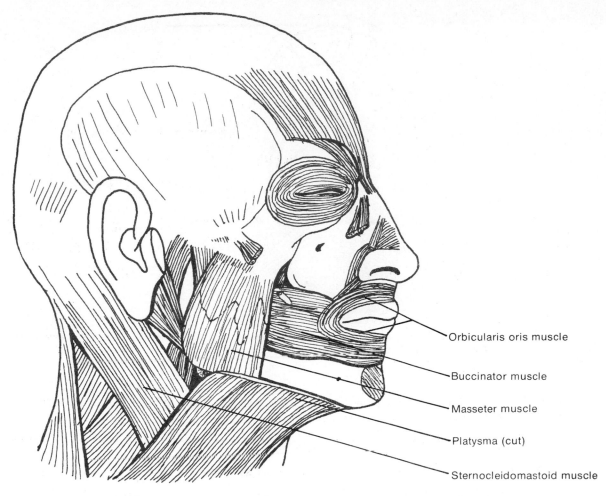

Figure 14–2. Cheek muscles in relationship to other muscles of the face and neck. (Redrawn from Wolf-Heidegger: Atlas of Systematic Human Anatomy. Vol. I. Basel, S. Karger A.G.)

THE CHEEK: THE VESTIBULAR SURFACE

ITEM 6

The vestibular surface of each cheek is bounded superiorly and inferiorly by the reflection of the mucous membrane onto the alveolar process. The posterior limit is a fold joining the posterior ends of the upper and lower alveolar processes. This fold is elevated by the *pterygomandibular raphe,* a connective tissue band between the pterygoid hamulus and the retromolar triangle. Observe the location of the pterygomandibular raphe on Figure 14–3.

Mucous membrane of the vestibule reflects superiorly and inferiorly onto the _____ processes.

QUESTION 13

---

alveolar

ANSWER

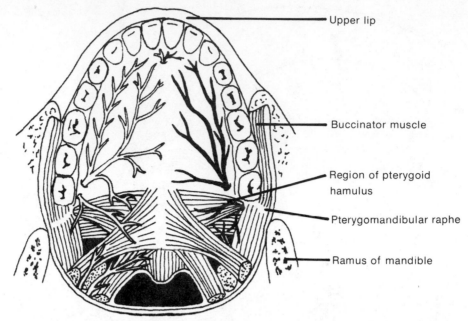

Figure 14-3. Roof of the mouth and pterygomandibular raphe. (Modified from Leeson and Leeson: Human Structure. Philadelphia, W. B. Saunders Co.)

QUESTION
14

The elevated band of connective tissue between the retromolar triangle and the pterygoid hamulus is called the _____ raphe.

ANSWER

pterygomandibular

ITEM
7

THE VESTIBULE

In the anterior midline of the vestibule are located folds of connective tissue covered by mucous membrane. These two folds, one anterior to maxillary incisors, one anterior to mandibular incisors, are called frenula.

QUESTION
15

The frenula in the anterior midline of the vestibule of the mouth are folds of _____ _____ with a mucous membrane covering.

ANSWER

connective tissue

THE VESTIBULE: THE ALVEOLAR MUCOSA

Alveolar mucosa in the uppermost and lowermost regions of the vestibule is thin, and loosely attached to connective tissue. It appears red due to the numerous underlying blood vessels. The thicker alveolar mucosa adjacent to teeth is firmly bound to the underlying bone, and is a pink color lighter than that of the mucosa at the top and bottom. This latter area is the *labial gingiva*. The line of demarcation between the two zones is the *mucogingival junction*.

The thicker alveolar mucosa is the _____ adjacent to the teeth.

gingiva

The demarcation between thin alveolar mucosa and the labial gingiva is called the _____ junction.

mucogingival

THE GINGIVAL PAPILLAE

Gingival papillae are projections of gingiva extending between teeth and forming the transition between vestibular mucosa and oral mucosa. Behind the last upper molar teeth, the mucosa is continuous over the alveolar tubercle in the *retromolar area*.

Gingival papillae extend between the _____ and mark the transition from vestibular _____ to oral _____.

teeth . . . mucosa . . . mucosa

The region posterior to molar teeth is the _____ area.

retromolar

ITEM
10

THE VESTIBULE: STRUCTURES

Gingiva covering the alveolar process immediately behind the last mandibular molar teeth is elevated to form a *retromolar papilla*. Posterior to the papilla is the retromolar pad, an accumulation of buccal glands called the *retromolar glands*.

The space between the retromolar alveolar processes is adequate to allow passage of a tube when the teeth are clenched, as in the case of tetanus or of the ankylosis of the temporomandibular joint.

The duct of the parotid gland extends medially through the buccinator muscle to reach the vestibule. This duct opens into the buccal mucosa at the level of the second maxillary molar tooth.

QUESTION
20

The retromolar pad is composed of _____ glands located behind the retromolar papilla.

ANSWER

buccal

QUESTION
21

The retromolar papilla consists of _____ covering the alveolar process behind the last _____ molar teeth.

ANSWER

gingiva . . . mandibular

QUESTION
22

The duct of the parotid gland penetrates the _____ muscle to enter the vestibule of the mouth at the level of the second _____ _____ tooth.

ANSWER

buccinator . . . maxillary molar

ITEM
11

THE ORAL CAVITY PROPER

The oral cavity proper is bounded by the alveolar process and the teeth peripherally, and the area formed by the *uvula* and *palatine folds* posteriorly. These latter structures can be seen on Figure 14–4. The hard and soft palate form the roof of the mouth; the mucosa covering the mylohyoid and hyoglossus muscles forms the floor.

QUESTION
23

The roof of the oral cavity proper is formed by the _____; the floor, by mucosa covering the _____ and _____ muscles.

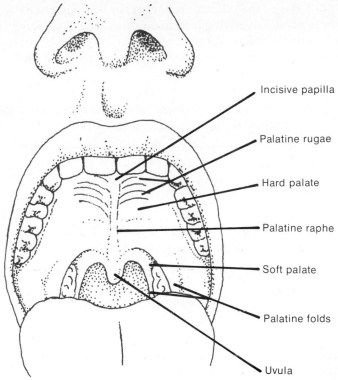

Incisive papilla

Palatine rugae

Hard palate

Palatine raphe

Soft palate

Palatine folds

Uvula

Figure 14–4. Interior of mouth, tongue extended, showing hard palate. (Redrawn from Wolf-Heidegger: Atlas of Systematic Human Anatomy. Vol. II. Basel, S. Karger AG.)

palate . . . mylohyoid . . . hyoglossus   *ANSWER*

The peripheral boundary of the oral cavity proper consists of the _____ and the _____ process; the posterior boundary, of the _____ and the _____ folds.   QUESTION **24**

teeth . . . alveolar . . . uvula . . . palatine   *ANSWER*

THE HARD PALATE   ITEM 12

The palate is composed of the bony hard palate and the muscular soft palate. The hard palate is formed by the palatine processes of the maxilla and the horizontal processes of the palatine bones, together with overlying mucosa. The mucous membrane is firmly attached by connective tissue strands to the periosteal covering of bone, and for this reason is termed *mucoperiosteum.*

Figure 14–4 shows the *palatine raphe* extending posteriorly in the midline from the *incisive papilla* overlying the incisive foramen. Extending laterally from the raphe are several ridges formed by underlying dense connective tissue. These ridges are called *transverse palatine folds,* or *palatine rugae.*

QUESTION
25

Bony parts of the hard palate include the palatine process of the _____ and the horizontal process of the _____ bone.

ANSWER

maxilla . . . palatine

QUESTION
26

The mucous membrane of the hard palate is called _____ because it attaches to the periosteal covering of bone.

ANSWER

mucoperiosteum

QUESTION
27

Transverse ridges of connective tissue, called palatine _____, extend laterally from the palatine_____.

ANSWER

rugae . . . raphe

ITEM 13   THE HARD PALATE: BLOOD SUPPLY

Figure 14–5 shows the main blood supply to the hard palate and adjacent gingiva. The arterial supply comes primarily from the *greater palatine branch* of the maxillary artery. This branch descends in the palatine canal and enters the roof of the mouth at the greater palatine foramen near the inner side of the third maxillary molar. The greater palatine artery passes forward in a groove at the base of the alveolar process to distribute to the gingiva, palatine glands, and mucoperiosteum of the hard palate. It joins the *sphenopalatine branch* of the maxillary artery at the incisive canal.

Additional blood supply to the gingiva is by way of the posterior, middle, and anterior superior alveolar branches of the maxillary artery.

QUESTION
28

Branches of the maxillary artery supplying the hard palate and adjacent gingiva are the _____ _____ and _____ branches, with

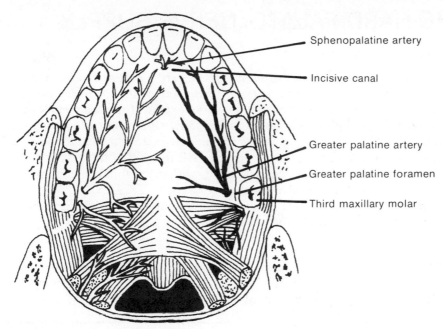

Figure 14–5. Blood supply to the hard palate. (Modified from Leeson and Leeson: Human Structure. Philadelphia, W. B. Saunders Co.)

additional supply to adjacent gingiva from the anterior, middle, and posterior _____ _____ arteries.

---

greater palatine . . . sphenopalatine . . . superior alveolar   *ANSWER*

The greater palatine foramen, through which branches of the maxillary artery enter the roof of the mouth, is situated medial to the third _____ _____ tooth.   QUESTION **29**

---

maxillary molar   *ANSWER*

Structures receiving blood from the greater palatine branches are the _____ membrane of the hard palate, the adjacent _____, and the _____ glands.   QUESTION **30**

---

mucous . . . gingiva . . . palatine   *ANSWER*

Branches of the greater palatine artery anastomose with the _____ _____ branch of the maxillary artery at the _____ canal.   QUESTION **31**

---

sphenopalatine . . . incisive   *ANSWER*

ITEM 14

THE HARD PALATE: NERVE SUPPLY

Figure 14–6 shows the nerve supply to the hard palate and adjacent gingiva: the *greater palatine* and the *nasopalatine branches* of the maxillary division of the trigeminal nerve. The greater palatine nerve extends from the pterygopalatine fossa downward in the palatine canals in company with the corresponding artery. Turning forward at the greater palatine foramen, it extends medial to the alveolar process, supplying the mucoperiosteum adjacent to most of the maxillary teeth.

The greater palatine nerve communicates with the nasopalatine branch of the maxillary division at the incisive canal.

The upper labial gingiva is also supplied by anterior, middle, and posterior superior alveolar branches of the maxillary nerve.

QUESTION
32

The main nerve supply to the hard palate is described by the same name as the main blood supply: it is called the _____ _____ nerve of the maxillary division of the trigeminal nerve.

ANSWER

greater palatine

QUESTION
33

The greater palatine nerve extends from the _____ fossa through the greater _____ foramen to reach the mucoperiosteum of the hard palate.

ANSWER

pterygopalatine . . . palatine

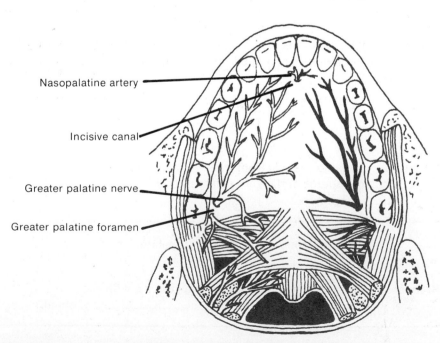

Nasopalatine artery

Incisive canal

Greater palatine nerve

Greater palatine foramen

Figure 14–6. Nerve supply to the hard palate. (Modified from Leeson and Leeson: Human Structure. Philadelphia, W. B. Saunders Co.)

The greater palatine nerve communicates with the _____ branch of the maxillary nerve at the incisive canal.

---

nasopalatine

Superior alveolar branches of the maxillary nerve also supply the maxillary _____ gingiva.

---

labial

THE SOFT PALATE   ITEM 15

The soft palate is composed of muscle and loosely woven connective tissue with a rich vascular composition overlaid with nonkeratinized epithelium. Underlying blood vessels and glands give the soft palate a red color, in contrast to the pale color of the hard palate. The free posterior border of the soft palate is bilaterally concave, with the uvula projecting downward in the midline.

The hard palate is composed of mucosa and dense connective tissue overlying _____; the soft palate, of mucosa and loose connective tissue overlying _____.

---

bone . . . muscle

The downward projection from the midline of the posterior soft palate is the _____.

---

uvula

THE SOFT PALATE: THE FOLDS   ITEM 16

Two folds which overlie muscles of the same name extend downward from the soft palate in a lateral direction. The *palatoglossal fold* and *palatoglossal muscle* are anterior; the *palatopharyngeal fold* and *muscle* are posterior. The *palatine tonsil* lies in the triangular groove between the two folds. These structures are shown in Figure 14–7.

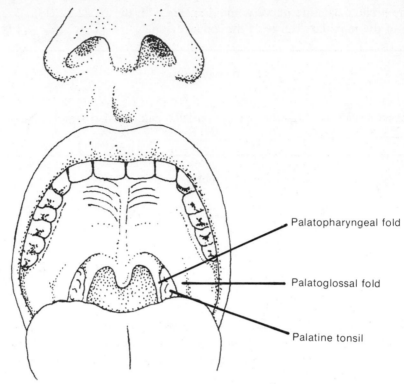

Figure 14–7.   Interior of mouth, tongue extended, showing palatoglossal and palatopharyngeal folds. (Redrawn from Wolf-Heidegger: Atlas of Systematic Human Anatomy. Vol. II. Basel, S. Karger AG.)

A third fold in the posterior region of the mouth, the pterygomandibular fold, was discussed in Item 6. The pterygomandibular fold is not considered part of the soft palate.

QUESTION 38

The three folds in the posterior portion of the mouth are called the _____ _____ fold, the _____ fold, and the _____ _____ fold.

ANSWER

palatoglossal . . . palatopharyngeal . . . pterygomandibular (in any order)

QUESTION 39

The palatine tonsil is situated in the groove between the _____ fold anteriorly and the _____ fold posteriorly.

ANSWER

palatoglossal . . . palatopharyngeal

QUESTION 40

Of the three folds in the posterior region of the mouth, one, the *palatoglossal/ palatopharyngeal/pterygomandibular* (circle one) fold, is not a palatine fold.

ANSWER

pterygomandibular

THE SOFT PALATE: THE MUSCLES   ITEM 17

Five palatine muscles can be seen in Figure 14–8. The *palatoglossus* muscle descends from the palate to the tongue; the *palatopharyngeal* muscle, from the palate to the pharynx. Two muscles descend to the soft palate from the base of the skull: the *levator veli palatini* and the *tensor veli palatini*. The fifth palatine muscle, the *musculus uvulae*, lies within the soft palate.

The palatine muscle within the soft palate is called the musculus _____.

QUESTION 41

uvulae

ANSWER

The palatoglossus muscle extends from the palate to the _____;
the palatopharyngeal, from the palate to the _____.

QUESTION 42

tongue . . . pharynx

ANSWER

The palatine muscles extending from the base of the skull to the palate are the
_____ _____ palatini and the _____ _____ palatini.

QUESTION 43

levator veli . . . tensor veli (in either order)

ANSWER

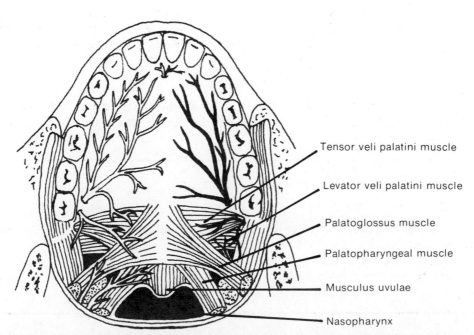

Tensor veli palatini muscle

Levator veli palatini muscle

Palatoglossus muscle

Palatopharyngeal muscle

Musculus uvulae

Nasopharynx

Figure 14–8. Muscles of the soft palate. (Modified from Leeson and Leeson: Human Structure. Philadelphia, W. B. Saunders Co.)

ITEM
18

THE LEVATOR VELI PALATINI MUSCLE

Note the position of the levator veli palatini muscle again on Figure 14–8. The levator veli palatini muscle originates on the undersurface of the skull at the apex of the petrous bone and the medial cartilage of the auditory tube and inserts into the palatine aponeurosis. Contraction of this muscle elevates the palate and pulls open the orifice of the auditory tube.

QUESTION
44

Contraction of the levator veli palatini does two things: it opens the orifice of the _____ _____ and it elevates the _____.

ANSWER

auditory tube . . . palate

ITEM
19

THE TENSOR VELI PALATINI MUSCLE

Refer to Figure 14–8 again, and note the position of the tensor veli palatini muscle. This muscle originates from the scaphoid fossa and the lateral cartilage of the auditory tube. Its fibers descend between the medial pterygoid muscle and the medial pterygoid plate, forming a tendon near the pterygoid hamulus. Contraction of the tensor veli palatini draws the palate tighter laterally and opens the orifice of the auditory tube.

QUESTION
45

Contraction of the _____ veli palatini muscle elevates the palate; contraction of the _____ veli palatini muscle draws the palate tighter in a lateral direction.

ANSWER

levator . . . tensor

QUESTION
46

The opening of the orifice of the auditory tube is accomplished by contraction of the (circle one)
A. levator veli palatini muscle
B. tensor veli palatini muscle
C. either of the above two muscles

ANSWER

The correct answer is C. Both the tensor veli palatini and the levator veli palatini muscles open the auditory tube when they contract.

THE PALATINE MUSCLES: CONTRACTIONS IN SWALLOWING

ITEM
20.

Look back to Figure 14–8 and observe the position of the palatoglossus and palatopharyngeal muscles in relation to the levator and tensor veli palatini muscles. When the latter muscles are relaxed, the soft palate extends downward into the anterior oropharynx. Contraction of the levator and tensor veli palatini muscles elevates the soft palate and carries it back toward the posterior pharyngeal wall. Contraction of the palatopharyngeal muscle brings the pharyngeal wall forward. These combined actions close off the nasopharynx to prevent food from entering the nasal cavity while being swallowed. During the act of swallowing, the palatoglossus muscle elevates the tongue toward the soft palate and the tensor veli palatini tenses the palate against this arching action of the tongue.

When swallowing, it is necessary to keep food from going into the nasal cavity. This preventive action is accomplished by the combined contractions of the palatopharyngeal muscle moving the pharyngeal wall *forward/backward* (circle one) and the levator and tensor veli palatini muscles moving the palate *forward/ backward* (circle one).

QUESTION
47

---

forward . . . backward

ANSWER

During the act of swallowing, the _____ muscle elevates the tongue and the _____ muscle elevates the pharynx.

QUESTION
48

---

palatoglossus . . . palatopharyngeal

ANSWER

It is necessary in swallowing to tense the palate against the arching action of the tongue; this tensing is accomplished by contraction of the _____ _____ _____ muscle.

QUESTION
49

---

tensor veli palatini

ANSWER

THE SOFT PALATE: NERVE SUPPLY

ITEM
21

The tensor veli palatini muscle is supplied by a branch of the mandibular division of the trigeminal nerve, called the *nerve to the tensor veli palatini*. All the other muscles of the soft palate are supplied by the vagus nerve through the pharyngeal plexus. Sensory innervation to the mucosa of the soft palate is by way of the lesser palatine branch of the maxillary nerve.

QUESTION
50

The vagus nerve supplies all the muscles of the soft palate except the _____ _____ palatini muscle, which receives motor innervation from a branch of the _____ division of the trigeminal nerve.

ANSWER

tensor veli . . . mandibular

QUESTION
51

The lesser palatine nerve, a branch of the _____ division of the trigeminal nerve, supplies sensory innervation to the _____ of the soft palate.

ANSWER

maxillary . . . mucosa

ITEM 22   THE SOFT PALATE: BLOOD SUPPLY

The *lesser palatine artery,* a branch of the maxillary artery, provides the blood supply to the soft palate and palatine folds. The lesser palatine artery descends along with the lesser palatine nerve through the palatine canal, exits through the lesser palatine foramen, and distributes to the soft palate and palatine arches. Figure 14–9 shows the lesser palatine artery and nerve after they enter the mouth through the lesser palatine foramen.

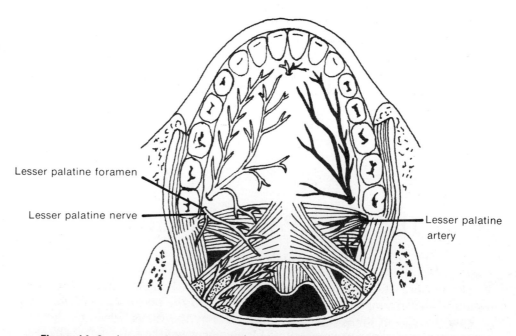

Figure 14–9. Lesser palatine artery and nerve. (Modified from Leeson and Leeson: Human Structure. Philadelphia, W. B. Saunders Co.)

The soft palate and palatine folds receive their blood supply from the _____ _____ branch of the maxillary artery.

QUESTION 52

lesser palatine

ANSWER

The lesser palatine artery enters the oral cavity through the _____ canal and _____ _____ foramen.

QUESTION 53

palatine . . . lesser palatine

ANSWER

THE SUBLINGUAL REGION OF THE MOUTH   ITEM 23

The sublingual region of the mouth, the *sublingual sulcus,* is a horseshoe shaped area surrounding the attachment of the tongue. A median fold of mucous membrane, the *lingual frenulum,* extends perpendicularly between the root of the tongue and the floor of the mouth. The floor of the mouth is supported by the *mylohoid, geniohyoid,* and *hyoglossus muscles,* shown in Figure 14–10. The muscular floor of the sublingual region is a part of the submandibular region of the neck. Between the floor and the sublingual mucosa are blood vessels, nerves, the sublingual gland, and the duct of the submandibular gland.

The three muscles supporting the floor of the mouth are the _____ muscle, the _____ muscle, and the _____ muscle.

QUESTION 54

mylohyoid . . . geniohyoid . . . hyoglossus (in any order)

ANSWER

The location of the nerves and blood vessels in the sublingual region of the mouth lies between the _____ of the floor of the mouth and the sublingual _____.

QUESTION 55

muscles . . . mucosa

ANSWER

The medial fold of membrane running from the base of the tongue to the floor of the mouth is called the lingual _____.

QUESTION 56

frenulum

ANSWER

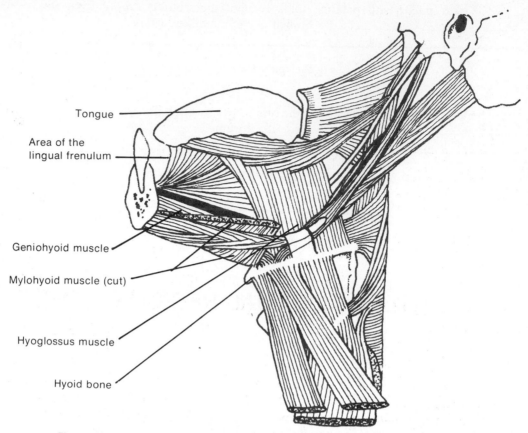

Tongue

Area of the
lingual frenulum

Geniohyoid muscle

Mylohyoid muscle (cut)

Hyoglossus muscle

Hyoid bone

Figure 14–10. Muscles supporting the floor of the mouth, lateral aspect. (Redrawn from Romanes,
Ed: Cunningham's Textbook of Anatomy. 10th Ed. New York, Oxford University Press.)

ITEM 24   THE MYLOHYOID MUSCLE

The *mylohyoid muscle* arises from the whole length of the mylohyoid line
of the mandible, from the symphysis anteriorly to the third mandibular molar tooth
posteriorly. The anterior and middle fibers of the mylohyoid muscle insert into the
fibrous mylohyoid raphe; its posterior fibers insert into the upper surface of the
hyoid bone. The mylohyoid muscle is innervated by the *nerve to the mylohyoid*,
a branch of the mandibular division of the trigeminal nerve.

QUESTION
57

The mylohyoid muscle originates at the _____ _____ of the
mandible.

ANSWER

mylohyoid line

QUESTION
58

The insertions of the mylohyoid muscle are the mylohyoid _____
and the _____ bone.

raphe . . . hyoid

The nerve to the mylohyoid muscle branches off the _____ division of the trigeminal nerve.

mandibular

THE GENIOHYOID MUSCLE   ITEM 25

The *geniohyoid muscle* lies superior to the mylohyoid muscle, as can be seen in Figure 14–10. The geniohyoid muscle arises from the *genial tubercles* (mental spine) on the posterior surface of the symphysis of the mandible; it inserts on the hyoid bone. The muscle is innervated by a branch of the first cervical nerve, which is conducted to the geniohyoid muscle by fibers of the hypoglossal nerve.

The mylohyoid muscle and the geniohyoid muscle both insert into the _____ bone.

hyoid

The geniohyoid muscle originates at the mental spine, which is also called the _____ tubercles.

genial

The motor nerve which supplies the geniohyoid muscle is a branch of the first _____ nerve conducted by the _____ nerve.

cervical . . . hypoglossal

THE HYOGLOSSUS MUSCLE   ITEM 26

Look back to Figure 14–10 and notice the *hyoglossus muscle* arising from the whole length of the greater horn of the hyoid bone. This muscle extends superiorly to insert at the side of the tongue. The hyoglossus is a retractor muscle which pulls the sides of the tongue downward. Innervation of the hyoglossus is by the hypoglossal nerve.

QUESTION
63

The function of the hyoglossus muscle is to retract the _____ of the _____ downward.

ANSWER

sides . . . tongue

QUESTION
64

The origin of the hyoglossus muscle is the greater horn of the _____ bone; the insertion, the lateral region of the _____ .

ANSWER

hyoid . . . tongue

QUESTION
65

The hyoglossus muscle receives motor impulses from the _____ nerve.

ANSWER

hypoglossal

ITEM
27

THE SUBLINGUAL REGION:
STRUCTURES

Examine Figure 14–11 and note the various structures located in the sublingual region of the mouth. The *sublingual glands* and *submandibular duct* lie between the sublingual mucosa and the muscular floor. The lingual and hypoglossal nerves and the lingual blood vessels approach inferiorly between the sublingual mucosa and muscular floor to supply the tongue.

QUESTION
66

Between the sublingual mucosa and muscular floor are found the _____ duct and the _____ gland.

ANSWER

submandibular . . . sublingual

QUESTION
67

Nerve supply to the tongue is carried by the _____ and _____ nerves; blood supply, by the _____ artery.

ANSWER

lingual . . . hypoglossal . . . lingual

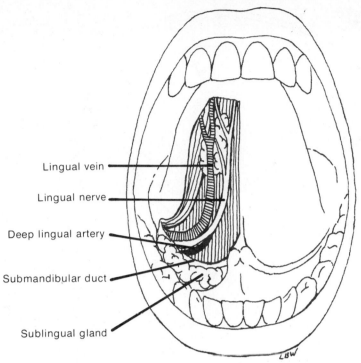

Lingual vein

Lingual nerve

Deep lingual artery

Submandibular duct

Sublingual gland

Figure 14–11. Inferior surface of the tongue, with right side removed to show structures in the sublingual region. (Redrawn from C. Goss, Ed: Gray's Anatomy of the Human Body. 29th Ed. Philadelphia, Lea & Febiger.)

THE SALIVARY GLANDS: THE PAROTID GLAND

ITEM 28

Three major salivary glands open into the mouth: the *parotid, submandibular,* and *sublingual* glands. The parotid is the largest of the three; it surrounds the posterior surface of the upper ramus of the mandible. In the retromandibular space, it extends irregularly downward from the zygomatic arch to the angle of the mandible. The deeper regions of the parotid gland extend almost to the muscles of the pharynx. Laterally it protrudes around the ramus of the mandible and partially overlaps the masseter muscle. Running within the parotid gland are the external carotid artery, the retromandibular vein, and the facial nerve. Find the locations of the salivary glands in Figure 14–12.

The vertical limits of the parotid gland are the _____ arch above, and the _____ of the mandible below.

QUESTION
68

---

zygomatic . . . angle

ANSWER

The parotid gland extends around the _____ of the mandible and covers part of the _____ muscle.

QUESTION
69

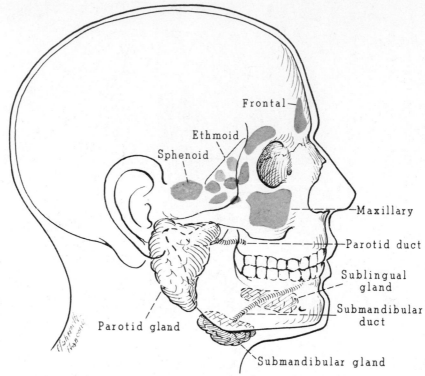

Figure 14–12.   The head, lateral view, showing salivary glands. (Modified from Jacob and Francone: Structure and Function in Man. 3rd Ed. Philadelphia: W. B. Saunders Company.)

ANSWER   ramus . . . masseter

QUESTION   Structures which pass through the parotid gland include the _____
70   nerve, the _____ vein, and the external _____ artery.

ANSWER   facial . . . retromandibular . . . carotid

ITEM 29   THE DUCT OF THE PAROTID GLAND

   The *parotid duct* leaves the glandular tissue lateral to the ramus of the mandible slightly below the zygoma. It courses lateral to the masseter muscle and around the buccal fat pad, then penetrates the buccinator muscle near its posterior limits. The duct opens into the vestibule at the parotid papilla, opposite the second maxillary molar tooth. Locate the parotid duct in Figure 14–12.

The parotid papilla, the site where the parotid duct enters the _____
of the mouth, is situated opposite the second _____ _____ tooth.

vestibule . . . maxillary molar

The route of the parotid duct runs lateral to the _____ muscle and
and through the _____ muscle.

masseter . . . buccinator

THE PAROTID FASCIA   ITEM 30

The fascia covering the parotid gland is an extension of the cervical fascia. As
it ascends, it splits into superficial and deep layers.

The *superficial parotid fascia* continues over the surface of the gland to the
zygomatic arch above and the masseter muscle anteriorly.

The *deep parotid fascia* extends to the styloid process where it thickens to
become the *stylomandibular ligament*. This ligament extends from the styloid
process to the posterior angle of the mandible, and separates the parotid gland from
the submandibular gland.

The superficial layer of fascia covering the parotid gland extends forward to
the _____ muscle and upward to the _____ arch.

masseter . . . zygomatic

The stylomastoid ligament is actually a thickening of the deep _____
fascia.

parotid

The stylomastoid ligament serves as a partition between the _____
gland and the _____ gland.

parotid . . . submandibular (in either order)

ITEM 31

THE SALIVARY GLANDS: THE SUBMANDIBULAR GLAND

The *submandibular gland* occupies that part of the submandibular triangle of the neck below and in front of the angle of the mandible. Most of the glandular tissue is superficial to the posterior border of the mylohyoid muscle, but a lesser portion extends around the mylohyoid and lies deep to that muscle. The facial artery, as it extends around the lower border of the mandible, grooves the medial and superficial surfaces of the submandibular gland. Locate the submandibular gland in Figure 14–12.

QUESTION 76

The medial and superior surfaces of the submandibular gland are grooved by the _____ artery.

ANSWER

facial

QUESTION 77

The submandibular gland lies mostly superficial to, but partially deep to, the _____ muscle.

ANSWER

mylohyoid

QUESTION 78

The submandibular gland lies *above/below* (circle one) and *behind/in front of* (circle one) the angle of the mandible.

ANSWER

below . . . in front of

ITEM 32

THE SUBMANDIBULAR DUCT

The *submandibular duct* arises from the deep part of the submandibular gland. It passes medially forward and upward superior to the hyoglossus and genioglossus muscles. The submandibular duct crosses the sublingual region medial to the sublingual fold to open, along with the major duct of the *sublingual gland,* into the *sublingual caruncle* at the midline of the floor of the mouth. Locate the submandibular duct in Figure 14–12.

QUESTION 79

From deep within its gland, the submandibular duct ascends forward, superior to the _____ and _____ muscles.

ANSWER

hyoglossus . . . genioglossus (in either order)

Two salivary ducts enter the mouth at the sublingual caruncle, the
_____ duct and the _____ duct.

submandibular . . . sublingual (in either order)

THE SUBLINGUAL GLAND: LOCATION   ITEM 33

The sublingual gland rests on the superior aspect of the mylohyoid muscle in the sublingual fossa of the mandible. Its mass forms an oblique elevation, the _sublingual fold_, along the floor of the mouth. Minor sublingual ducts open along the crest of the fold. Note the location of the sublingual gland in Figure 14–12.

The sublingual fold is an elevation formed by the _____ gland at the floor of the mouth.

sublingual

Structures which open on the crest of the sublingual fold are small _____ ducts.

sublingual

The sublingual gland is located in the sublingual fossa of the _____, lying on the anterior part of the _____ muscle.

mandible . . . mylohyoid

THE SALIVARY GLANDS: BLOOD SUPPLY   ITEM 34

The blood supply to the parotid gland is from three branches of the external carotid artery: the _posterior auricular, superficial temporal,_ and _transverse facial_ arteries. Blood supply to the submandibular gland is from branches of the _facial artery_. Blood supply to the sublingual gland is from the _sublingual branch_ of the lingual artery and the _submental branch_ of the facial artery.

QUESTION
84

Three arteries supply blood to the parotid gland: the posterior _____, the superficial _____, and the transverse _____.

ANSWER

auricular . . . temporal . . . facial

QUESTION
85

The facial artery supplies blood to two salivary glands, the _____ gland and the _____ gland.

ANSWER

submandibular . . . sublingual (in either order)

QUESTION
86

The sublingual gland receives blood supply from the sublingual branch of the _____ artery and from the submental branch of the _____ artery.

ANSWER

lingual . . . facial

ITEM 35   THE PAROTID GLAND: NERVE SUPPLY

Salivary glands receive both a sympathetic and a parasympathetic nerve supply. Sympathetic nerves are vasoconstrictor in nature, and reach the respective glands as plexi surrounding incoming blood vessels. The parotid gland receives its sensory innervation from the auriculotemporal nerve. Parasympathetic fibers originate in the glossopharyngeal nerve, synapse at the otic ganglion, and travel with the auriculotemporal nerve to the gland.

QUESTION
87

Plexi which constrict the blood vessels entering the salivary glands are *sympathetic/parasympathetic* (circle one) nerves.

ANSWER

sympathetic

QUESTION
88

The afferent nerve supply of the parotid gland is from the _____ nerve; the efferent supply, from the _____ nerve.

ANSWER

auriculotemporal . . . glossopharyngeal

Preganglionic parasympathetic fibers to the parotid gland synapse in the _____ ganglion; the postganglionic fibers travel to the gland along with sensory fibers of the _____ nerve.

QUESTION
89

---

otic . . . auriculotemporal

ANSWER

THE SUBMANDIBULAR AND SUBLINGUAL GLANDS: NERVE SUPPLY

ITEM
36

Parasympathetic fibers from the facial nerve enter the chorda tympani branch and travel with the lingual nerve of the mandibular division to the submandibular ganglion. This ganglion lies between the hyoglossus and mylohyoid muscles. Here, preganglionic fibers synapse with postganglionic fibers which distribute to both submandibular and sublingual glands.

Preganglionic parasympathetic nerves to the submandibular and sublingual glands are fibers of the _____ nerve which synapse in the _____ _____ ganglion, from which postganglionic fibers distribute to the two glands.

QUESTION
90

---

facial . . . submandibular

ANSWER

The submandibular ganglion lies between the _____ muscle and the _____ muscle.

QUESTION
91

---

hyoglossus . . . mylohyoid (in either order)

ANSWER

Preganglionic fibers which supply parasympathetic innervation to the submandibular and sublingual glands travel in the _____ _____ branch of the facial nerve together with the lingual branch of the _____ nerve.

QUESTION
92

---

chorda tympani . . . mandibular

ANSWER

ITEM 37

THE LESSER SALIVARY GLANDS: LABIAL AND BUCCAL

Labial glands are isolated lesser glands in the submucosa of the lips whose ducts reach the vestibule singly or in small groups. These are especially numerous near the midline. *Buccal glands* are similarly arranged, and are more numerous in the posterior region of the buccal mucosa.

QUESTION 93

Labial glands are located in the submucosa of the _____; buccal glands, in the posterior region of the _____ mucosa.

ANSWER

lips . . . buccal

ITEM 38

THE LINGUAL, INCISIVE, AND PALATINE GLANDS

Three additional groups of lesser salivary glands are the lingual, the incisive, and the palatine. *Lingual glands* are found on the undersurface of the tongue and on the dorsal surface of the base of the tongue. *Incisive glands* are in the floor of the mouth behind the lower incisors. *Palatine glands* are numerous in the entire region of the soft palate and the posterior region of the hard palate.

QUESTION 94

Additional lesser salivary glands include the _____, the _____, and the _____ glands.

ANSWER

lingual . . . incisive . . . palatine (in any order)

ITEM 39

THE TONGUE: STRUCTURE

The tongue is composed principally of muscle tissue, with a mucous membrane covering the inferior surface and a specialized epithelium covering the upper and posterior surfaces.

The anterior two thirds of the tongue develop in the embryo from the first branchial arch. The posterior third of the tongue develops from the second and third branchial arches. Because of their diverse embryonic origins, the two regions have a different appearance and a different nerve supply.

The anterior two thirds of the tongue are derived from the _____ branchial arch; the posterior third is derived from the _____ and _____ branchial arches.

QUESTION
95

---

first . . . second . . . third

ANSWER

The explanation of the two different nerve supplies to the two different parts of the tongue is to be found in the different _____ derivation of the two parts.

QUESTION
96

---

embryonic

ANSWER

The undersurface of the tongue is covered by _____ membrane; the top surface, by a highly specialized _____.

QUESTION
97

---

mucous . . . epithelium

ANSWER

SULCI ON THE TONGUE   ITEM 40

Examine Figure 14–13 and notice how the anterior two thirds of the tongue are delimited from the posterior third on the dorsal surface by an inverted V-shaped sulcus, the *sulcus terminalis.* At the posterior end of the sulcus terminalis is a pit, the *foramen cecum,* which marks the site of origin of the thyroid gland in the embryo. The *median lingual sulcus,* the longitudinal depression down the midline of the tongue, may be noted in Figure 14–13.

The demarcation between the anterior two thirds and the posterior third of the tongue is called the _____ _____.

QUESTION
98

---

sulcus terminalis

ANSWER

The foramen cecum, found at the posterior end of the _____ _____, is a point at which the _____ gland originated embryonically.

QUESTION
99

---

sulcus terminalis . . . thyroid

ANSWER

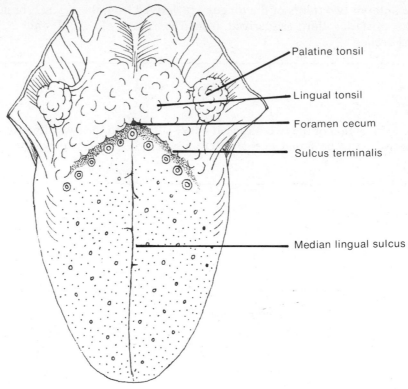

Figure 14–13.   Dorsum of tongue, showing sulci and lingual tonsil. (Redrawn from Woodburne: Essentials of Human Anatomy. 4th Ed. New York, Oxford University Press.)

QUESTION
100

The depression down the midline of the dorsum of the tongue is called the median _____ sulcus.

ANSWER

lingual

ITEM 41   THE TONGUE: THE DORSAL SURFACE

The mucous membrane of the dorsal surface of the body of the tongue is ·closely attached to underlying muscle. The dorsum of the base of the tongue is more loosely attached and contains, under the mucosa, two aggregates of _lymphoid tissue_, each making up a _lingual tonsil_. Each nodule surrounds a narrow crypt, which projects upward to the surface. The lingual tonsils extend laterally to become almost continuous with the palatine tonsils. Refer to Figure 14–13 to note the position of the lingual and palatine tonsils.

The lingual tonsils are aggregations of _____ tissue under the _____ of the base of the tongue.

---

lymphoid . . . mucosa

The dorsal mucosa of the _____ of the tongue is loosely attached to the muscle beneath, while that of the _____ of the tongue is closely attached.

---

base . . . body

In their lateral extension, the _____ tonsils and the _____ tonsils are nearly continuous.

---

lingual . . . palatine

THE TONGUE: THE INFERIOR SURFACE

ITEM 42

The mucous membrane on the undersurface of the tongue is thin and vascular and continues onto the sublingual floor of the mouth. The lingual vein is visible through the translucent epithelium of the inferior surface. A fold of mucosa, the *fimbriated fold*, runs anteriorly lateral to the lingual vein. This fold marks the location of the deeper lingual artery. Glance back at Figure 14–11 to see the position of the lingual vein and deep artery on the inferior surface of the tongue.

The mucous membrane of the undersurface of the tongue is *thicker/thinner* (circle one) than that of the dorsal surface.

---

thinner

The fold of mucosa separating the lingual vein from the deeper lingual artery is the _____ fold.

---

fimbriated

ITEM 43

THE VALLATE PAPILLAE

Four kinds of papillae containing receptors for taste are found on the tongue: vallate, fungiform, filiform, and foliate papillae. Locate these groups of papillae on Figure 14–14. These papillae give the anterior two thirds of the dorsum of the tongue their characteristic rough surface.

Vallate papillae, 8 to 12 in number, are flattened structures surrounded by circular sulci which enclose taste buds. The vallate papillae are arranged in a line anterior and parallel to the V-shaped sulcus terminalis. Serous glands open into the troughs of the vallate papillae.

QUESTION
106

The roughness of the tongue is due to the _____ covering the dorsal surface of the anterior two thirds.

ANSWER

papillae

QUESTION
107

Vallate papillae are located parallel to the anterior side of the V-shaped _____ _____.

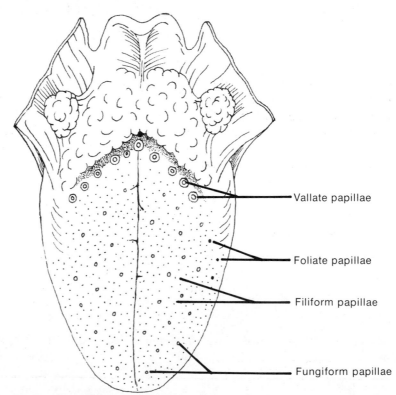

Figure 14–14.   Papillae on the dorsum of the tongue. (Redrawn from Woodburne: Essentials of Human Anatomy. 4th Ed. New York, Oxford University Press.)

sulcus terminalis

The circular sulci surrounding each of the 8 to 12 vallate papillae enclose
_____ _____ within their walls.

QUESTION
108

ANSWER

taste buds

Serous glands empty into the sulci surrounding the _____ papillae.

QUESTION
109

ANSWER

vallate

THE FUNGIFORM, FILIFORM, AND FOLIATE PAPILLAE

ITEM 44

Fungiform papillae are globular, bright red projections on the apex and sides of the tongue. *Filiform papillae* are minute conical elevations on the dorsum of the body of the tongue. A few *foliate papillae* are located on the posterior region of the sides of the tongue. The latter papillae are vestigial in man.

The fungiform papillae are located on the _____ and _____ of the tongue; filiform papillae, on the _____ of the tongue; the vestigial foliate papillae, on the posterior region of the _____ of the tongue.

QUESTION
110

---

tip (apex) . . . sides . . . dorsum (body) . . . sides

ANSWER

THE TYPES OF TONGUE MUSCLES

ITEM 45

Muscles of the tongue are of two types, *intrinsic* and *extrinsic*. Intrinsic muscles are contained within the tongue inself. Extrinsic muscles suspend and anchor the tongue to the mandible, the styloid process, and the hyoid bone. Intrinsic muscles are oriented longitudinally, vertically, and transversely, with extensive interdigitation of fibers.

QUESTION
111

The muscles which suspend and anchor the tongue are referred to collectively as the _____ muscles of the tongue; muscles making up the bulk of the tongue itself, the _____ muscles of the tongue.

ANSWER

extrinsic . . . intrinsic

QUESTION
112

Structures to which the tongue is anchored include the _____, the _____ process, and the _____ bone.

ANSWER

mandible . . . styloid . . . hyoid

QUESTION
113

Fibers of the intrinsic muscles of the tongue are oriented in three directions: _____, _____, and _____.

ANSWER

longitudinally . . . horizontally . . . vertically (in any order)

ITEM 46   THE EXTRINSIC MUSCLES OF THE TONGUE

The extrinsic muscles of the tongue include the *styloglossus,* the *hyoglossus,* the *genioglossus,* and the *palatoglossus*. Locate these muscles in Figure 14–15.

The styloglossus muscle originates at the styloid process and the stylo-mandibular ligament. Notice how its fibers extend downward and anteriorly. The hyoglossus muscle extends from the upper border of the hyoid bone to the body of the tongue. The genioglossus muscle extends from the mental spine to the entire area of the tongue from apex to base. The palatoglossus muscle, usually considered a muscle of the palate, extends from the palatine aponeurosis to the side of the tongue and forms the anterior tonsillar pillar.

QUESTION
114

The styloglossus muscle originates at the _____ process and the _____ ligament and inserts into the tongue.

ANSWER

styloid . . . stylomandibular

QUESTION
115

The hyoglossus muscle originates on the upper border of the _____ bone and extends superiorly and anteriorly to reach the _____.

ANSWER

hyoid . . . tongue

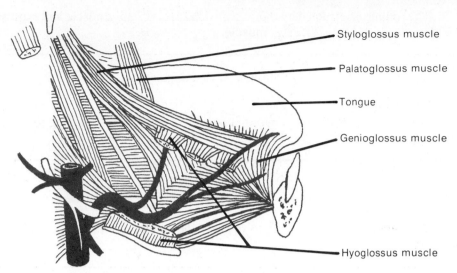

Figure 14–15. Extrinsic muscles of the tongue, lateral aspect. (Redrawn from Leeson and Leeson: Human Structure. Philadelphia, W. B. Saunders Co.)

The genioglossus muscle extends from the _____ spine to the _____.

QUESTION
116

mental . . . tongue

ANSWER

The point of origin of the palatoglossus muscle is the _____ aponeurosis and the point of termination is on the _____ surface of the tongue.

QUESTION
117

palatine . . . lateral

ANSWER

THE TONGUE: MUSCULAR ACTION IN MOVEMENT

ITEM 47

Complex movements of the tongue, such as those which occur during phonation, result from the combined action of several muscle groups. As the action of each of the four extrinsic muscles is described, look at that muscle in Figure 14–15 and visualize the tongue movement which the muscle effects.

The styloglossus muscle retracts the tongue, and the hyoglossus muscle depresses it. The genioglossus muscle protrudes the tongue or depresses it into the floor of the mouth; the palatoglossus elevates the root of the tongue.

QUESTION
118

The tongue is retracted by the _____ muscle and protruded by the _____ muscle.

ANSWER

styloglossus . . . genioglossus

QUESTION
119

The function of the palatoglossus muscle is to _____ the root of the tongue.

ANSWER

elevate

QUESTION
120

The two muscles which act to depress the tongue are the _____ and the _____.

ANSWER

hyoglossus . . . genioglossus (in either order)

ITEM 48   THE TONGUE: BLOOD SUPPLY

The blood supply to the tongue is carried by the lingual artery, a branch of the external carotid artery. The origin and course of the lingual artery in the tongue can be seen in Figure 14–16. The lingual artery arises between the superior thyroid artery and the facial artery. It turns forward under the hyoglossus muscle, at which point it is crossed laterally by the hypoglossal nerve. After entering the tongue, the lingual artery courses forward to the apex as the *deep lingual artery*. The lingual artery gives off the *dorsal lingual branch* which distributes to the tonsil, soft palate, and dorsum of the tongue. The *sublingual branch* is given off in the floor of the mouth to supply the sublingual gland and the mylohyoid muscle. A lingual branch of the maxillary artery supplies the sublingual mucosa.

QUESTION
121

The lingual artery branches off the _____ _____ artery.

ANSWER

external carotid

QUESTION
122

In its forward route, the lingual artery is crossed by the _____ nerve before disappearing deep to the hyoglossus muscle.

ANSWER

hypoglossal

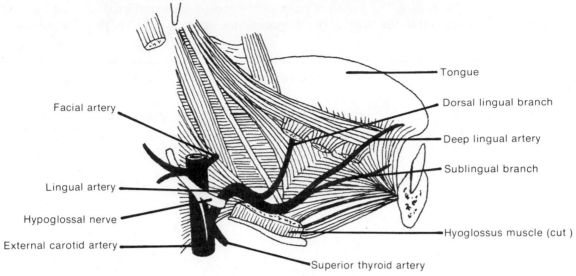

Figure 14-16. Branches of the lingual artery supplying the tongue and adjacent structures. (Redrawn from Leeson and Leeson: Human Structure. Philadelphia, W. B. Saunders Co.)

The forward continuation of the lingual artery to the apex of the tongue is the _____ lingual artery.

QUESTION
123

---

deep

ANSWER

The branch of the lingual artery supplying the soft palate, tonsil, and dorsum of the tongue is the _____ lingual artery; the branch supplying the mylohyoid muscle and the sublingual gland is the _____ branch.

QUESTION
124

---

dorsal . . . sublingual

ANSWER

NERVE SUPPLY TO PARTS OF THE TONGUE AND EPIGLOTTIC REGION

ITEM 49

The anterior two thirds and the posterior third of the tongue have different embryonic origins and, consequently, different afferent nerve supplies. Both anterior and posterior parts of the tongue are supplied with general somatic afferent (GSA) fibers for general sensation and special visceral afferent (SVA) fibers for taste. A third area immediately behind the tongue, the epiglottic region, also is supplied with GSA fibers for general sensation and SVA fibers for taste.

QUESTION
125

The reason that different parts of the tongue have different afferent nerve supplies is that the anterior two thirds and the posterior third of the tongue have different _____ _____.

ANSWER

embryonic origins

QUESTION
126

The functional component of fibers which convey general sensation from the tongue and epiglottic region is _____ _____ afferent; the component of fibers which convey taste is _____ _____ afferent.

ANSWER

general somatic . . . special visceral

ITEM 50

THE CRANIAL NERVES TO THE TONGUE AND EPIGLOTTIC REGION

General somatic afferent fibers for the anterior two thirds of the tongue come from a branch of the *trigeminal* (fifth cranial) nerve; special visceral afferent fibers for the anterior two thirds come from a branch of the *facial* (seventh cranial) nerve. Both GVA and SVA fibers for the posterior third of the tongue come from the *glossopharyngeal* (ninth cranial) nerve. GVA and SVA fibers for the epiglottic region come from a branch of the *vagus* (tenth cranial) nerve.

General somatic efferent motor fibers from the *hypoglossal* (twelfth cranial) nerve supply all the intrinsic and extrinsic muscles of the tongue except the palatoglossus muscle. GSE fibers to the palatoglossus muscle come from the *vagus* nerve.

QUESTION
127

In the numbered blanks below, write the names of the various cranial nerves which supply the corresponding numbered areas of the tongue shown in the diagram, page 579. It may be necessary for you to reread Item 50 before you can answer this question.

Labels

1. _____ nerve
2. _____ nerve
3. _____ nerve
4. _____ nerve
5. _____ nerve
6. _____ nerve

ANSWER

1. vagus
2. glossopharyngeal
3. trigeminal

4. facial
5. vagus
6. hypoglossal

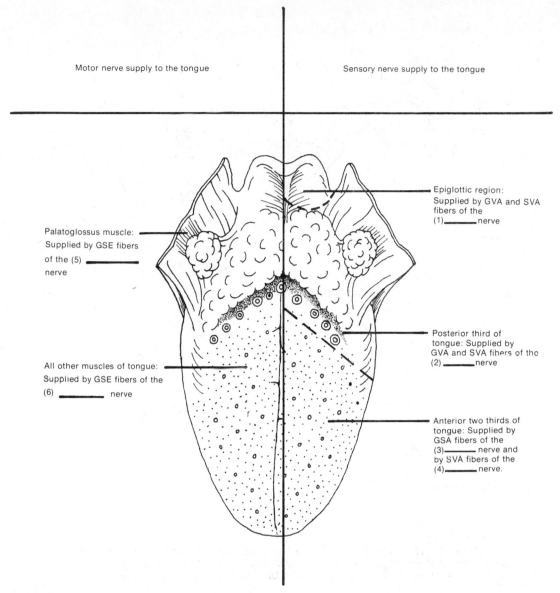

Motor nerve supply to the tongue

Sensory nerve supply to the tongue

Epiglottic region:
Supplied by GVA and SVA
fibers of the
(1)_____nerve

Palatoglossus muscle:
Supplied by GSE fibers
of the (5) _____
nerve

Posterior third of
tongue: Supplied by
GVA and SVA fibers of the
(2) _____nerve

All other muscles of tongue:
Supplied by GSE fibers of the
(6) _____ nerve

Anterior two thirds of
tongue: Supplied by
GSA fibers of the
(3)_____ nerve and
by SVA fibers of the
(4)_____nerve.

(Redrawn from Woodburne: Essentials of Human Anatomy. 4th Ed. New York, Oxford University Press.)

THE ANTERIOR TWO THIRDS OF THE TONGUE: SENSORY NERVE SUPPLY   ITEM 51

The afferent nerve supply to the anterior two thirds of the tongue is illustrated in Figure 14–17. GSA fibers for general sensation from the anterior two thirds of the tongue are carried by the lingual branch of the mandibular division of the trigeminal nerve (V).

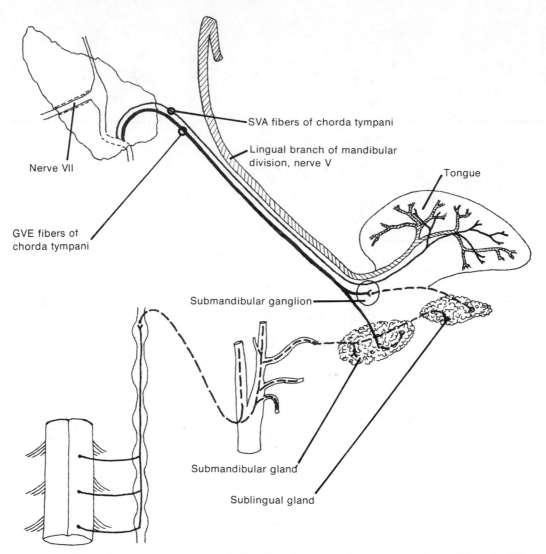

Figure 14–17. Lingual branch of the trigeminal nerve (V) and chorda tympani branch of the facial nerve (VII), which supply the anterior two thirds of tongue. (Redrawn from Woodburne: Essentials of Human Anatomy. 4th Ed. New York, Oxford University Press.)

QUESTION
128
The lingual nerve, which conveys general sensation from the anterior two thirds of the tongue, is a branch of the _____ division of the _____ nerve.

ANSWER
mandibular . . . trigeminal

QUESTION
129
The functional component of the lingual nerve is _____ _____ _____.

ANSWER
general somatic afferent

THE CHORDA TYMPANI NERVE: STRUCTURES INNERVATED

Special visceral afferent fibers for taste from the anterior two thirds of the tongue are carried by the chorda tympani branch of the facial nerve (VII). Observe the route of the chorda tympani in Figure 14–17. After branching from the facial nerve at the stylomastoid foramen, the chorda tympani joins the lingual branch of the mandibular nerve in the infratemporal fossa and travels with the lingual nerve to the tongue.

In addition to carrying fibers for taste from the anterior part of the tongue, the chorda tympani carries motor fibers (GVE) which synapse in the submandibular ganglion for parasympathetic innervation of the submandibular and sublingual glands.

Nerve impulses for taste from the anterior portion of the tongue are carried by the _____ _____ branch of the _____ nerve.

QUESTION
130

---

chorda tympani . . . facial

ANSWER

The chorda tympani branches off the facial nerve at the _____ foramen and joins the lingual nerve in the _____ fossa.

QUESTION
131

---

stylomastoid . . . infratemporal

ANSWER

The chorda tympani carries two visceral components: (1) special visceral afferent fibers from the _____, and (2) general visceral efferent fibers to the _____ and _____ glands.

QUESTION
132

---

tongue . . . submandibular . . . sublingual

ANSWER

THE TONGUE: SENSORY NERVE SUPPLY TO THE POSTERIOR PART

The afferent nerve supply to the posterior third of the tongue is shown in Figure 14–18. Both the GVA fibers for general sensation and the SVA fibers for taste are carried by the glossopharyngeal nerve (IX). After descending from the inferior glossopharyngeal ganglion and passing between the external and internal carotid arteries, the glossopharyngeal nerve runs forward to cross the stylopharyngeus muscle and then goes deep to the hyoglossus muscle to reach the posterior part of the tongue.

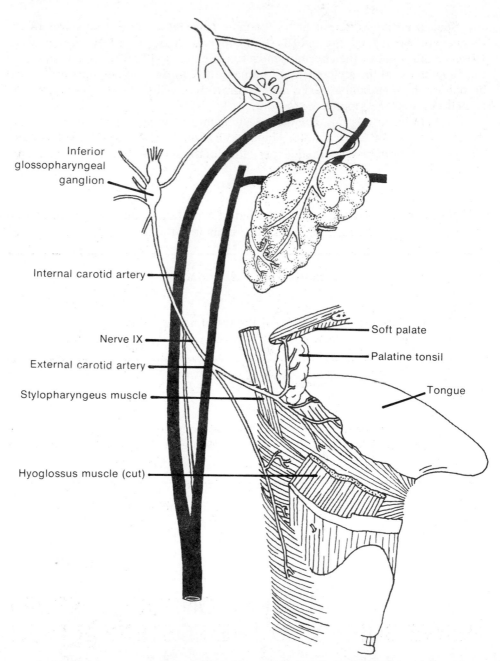

Figure 14–18. Glossopharyngeal nerve (IX) supply to the posterior third of the tongue. (Modified from Woodburne: Essentials of Human Anatomy. 4th Ed. New York, Oxford University Press.)

The glossopharyngeal nerve carries sensory fibers both for general _____ and for _____ from the posterior part of the tongue.

QUESTION
133

sensation . . . taste

ANSWER

The glossopharyngeal nerve passes between the external and internal _____ _____ on its way to the tongue.

QUESTION
134

carotid arteries

ANSWER

The glossopharyngeal nerve crosses the _____ muscle before going deep to the _____ muscle in its route to the tongue.

QUESTION
135

stylopharyngeus . . . hyoglossus

ANSWER

THE EPIGLOTTIC REGION: SENSORY NERVE SUPPLY   ITEM 54

The sensory nerve supply to the epiglottic region is shown in Figure 14–19. The *superior laryngeal branch* of the vagus nerve (X) carries both the GVA fibers for general sensation and the SVA fibers for taste from the epiglottic region. After passing obliquely downward from the inferior ganglion of the vagus nerve, the superior laryngeal branch divides into an external and an internal branch. The *internal branch* penetrates the thyrohyoid membrane and distributes both GVA and SVA fibers to the epiglottis, the base of the tongue, and the larynx.

The superior laryngeal nerve, which provides sensory innervation to the epiglottic region, is a branch of the _____ nerve.

QUESTION
136

vagus

ANSWER

General sensation and taste from the epiglottic region are conveyed by the *external/internal* (circle one) branch of the superior laryngeal nerve.

QUESTION
137

internal

ANSWER

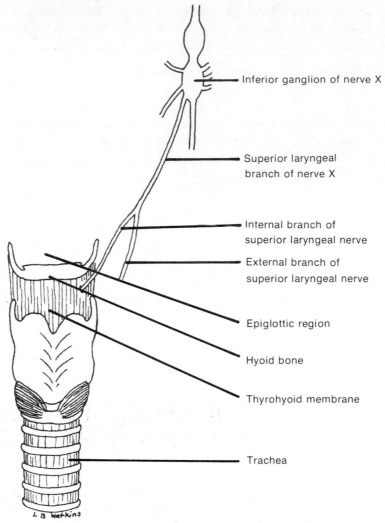

— Inferior ganglion of nerve X

— Superior laryngeal
branch of nerve X

— Internal branch of
superior laryngeal nerve

— External branch of
superior laryngeal nerve

— Epiglottic region

— Hyoid bone

— Thyrohyoid membrane

— Trachea

Figure 14–19. Course of the internal branch of the superior laryngeal nerve to the epiglottic region. (Modified from Woodburne: Essentials of Human Anatomy. 4th Ed. New York, Oxford University Press.)

ITEM   THE MUSCLES OF THE TONGUE:
55   MOTOR NERVE SUPPLY

Figure 14–20 shows the distribution of the general somatic efferent (GSE) fibers of the hypoglossal nerve (XII) to muscles of the tongue. The hypoglossal nerve supplies all the intrinsic muscles of the tongue as well as the following three extrinsic muscles: the styloglossus, the hyoglossus, and the genioglossus. The fourth extrinsic tongue muscle, the palatoglossus, receives its motor innervation from the pharyngeal plexus of the vagus nerve (X).

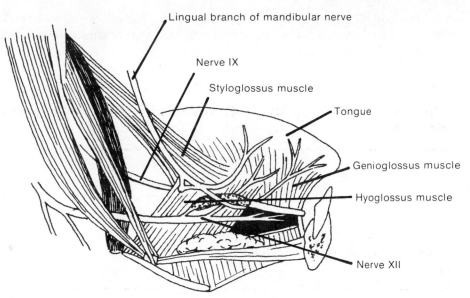

Lingual branch of mandibular nerve

Nerve IX

Styloglossus muscle

Tongue

Genioglossus muscle

Hyoglossus muscle

Nerve XII

Figure 14–20. Hypoglossal nerve (XII) branches to muscles of the tongue. (Redrawn from Leeson and Leeson: Human Structure. Philadelphia, W. B. Saunders Co.)

The extrinsic muscles of the tongue supplied by the hypoglossal nerve include the _____, the _____, and the _____ muscles.

QUESTION 138

hyoglossus . . . styloglossus . . . genioglossus (in any order)

ANSWER

The pharyngeal plexus of the vagus nerve supplies efferent innervation of the _____ muscle.

QUESTION 139

palatoglossus

ANSWER

THE TEETH: BLOOD SUPPLY ITEM 56

The blood supply to the teeth has been dealt with in Unit 11 and nerve supply to the teeth was considered in Unit 6. However, as a review, this item will consider the blood supply to the teeth in a regional context, and the next three items will discuss the nerve supply to the teeth.

The posterior, middle, and anterior superior alveolar branches of the maxillary artery provide blood supply to the maxillary teeth. The inferior alveolar branch of the maxillary artery supplies the mandibular teeth. Branches of these vessels also supply adjacent gingiva and alveolar bone.

QUESTION
140
The blood supply to maxillary and mandibular teeth is provided by various branches of the _____ artery.

ANSWER
maxillary

QUESTION
141
The anterior, middle, and posterior _____ _____ arteries supply maxillary teeth; the _____ _____ artery supplies mandibular teeth.

ANSWER
superior alveolar . . . inferior alveolar

ITEM 57   THE MAXILLARY TEETH: NERVE SUPPLY

General somatic afferent fibers of the maxillary division of the trigeminal nerve supply maxillary teeth. Maxillary molars are supplied by the posterior superior alveolar nerve; premolars, by the middle superior alveolar nerve; canines and incisors, by the anterior superior alveolar nerve.

QUESTION
142
The posterior superior alveolar branch of the maxillary nerve supplies the maxillary _____ teeth; the middle superior alveolar nerve, the maxillary _____ teeth.

ANSWER
molar . . . premolar

QUESTION
143
The maxillary canine and incisor teeth are innervated by the _____ _____ nerve.

ANSWER
anterior superior alveolar

THE MAXILLARY GINGIVAE: NERVE SUPPLY

ITEM 58

Posterior, middle, and anterior superior alveolar nerves supply the buccal gingiva of the maxillary teeth. The infraorbital branch of the maxillary nerve supplies additional innervation to the buccal gingiva of the incisor, canine, and premolar teeth. The greater palatine branch of the maxillary nerve provides innervation of the palatine gingiva opposite the maxillary canine, premolar, and molar teeth. The nasopalatine nerve supplies palatine gingiva of the incisors.

Buccal gingiva of the maxillary premolar, canine, and incisor teeth is innervated both by superior alveolar branches and by the _____ branch of the maxillary nerve.

QUESTION **144**

infraorbital

ANSWER

The palatine gingiva of the maxillary incisor teeth is supplied by the _____ _____ nerve; palatine gingiva of maxillary canine, premolar, and molar teeth is supplied by the _____ ____ _____ nerve.

QUESTION **145**

nasopalatine . . . greater palatine

ANSWER

THE MANDIBULAR TEETH AND GINGIVAE: NERVE SUPPLY

ITEM 59

The inferior alveolar branch of the mandibular division of the trigeminal nerve innervates all of the mandibular teeth. The lingual branch of the mandibular nerve supplies the whole lingual surface of the mandibular gingiva. The buccal branch of the mandibular nerve supplies the buccal gingiva of the mandibular molars. The mental nerve supplies the buccal gingiva of the mandibular incisor, canine, and premolar teeth.

Mandibular teeth are innervated by the _____ _____ branch of the _____ division of the trigeminal nerve.

QUESTION **146**

inferior alveolar . . . mandibular

ANSWER

The lingual gingiva of the mandibular teeth is innervated by the _____ branch of the _____ nerve.

QUESTION **147**

ANSWER   lingual . . . mandibular

QUESTION
148
The buccal branch of the mandibular nerve supplies buccal gingiva of the mandibular _____ teeth.

ANSWER   molar

QUESTION
149
Gingiva related to the mandibular incisor, canine, and premolar teeth is innervated by the _____ branch of the mandibular nerve.

ANSWER   mental

SUMMARY OF UNIT FOURTEEN

THE REGIONS OF THE MOUTH

The oral cavity is bounded above by the hard and soft palates, below by the tongue and muscular floor, anteriorly by the lips, and posteriorly by the pharynx. The mouth has two parts: the narrow vestibule between the lips and the teeth and gums, and the oral cavity proper.

The lips are mobile muscular folds containing closely packed labial glands between muscle and inner mucosa. Lateral borders of the upper lip are the naso-labial sulci. The vertical groove below the nose is the philtrum. The labiomental groove separates lower lip from chin. The connections between lower and upper lips at the corners of the mouth are the labial commissures. The red zone is the margin between the skin and mucosa of the lips.

The cheeks are formed from the horizontal buccinator muscles and the vertical masseter muscle. They contain buccal glands under their inner mucosal lining. The posterior limit of the vestibular side of the cheek is the pterygomandibular raphe, a connective tissue band extending from the pterygoid hamulus to the retromolar area. The duct from the parotid gland goes through the buccinator muscle to enter the mouth above the second maxillary molar.

The gingivae are mucous membranes overlying dense connective tissue attached firmly to alveolar bone. Gingivae surround the necks of the teeth, with gingival papillae extending between the teeth. The retromolar papilla is an elevation of gingiva behind the last mandibular molar tooth, posterior to which is an accumulation of buccal glands called the retromolar pad.

The hard palate, formed from processes of the maxilla and the palatine bones, and the muscular soft palate constitute the arched roof of the mouth. Palatine rugae are lateral ridges extending from the midline palatine raphe of the hard palate. Blood and nerve supply to the hard palate are provided by the greater palatine artery and nerve, respectively. The greater palatine artery is a branch of the maxillary artery; the greater palatine nerve, a branch of the maxillary nerve.

The soft palate terminates in the uvula. The palatine arches, between which lies the palatine tonsil, are folds overlying the palatoglossal and palatopharyngeal muscles. The musculus uvulae is within the soft palate; the palatoglossus, palatopharyngeal, and levator and tensor veli palatini muscles attach to the soft palate. The nerve supply to the soft palate comes from the vagus nerve through the pharyngeal plexus, except for the supply to the tensor veli palatini, which comes by way of a branch of the mandibular nerve. Blood supply to the soft palate is through the lesser palatine branch of the maxillary artery.

The sublingual region of the mouth is the area surrounding the attachment of the tongue in the floor of the mouth. The mylohyoid, geniohyoid, and hyoglossus muscles support the floor of the mouth. Between these muscles and the sublingual mucosa are found the sublingual glands, the submandibular duct, and nerves and blood vessels.

THE SALIVARY GLANDS

Salivary glands opening into the mouth are the parotid, submandibular, and sublingual. Lesser salivary glands are the lingual, incisive, and palatine glands. The parotid, the largest salivary gland, is located around the ramus of the mandible.

The deep parotid fascia covering the gland extends to the styloid process, where it thickens to become the stylomandibular ligament separating the parotid from the submandibular gland. The submandibular gland occupies a triangle of the neck below and anterior to the angle of the mandible. The sublingual gland rests on the anterior surface of the mylohyoid muscle in the sublingual fossa of the mandible.

Blood supply to the parotid gland is from the posterior auricular, superficial temporal, and transverse facial arteries; to the submandibular gland, from the facial artery; to the sublingual gland, from the facial and lingual arteries. The salivary glands receive both sympathetic and parasympathetic nerve supplies in addition to sensory innervation. Sensory innervation of the parotid gland is from the auriculotemporal nerve, along with which travel parasympathetic fibers from the otic ganglion of the glossopharyngeal nerve. The submandibular and sublingual glands receive parasympathetic fibers from the chorda tympani branch of the facial nerve.

THE TONGUE

The tongue is composed of muscle with an undercover of mucous membrane and a specialized epithelial dorsal covering. The anterior two thirds of the tongue and the posterior third have different embryonic origins and therefore different nerve supplies. The posterior limit of the anterior part of the tongue is the sulcus terminalis, at the posterior tip of which is a pit called the foramen cecum. The median lingual sulcus is a depression down the midline of the dorsum of the tongue. The lingual tonsils, aggregates of lymphoid tissue under the mucosa at the base of the tongue, are almost continuous with the palatine tonsils. Papillae containing receptors for taste give the tongue its characteristic rough surface. Vallate papillae are anterior and parallel to the V-shaped sulcus terminalis and are surrounded by tiny moats containing taste buds. Other papillae on the tongue are the fungiform, filiform, and foliate papillae.

The intrinsic muscles of the tongue are longitudinal, vertical, and transverse muscles which make up the bulk of the tongue itself. Movements of the tongue, as in phonation, for example, involve the coordinated contraction of the four extrinsic muscles of the tongue: the styloglossus, hyoglossus, genioglossus, and palatoglossus. These four muscles also suspend the tongue and anchor it to the mandible, styloid process, and hyoid bone. Blood supply to the tongue is through branches of the lingual artery.

The hypoglossal nerve supplies the motor innervation of all muscles of the tongue except the palatoglossus muscle, which is innervated by the vagus nerve. SVA fibers for taste from the anterior of the tongue come from the facial nerve; fibers for taste from the posterior part of the tongue come from the glossopharyngeal nerve; taste fibers in the epiglottic region, from the vagus nerve. Fibers for general sensation in the anterior part of the tongue are carried by a branch of the trigeminal nerve; in the posterior part, by the glossopharyngeal nerve; in the epiglottic region, by the vagus nerve.

BLOOD AND NERVE SUPPLY TO THE TEETH

Blood supply to the teeth is provided by branches of the maxillary artery. Posterior, middle, and anterior superior alveolar arteries supply the maxillary teeth; the inferior alveolar artery supplies the mandibular teeth.

The posterior superior alveolar nerve supplies maxillary molar teeth; the middle superior alveolar nerve, maxillary premolars; the anterior superior alveolar nerve, maxillary canines and incisors. The inferior alveolar nerve supplies the mandibular teeth.

The anterior and middle superior alveolar nerves and the infraorbital nerve supply buccal gingiva of the maxillary incisors, canines, and premolars; the posterior superior alveolar nerve, the buccal gingiva of the maxillary molars. The nasopalatine nerve supplies palatine gingiva of the maxillary incisors; the greater palatine nerve, the palatine gingiva of maxillary canines, premolars, and molars. Buccal gingiva of mandibular molars is innervated by the buccal nerve; buccal gingiva of mandibular premolars, canines and incisors is innervated by the mental nerve. Lingual gingiva of the mandibular teeth is innervated by the lingual nerve.

The fauces is the opening of the oral cavity into the _____.

QUESTION
150

pharynx

ANSWER

The mucosa-lined area between the cheeks and lips and the teeth is the _____ of the mouth.

QUESTION
151

vestibule

ANSWER

The lateral grooves between the upper lip and the wing of the nose are called the _____ sulci.

QUESTION
152

nasolabial

ANSWER

The labiomental groove separates the _____ lip from the _____.

QUESTION
153

lower . . . chin

ANSWER

Muscles which make up the cheek are the _____ muscle anteriorly and the _____ muscle posteriorly.

QUESTION
154

buccinator . . . masseter

ANSWER

The line of connective tissue extending between the pterygoid hamulus and the retromolar area is the _____ raphe.

QUESTION
155

pterygomandibular

ANSWER

QUESTION
156

The roots of the teeth are surrounded by _____ which is firmly attached to alveolar bone.

ANSWER

gingiva

QUESTION
157

The retromolar papilla is an elevation of _____; the retromolar pad behind the retromolar papilla is an aggregation of _____.

ANSWER

gingiva . . . glands

QUESTION
158

Ridges extending laterally across the hard palate are termed palatine _____.

ANSWER

rugae

QUESTION
159

Blood supply to the hard palate is from the greater _____ artery; nerve supply to the hard palate is from the greater _____ nerve.

ANSWER

palatine . . . palatine

QUESTION
160

Blood supply to the soft palate is from the _____ palatine branch of the maxillary artery.

ANSWER

lesser

QUESTION
161

The palatine tonsil is situated between the _____ arch anteriorly and the _____ arch posteriorly.

ANSWER

palatoglossal . . . palatopharyngeal

QUESTION
162

The tensor and levator veli palatini muscles attach to the _____ _____.

ANSWER

soft palate

QUESTION
163

Except for the tensor veli palatini muscle, all the muscles of the soft palate are innervated by the _____ nerve.

ANSWER

vagus

The three muscles supporting the floor of the mouth are the _____, the _____, and the _____ muscles.

QUESTION 164

---

mylohyoid . . . geniohyoid . . . hyoglossus (in any order)

ANSWER

The parotid gland is located deep to the _____ of the mandible; the submandibular gland, anterior and inferior to the _____ of the mandible.

QUESTION 165

---

ramus . . . angle

ANSWER

The duct of the parotid gland passes through the _____ muscle on its way to the mouth.

QUESTION 166

---

buccinator

ANSWER

The sublingual gland is located on the anterior aspect of the _____ muscle.

QUESTION 167

---

mylohyoid

ANSWER

The stylomandibular ligament separates the _____ gland from the submandibular gland.

QUESTION 168

---

parotid

ANSWER

The submandibular and sublingual glands both receive blood supply from the _____ artery; the sublingual gland receives additional supply from the _____ artery.

QUESTION 169

---

facial . . . lingual

ANSWER

The posterior auricular, superficial temporal, and transverse facial arteries all contribute blood supply to the _____ gland.

QUESTION 170

---

parotid

ANSWER

The chorda tympani nerve brings _____ nerve supply to the submandibular and sublingual glands.

QUESTION 171

---

parasympathetic

ANSWER

QUESTION
172

The sulcus _____ is a V-shaped groove on the dorsum of the tongue; the _____ _____ sulcus extends down the midline of the tongue.

ANSWER

terminalis . . . median lingual

QUESTION
173

Along the anterior margin of the sulcus terminalis are found the _____ papillae, which contain receptors for _____.

ANSWER

vallate . . . taste

QUESTION
174

The lingual tonsils are aggregates of _____ tissue.

ANSWER

lymphoid

QUESTION
175

The intrinsic muscles constituting the bulk of the tongue itself run in three different directions within the tongue: _____, _____, and _____.

ANSWER

longitudinally . . . vertically . . . transversely (in any order)

QUESTION
176

The styloglossus, hyoglossus, genioglossus, and palatoglossus muscles are _____ muscles of the tongue.

ANSWER

extrinsic

QUESTION
177

The structures to which the tongue is anchored by the four extrinsic tongue muscles are the _____, the _____ bone, and the _____ process.

ANSWER

mandible . . . hyoid . . . styloid

QUESTION
178

Special visceral afferent fibers conveying taste from various parts of the tongue emanate from the following cranial nerves: SVA fibers from the anterior part of the tongue come from the _____ nerve; those from the posterior part of the tongue, from the _____ nerve; those from the base of the tongue and the epiglottic region, from the _____ nerve.

ANSWER

facial . . . glossopharyngeal . . . vagus

General sensation from the various parts of the tongue is conveyed by various cranial nerves as follows: sensation from the anterior part of the tongue is carried by the _____ nerve; sensation from the posterior part, by the _____ nerve; sensation from the epiglottic region, by the _____ nerve.

QUESTION 179

---

trigeminal . . . glossopharyngeal . . . vagus

ANSWER

All tongue muscles except the palatoglossus receive motor innervation by the _____ nerve.

QUESTION 180

---

hypoglossal

ANSWER

The blood supply to the tongue comes from the _____ artery.

QUESTION 181

---

lingual

ANSWER

Blood supply to the teeth is derived from the superior _____ branches and the inferior _____ branch of the maxillary artery.

QUESTION 182

---

alveolar . . . alveolar

ANSWER

Match the names of the teeth from Column B with the appropriate supplying nerves in Column A.

QUESTION 183

Column A	Column B
( ) 1. anterior superior alveolar nerve	A. mandibular teeth
( ) 2. inferior alveolar nerve	B. maxillary canines and incisors
( ) 3. middle superior alveolar nerve	C. maxillary molars
( ) 4. posterior superior alveolar nerve	D. maxillary premolars

---

1—(B); 2—(A); 3—(D); 4—(C)

ANSWER

QUESTION
184

Match the gingivae in Column B with the appropriate supplying nerves in Column A.

Column A

( ) 1. buccal nerve
( ) 2. greater palatine nerve
( ) 3. infraorbital nerve
( ) 4. lingual nerve
( ) 5. mental nerve
( ) 6. nasopalatine nerve
( ) 7. posterior superior alveolar
    nerve

Column B

A. buccal gingiva of mandibular incisors, canines, and premolars
B. buccal gingiva of mandibular molars
C. buccal gingiva of maxillary molars
D. buccal gingiva of maxillary pre-molars, canines, and incisors
E. lingual gingiva of mandibular teeth
F. palatine gingiva of maxillary incisors
G. palatine gingiva of maxillary molars, premolars, and canines

ANSWER

1—(B); 2—(G); 3—(D); 4—(E); 5—(A); 6—(F); 7—(C)

Unit Fifteen □ THE NOSE AND THE PARANASAL SINUSES

THE EXTERNAL NOSE

The external nose, shown in Figure 15–1, is a bony and cartilaginous structure projecting from the external *nares,* or nostrils. The upper part, referred to as the *root of the nose,* overlies the nasal bones. The lower cartilaginous region is composed of two *alae,* or wings, which extend to the midline of the nose. The tip of the nose is called the *apex.*

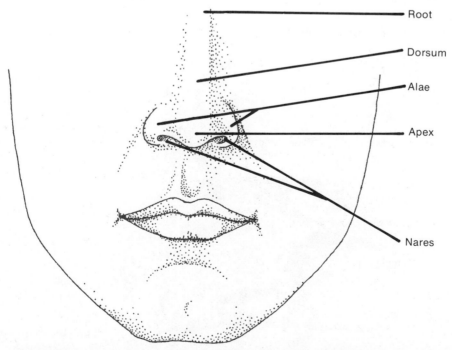

Figure 15–1. Lower part of the face, showing the external nose. (Redrawn from Wolf-Heidegger: Atlas of Systematic Human Anatomy. Vol. II. Basel, S. Karger AG.)

QUESTION
1

The root of the nose is *bony/cartilaginous* (circle one).

ANSWER

bony

QUESTION
2

External openings of the nose are the _____.

ANSWER

nares (nostrils)

QUESTION
3

The alae are the two cartilaginous _____ of the nose.

ANSWER

wings

ITEM 2

THE NASAL CAVITY AND SEPTUM

The nasal cavity is a triangular area made up of two wedge shaped cavities separated by a perpendicular *septum*. The nasal cavity extends from the external nares to the internal nares, or *choanae,* where it is continuous with the nasopharynx.

The nasal septum is formed by cartilage and bone, as shown in Figure 15–2.

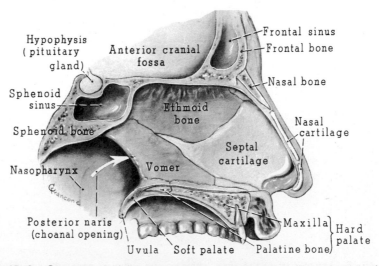

Figure 15–2. Components of the nasal septum, sagittal section. (From Jacob and Francone: Structure and Function in Man. 3rd Ed. Philadelphia, W. B. Saunders Co.)

The *perpendicular plate of the ethmoid bone* partitions the nasal cavity from above; the *vomer,* from below. Septal cartilage extends between the two bones and projects forward into the anteriormost region of the nose, the *vestibule.*

The choanae are *external/internal* (circle one) nares.

internal

The nasal septum is partitioned from above by the _____ bone and from below by the _____.

ethmoid . . . vomer

The vestibule is the *anterior/posterior* (circle one) portion of the nasal cavity.

anterior

The cartilaginous portion of the nasal septum is situated between the two _____ parts of the septum.

bony

THE CONCHAE AND MEATUSES   ITEM 3

The lateral nasal wall presents three scroll shaped folds of thin bone covered by mucosa. These folds are called the *superior, middle,* and *inferior conchae,* illustrated in Figure 15–3. The cavities formed by the overlying conchae are the *superior, middle,* and *inferior meatuses.* The meatuses are the sites where openings of the paranasal sinuses and other apertures in the lateral nasal wall are found.

The three scroll shaped conchae are folds of _____, covered by mucosa, situated in the _____ nasal wall.

bone . . . lateral

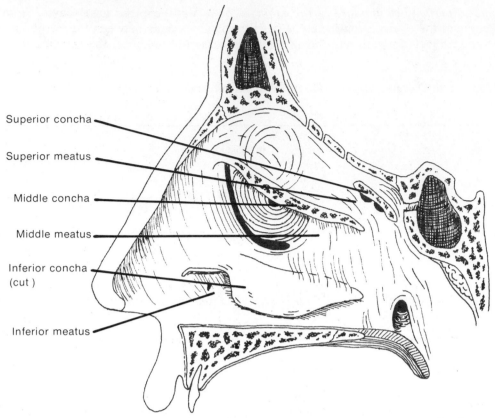

Superior concha

Superior meatus

Middle concha

Middle meatus

Inferior concha
(cut)

Inferior meatus

Figure 15-3. Conchae and meatuses of the lateral nasal wall. (Redrawn from Woodburne: Essentials of Human Anatomy. 4th Ed. New York, Oxford University Press.)

QUESTION
9
The superior, middle, and inferior conchae overlie three cavities in the lateral nasal wall called the nasal _____.

ANSWER
meatuses

QUESTION
10
Through openings in the lateral nasal wall the paranasal _____ communicate with the nasal cavity.

ANSWER
sinuses

QUESTION
11
The openings of the paranasal sinuses are found in the *conchae/meatuses* (circle one) on the lateral nasal wall.

ANSWER
meatuses

BLOOD SUPPLY TO THE NASAL CAVITY: THE SPHENOPALATINE ARTERY

ITEM 4

Blood supply to the nose runs together with nerve supply along the septum and the lateral nasal wall. The principal arteries supplying the nose may be seen from the medial aspect on Figure 15–4, which includes the septum.

The *sphenopalatine artery,* a branch of the maxillary artery, provides the main arterial supply to the nose. It enters the posterolateral part of the nasal cavity through the sphenopalatine foramen on the lateral wall. Upon entering the nasal cavity, the sphenopalatine artery divides into two branches: the *lateral nasal branch* and the *posterior septal branch*. The lateral branch is not visible on the medial aspect, but the posterior septal branch may be seen descending the septum in Figure 15–4.

The sphenopalatine artery runs along the vomer downward and forward to the incisive canal, where it anastomoses with terminal branches of the greater palatine artery.

The sphenopalatine artery supplying the nose is a branch of the _____ artery; it enters the nasal cavity through the _____ foramen.

QUESTION 12

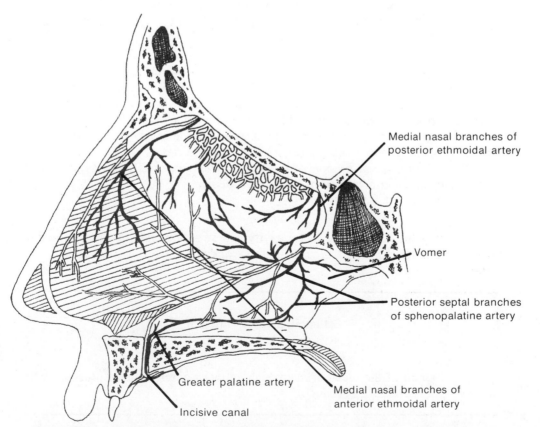

Figure 15–4. Blood supply to the nasal cavity, medial aspect. (Redrawn from Woodburne: Essentials of Human Anatomy. 4th Ed. New York, Oxford University Press.)

ANSWER   maxillary . . . sphenopalatine

QUESTION
13
The posterior lateral nasal branch of the sphenopalatine artery travels on the _____ wall of the nasal cavity; the posterior septal branch, on the _____.

ANSWER   lateral . . . septum

QUESTION
14
The sphenopalatine artery anastomoses with the _____ _____ artery at the incisive foramen.

ANSWER   greater palatine

ITEM 5

BLOOD SUPPLY TO THE NASAL CAVITY: THE ETHMOIDAL AND FACIAL ARTERIES

The *anterior* and *posterior ethmoidal arteries,* which are branches of the ophthalmic artery, enter the roof of the nasal cavity and branch over the lateral wall and septum. Re-examine Figure 15–4 and observe the medial nasal branches of the anterior and posterior ethmoidal arteries on the septum. Also note how the posterior septal branches of the sphenopalatine artery anastomose with the medial branches of the anterior and posterior ethmoidal arteries.

The *superior labial branch* of the *facial artery,* not visible in Figure 15–4, extends to the anterior region of the nasal mucosa.

QUESTION
15
Entering the roof of the nasal cavity are two branches of the ophthalmic artery: the anterior _____ artery and the posterior _____ artery.

ANSWER   ethmoidal . . . ethmoidal

QUESTION
16
The branch of the facial artery which supplies anterior nasal mucosa is the superior _____ branch.

ANSWER   labial

BLOOD SUPPLY TO THE NASAL CAVITY: THE GREATER PALATINE ARTERY

The *greater palatine branch* of the *maxillary artery,* which primarily supplies the hard palate, turns upward at the incisive canal to enter the nasal cavity. Look back to Figure 15–4 and locate the termination of the greater palatine artery in the nasal cavity as it anastomoses with branches of the sphenopalatine artery on the nasal septum.

The greater palatine artery is a branch of the _____ artery.

QUESTION
17

---

maxillary

ANSWER

The opening in the roof of the mouth through which the greater palatine artery enters the nasal cavity is the _____ canal.

QUESTION
18

---

incisive

ANSWER

NERVE SUPPLY TO THE NASAL CAVITY: THE OLFACTORY NERVES

Figure 15–5 shows the nerve supply to the nasal cavity. Notice the olfactory nerves at the top of the illustration. The *olfactory nerves* are small bundles of special visceral afferent (SVA) fibers conveying the sensation of smell. They arise from the olfactory mucosa in the uppermost part of the nasal cavity. Olfactory nerves ascend through the *cribriform plate* on the ethmoid bone and almost immediately enter the *olfactory bulb* on the undersurface of the frontal lobe of the brain. The remaining nerves in the nasal cavity run with arteries, usually with those having the same names.

Olfactory nerves carry _____ / _____ afferent fibers for smell.

QUESTION
19

---

special visceral

ANSWER

The olfactory nerves are located in the *upper/lower* (circle one) part of the nasal cavity.

QUESTION
20

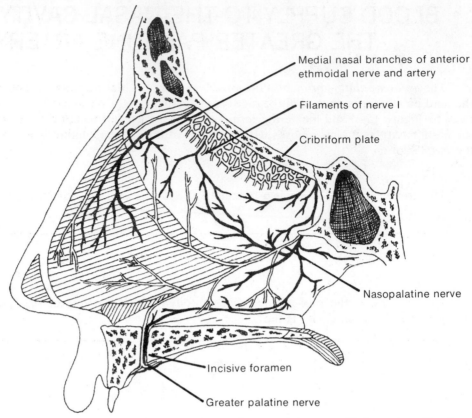

Figure 15–5. Nerve supply to the nasal cavity, medial aspect. (Redrawn from Woodburne: Essentials of Human Anatomy. 4th Ed. New York, Oxford University Press.)

ANSWER   upper

QUESTION   The olfactory nerves, en route from the nasal cavity to the brain, pass through
21   the _____ plate of the _____ bone.

―――

ANSWER   cribriform . . . ethmoid

QUESTION   The olfactory nerves enter the olfactory bulbs on the undersurface of the
22   _____ lobes of the brain.

―――

ANSWER   frontal

QUESTION   With the exception of the olfactory nerves, the nerves of the nasal cavity
23   follow the routes of _____ of the same names.

―――

ANSWER   arteries

NERVE SUPPLY TO THE NASAL CAVITY: THE NASOPALATINE NERVE

ITEM
8

Examine Figure 15–5 again and locate the position of the nasopalatine nerve. The *nasopalatine nerve,* a branch of the maxillary division of the trigeminal nerve, enters the posterior lateral nasal wall at the sphenopalatine foramen along with the sphenopalatine artery. The main trunk of the nasopalatine nerve extends medially over the roof of the nose to the septum, which it supplies. Notice how the nasopalatine nerve runs obliquely down and forward to the incisive canal, where it joins branches of the greater palatine nerve to innervate the upper incisive teeth and adjacent gingiva. The nasopalatine nerve supplies general somatic afferent innervation, but carries with it some postganglionic parasympathetic fibers from the pterygopalatine ganglion.

Also in Figure 15–5, notice the medial nasal branches of the anterior ethmoidal nerve traveling on the septum with the artery of the same name.

The artery and nerve which enter the nasal cavity together through the sphenopalatine foramen are the _____ artery and the _____ nerve.

QUESTION
24

---

sphenopalatine . . . nasopalatine

ANSWER

Fibers of the nasopalatine nerve convey general sensation from the nasal _____ and from the upper _____ teeth and adjacent _____.

QUESTION
25

---

septum . . . incisive . . . gingiva

ANSWER

The nasopalatine nerve is a branch of the _____ division of the _____ nerve.

QUESTION
26

---

maxillary . . . trigeminal

ANSWER

The functional component of the nasopalatine fibers themselves is _____ _____ afferent, but the nerve also carries with it postganglionic _____ fibers from the pterygopalatine ganglion.

QUESTION
27

---

general somatic . . . parasympathetic

ANSWER

ITEM
9

THE PARANASAL SINUSES

The *paranasal sinuses* are paired airfilled cavities in bone, lined with mucous membrane. These sinuses communicate with the nasal cavity through small openings, or *ostia,* in the lateral nasal wall. The paranasal sinuses serve several purposes: they lighten the bones of the skull, act as sound resonators, and provide mucus for the nasal cavity.

The paranasal sinuses, the locations of which appear in Figure 15–6, include the frontal, maxillary, ethmoid, and sphenoid sinuses. The names of the sinuses are derived from the bones in which they are located.

QUESTION
28

The paranasal sinuses are airfilled cavities in certain _____ of the skull.

ANSWER

bones

QUESTION
29

The principal functions of the paranasal sinuses are to _____ the bones of the skull, to provide _____, and to supply _____ for the nasal cavity.

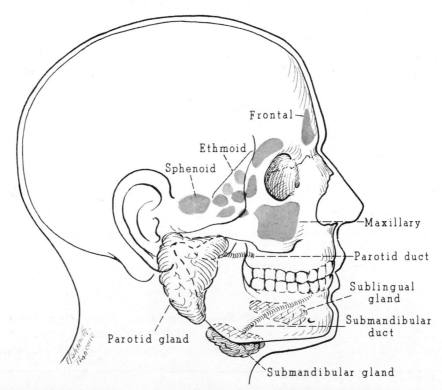

Figure 15–6. Locations of the paranasal sinuses. (Modified from Jacob and Francone: Structure and Function in Man. 3rd Ed. Philadelphia, W. B. Saunders Co.)

lighten . . . resonance . . . mucus

The four bones of the skull in which paranasal sinuses are located are the
_____, the _____, the _____, and the _____
bones.

frontal . . . maxillary . . . ethmoid . . . sphenoid (in any order)

THE PARANASAL SINUSES: GROWTH AND DEVELOPMENT

The ethmoid sinuses, called *ethmoid air cells,* begin development during the third month of fetal life. The sphenoid sinuses are rudimentary at birth, but develop rapidly during the first several years. The maxillary sinuses, also rudimentary at birth, do not develop significantly until after the permanent teeth have erupted. Development of the frontal sinuses is insignificant until the sixth or eighth year and is not complete until after puberty.

The earliest of the paranasal sinuses to develop are the _____ air cells; the latest, the _____ sinuses.

ethmoidal . . . frontal

The sphenoid and the maxillary sinuses are both rudimentary at birth, but during early childhood the sphenoid sinuses develop *more rapidly/more slowly* (circle one) than the maxillary sinuses.

more rapidly

THE MAXILLARY SINUS: SIGNIFICANCE IN DENTISTRY

The maxillary sinus, occupying much of the interior of the maxilla, is the largest of the paranasal sinuses. Because of its size and its proximity to, and relationship with, the maxillary teeth and jaw, the maxillary sinus is the most significant to the study of dentistry of all the paranasal sinuses.

Continuing its growth throughout adult life, the maxillary sinus becomes larger as stresses on bone are diminished. In extreme cases, the sinus may expand deep into the alveolar process after teeth have been lost, so that the roots of remaining teeth project inward toward the sinus and are separated from it only by the sinus mucosa and a thin sheet of bone called the *periapical tissue*.

QUESTION
33

One reason why the maxillary sinus is more relevant to the study of dentistry than the other paranasal sinuses is its closeness to the _____ _____ and _____.

ANSWER

maxillary teeth . . . jaw

QUESTION
34

A major factor contributing to the enlargement and expansion of the maxillary sinus is a lessening of the stress on _____ brought about by loss of _____.

ANSWER

bone . . . teeth

QUESTION
35

Periapical tissue is a thin sheet of _____ separating the roots of teeth from the floor of the _____ _____ in exaggerated cases of encroachment of the maxillary sinus into the alveolar process.

ANSWER

bone . . . maxillary sinus

ITEM 12   THE MAXILLARY SINUS: BOUNDARIES, BLOOD SUPPLY, AND INNERVATION

Figure 15–7 shows the boundaries of the maxillary sinus as viewed from the front. The roof of the sinus is the *orbital process of the maxilla;* the floor, the upper surface of the *alveolar process.* The medial boundary is the *lateral nasal wall;* the lateral boundary, the *zygomatic process of the maxilla.* The maxillary sinus opens into the nasal cavity at the middle meatus into a deep groove called the *hiatus semilunaris.*

Blood supply to the lining of the maxillary sinus is from the superior alveolar and infraorbital branches of the maxillary artery; innervation, from the corresponding branches of the maxillary division of the trigeminal nerve.

QUESTION
36

The hiatus semilunaris is a deep groove in the _____ meatus into which the maxillary sinus opens.

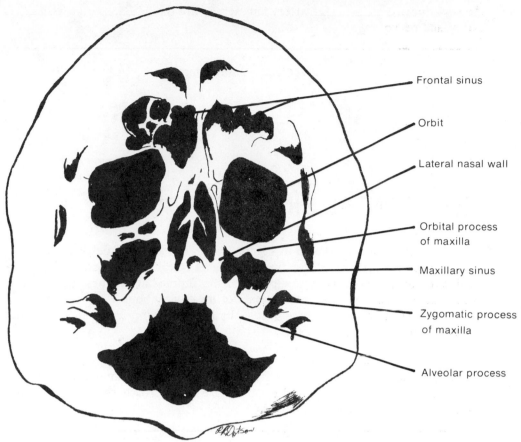

Figure 15–7. Boundaries of the maxillary sinus. Radiograph, Water's projection. (Redrawn from Woodburne: Essentials of Human Anatomy. 4th Ed. New York, Oxford University Press.)

middle

ANSWER

Match the boundaries of the maxillary sinus listed in Column A with the bony processes listed in Column B.

QUESTION
37

Column A	Column B
( ) 1. superior	A. zygomatic process of the maxilla
( ) 2. inferior	B. orbital process of the maxilla
( ) 3. medial	C. superior surface of the alveolar process
( ) 4. lateral	D. lateral nasal wall

If you are unable to visualize the boundaries clearly enough to match the columns, look at Figure 15–7 while you work out the answers.

1—(B); 2—(C); 3—(D); 4—(A)

ANSWER

Blood supply and innervation of the lining of the maxillary sinus are furnished by identically named branches of the maxillary artery and the maxillary nerve:

QUESTION
38

the superior _____ artery and nerve, and the _____ artery and nerve.

ANSWER

alveolar . . . infraorbital

ITEM 13

THE FRONTAL SINUSES

The *frontal sinuses,* shown in Figure 15–7, are two asymmetrical apertures located near the midline of the frontal bone. Typically, these cavities have a vertical extension posterior and superior to the supraciliary arches, and a lower horizontal extension into the orbital plate of the frontal bone.

The opening to the frontal sinuses, the *frontonasal duct,* is located in the anterior part of the middle meatus.

QUESTION 39

The perpendicular extension of the frontal sinuses runs above and behind the _____ arches; the horizontal extension of these sinuses runs into the _____ plate of the frontal bone.

ANSWER

supraciliary . . . orbital

QUESTION 40

The frontal sinus opens into the nasal cavity through the _____ duct, which is located in the anterior part of the _____ meatus.

ANSWER

frontonasal . . . middle

ITEM 14

THE ETHMOID AIR CELLS

The ethmoid sinuses, also called the *ethmoid air cells,* consist of a variable number of small cavities in the lateral mass of the ethmoid bone. These air spaces are roughly divided into anterior, middle, and posterior groups.

The *anterior ethmoid air cells* open into a curved groove in the middle meatus, the hiatus semilunaris; the *middle ethmoid air cells,* into a conical projection of bone in the middle meatus known as the *bulla ethmoidalis;* the *posterior ethmoid air cells,* into the superior meatus.

The curved groove in the middle meatus is the _____ _____.

QUESTION 41

hiatus semilunaris

ANSWER

The bulla ethmoidalis is a bulge in the _____ meatus into which the _____ group of ethmoid air cells opens into the nasal cavity.

QUESTION 42

middle . . . middle

ANSWER

The anterior ethmoid air cells open into the _____ meatus; the posterior group opens into the _____ meatus.

QUESTION 43

middle . . . superior

ANSWER

THE SPHENOID SINUS   ITEM 15

The *sphenoid sinus,* sometimes paired, is located in the body of the sphenoid bone. The sphenoid sinus opens into a deep groove of the lateral nasal wall known as the sphenoethmoidal recess, located superior and posterior to the superior conchae. Infections in the sphenoid sinus, like infections in the ethmoid sinuses, are dangerous because of the close proximity of the cavernous sinus and the optic nerve.

The groove into which the sphenoid sinus opens is called the _____ recess.

QUESTION 44

sphenoethmoidal

ANSWER

The structures which are particularly vulnerable to invasion by infection from the sphenoid sinus are the _____ sinus and the _____ nerve.

QUESTION 45

cavernous . . . optic

ANSWER

ITEM 16   THE OSTIA OF THE PARANASAL SINUSES

The cavities of the paranasal sinuses communicate with the nasal cavity through their openings, which are called *ostia*. Ventilation of the sinuses normally occurs with respiration. The locations of the ostia are shown in Figure 15–8. Although these sites have been mentioned in preceding items, they are recapitulated here as a review.

The sphenoethmoidal recess, located above and behind the superior concha, contains the ostium of the sphenoid sinus. The superior meatus contains the ostium of the posterior ethmoid air cells. The hiatus semilunaris, a groove in the middle meatus, contains ostia of the frontonasal duct, the anterior ethmoidal air cells, and the maxillary sinus. Middle ethmoidal air cells open into the bulla ethmoidalis, the bulging mass in the middle meatus.

To answer the following questions, refer to Figure 15–8 as well as to the text of Item 16.

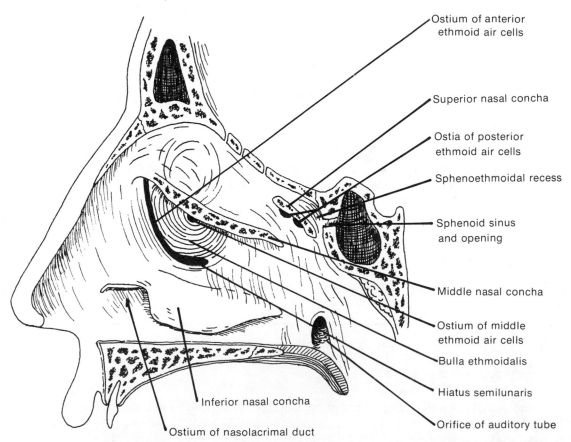

Figure 15–8. Ostia of the paranasal sinuses. (Redrawn from Woodburne: Essentials of Human Anatomy. 4th Ed. New York, Oxford University Press.)

Place check marks before the paranasal sinuses which open into the middle nasal meatus.

      (   ) A. anterior ethmoid sinuses
      (   ) B. frontal sinus
      (   ) C. maxillary sinus
      (   ) D. middle ethmoid sinuses
      (   ) E. posterior ethmoid sinuses
      (   ) F. sphenoid sinus

You should have placed check marks before A, B, C, and D.

The ostia located in the superior nasal meatus are those of the *sphenoid/ posterior ethmoid* (circle one) sinuses; those located above and behind the superior concha are those of the *sphenoid/posterior ethmoid* (circle one) sinuses.

posterior ethmoid . . . sphenoid

Ostia in the sphenoethmoidal recess are those of the *sphenoid/ethmoid* (circle one) sinuses.

sphenoid

The anterior ethmoid and the maxillary sinuses open into the hiatus _____ in the middle meatus.

semilunaris

The frontal sinus opens into the middle meatus through the _____ duct; the middle ethmoid sinuses open through the bulla _____.

frontonasal . . . ethmoidalis

The paranasal sinuses, under normal conditions, are ventilated by _____.

respiration (breathing)

ITEM 17

THE NASOLACRIMAL DUCT AND THE AUDITORY TUBE

If you look back to Figure 15–8, you can see, in addition to the openings of the paranasal sinuses, two other important apertures in the lateral nasal wall. In the inferior meatus, where the front part of the inferior concha has been cut away, there is a slitlike opening called the *nasolacrimal duct*. This duct drains tears, which constantly wash the eyeball, into the nasal cavity.

Adjacent to the nasopharynx in Figure 15–8 is the orifice of the *auditory tube,* through which the nasal portion of the pharynx communicates with the tympanic cavity.

QUESTION 52

The opening in the anterior region of the inferior nasal meatus is the _____ duct, which drains _____.

ANSWER

nasolacrimal . . . tears

QUESTION 53

The auditory tube is a passage from the nasal part of the _____ to the _____ cavity.

ANSWER

pharynx . . . tympanic

ITEM 18

THE PARANASAL SINUSES: DRAINAGE

The mucous membrane lining the paranasal sinuses has cilia which beat in the direction of the ostia, promoting drainage of accumulating fluids. The locations of the ostia do not favor drainage in the upright position, except in the case of the frontal sinus.

Congestion of the mucosa can occlude the openings, block exchange of air and normal drainage, and produce an inflammatory reaction known as *sinusitis*. In extreme cases of sinusitis it may be necessary to surgically extend the openings in the lateral nasal wall so that adequate drainage can take place.

QUESTION 54

Drainage of the paranasal sinuses is effected by the movement of _____ beating in the direction of the _____ in the lateral nasal wall.

ANSWER

cilia . . . ostia

The single paranasal sinus which will drain easily while one is standing erect is the _____ sinus.

frontal

Inflammation of the mucosa of the paranasal sinuses is called _____.

sinusitis

When mucous congestion of the paranasal sinuses blocks drainage in aggravated cases of sinusitis, surgery can be performed to _____ the ostia in the lateral nasal wall.

enlarge

SUMMARY OF UNIT FIFTEEN

THE NOSE

Externally, the nose is a bony and cartilaginous structure; internally, it is a triangular area comprising two wedgeshaped cavities separated by a septum. The septum is made up of the vomer below and the perpendicular plate of the ethmoid bone above, with cartilage between. Three folds of thin bone on the lateral walls, the conchae, overlie three cavities called the meatuses.

The main arterial blood supply to the nasal cavity is the sphenopalatine artery. After giving off posterior lateral nasal and posterior septal branches, the spheno-palatine artery supplies the septum as it makes its way downward and forward to anastomose with the greater palatine artery at the incisive foramen. The anterior part of the nasal cavity is supplied by ethmoidal branches of the ophthalmic artery and by the superior labial branch of the facial artery.

The nerves to the nasal cavity include the olfactory nerves located in the uppermost part of the cavity; the nasopalatine branch of the maxillary nerve, which runs with the sphenopalatine artery; and other nerves which run with arteries of the same name.

PARANASAL SINUSES

The paranasal sinuses are membrane-lined cavities which lighten bone, serve as resonators, and provide mucus for the nasal cavity. These sinuses communicate with the nasal cavity through small ostia in the lateral nasal wall. The rate of development of the paranasal sinuses is variable.

Of the four paranasal sinuses, the maxillary sinus is most significant in dentistry because of its proximity to the maxillary teeth and jaw. Following loss of teeth, the maxillary sinus can invade the alveolar process until only a thin sheet of bone separates it from the roots of the teeth.

The two frontal sinuses are near the lower midline of the frontal bone. The ethmoid sinuses, or air cells, are divided into anterior, middle, and posterior groups. The sphenoid sinus is located in the sphenoid bone above and behind the nasal cavity.

The ostia of the paranasal sinuses are in the middle and superior meatuses and behind the superior concha. The maxillary sinus opens into the hiatus semilunaris in the middle meatus; the frontal sinus, through the frontonasal duct into the anterior part of the middle meatus; the sphenoid sinus, into the sphenoethmoidal recess above and behind the superior concha. The anterior ethmoid air cells open into the hiatus semilunaris in the middle meatus; the middle air cells, into the bulla ethmoidalis, also in the middle meatus; the posterior air cells, into the superior meatus. Besides the paranasal ostia, the nasal cavity also contains the opening for the nasolacrimal duct through which tears drain, and the orifice of the auditory tube at the beginning of the nasopharynx.

QUESTION
58

The lower bone of the nasal septum is the _____; the upper bone is the perpendicular plate of the _____ bone; the space between the two septal bones is filled out with _____.

vomer . . . ethmoid . . . cartilage

ANSWER

The main blood supply to the nasal cavity is provided by the _____ _____ artery.

QUESTION **59**

---

sphenopalatine

ANSWER

In addition to receiving blood from branches of the sphenopalatine artery, the septum is also supplied by the _____ _____ artery.

QUESTION **60**

---

greater palatine

ANSWER

The terminal organs for transmitting the sense of smell are the _____ nerves in the _____ part of the nasal cavity.

QUESTION **61**

---

olfactory . . . superior

ANSWER

The nerve which travels in the nasal cavity in company with the sphenopalatine artery is the _____ nerve.

QUESTION **62**

---

nasopalatine

ANSWER

The main functions of the paranasal sinuses are to _____ bones of the skull, to serve as a _____ cavity for sound, and to provide _____ for the nasal cavity.

QUESTION **63**

---

lighten . . . resonator . . . mucus

ANSWER

The paranasal sinus which has the greatest significance in dentistry is the _____ sinus.

QUESTION **64**

---

maxillary

ANSWER

Paranasal ostia in the hiatus semilunaris are those of the _____ sinus and those of the _____ ethmoid sinuses.

QUESTION **65**

---

maxillary . . . anterior

ANSWER

The ostium of the frontal sinus is in the anterior part of the _____ meatus; the sphenoid sinus opens into the _____ recess.

QUESTION **66**

ANSWER

middle . . . sphenoethmoidal

QUESTION 67

The ostium of the middle ethmoid air cells is located in the summit of the _____ _____; the ostia of the posterior ethmoid air cells, in the _____ meatus.

ANSWER

bulla ethmoidalis . . . superior

QUESTION 68

The nasolacrimal duct opens into the *superior/middle/inferior* (circle one) meatus.

ANSWER

inferior

QUESTION 69

Sinusitis is inflammation of the _____ of the paranasal sinuses, which sometimes requires surgical enlargement of the _____ in the lateral nasal wall.

ANSWER

mucosa . . . ostia

Unit Sixteen □ THE NECK, PHARYNX, AND LARYNX

AN OVERVIEW OF THE NECK: THE ANTERIOR HALF

Unit Sixteen covers two main topics concerning the neck: the muscles related to the skull and lower jaw, and the structural features of the pharynx and larynx. A cross section of the neck is shown in Figure 16–1 to provide an overview for locating the principal neck structures.

The anterior portion of the neck is illustrated in the lower part of Figure 16–1. As your examination of the neck proceeds from superficial to deep portions, you will see four successive muscle layers before you come to the *thyroid gland*. These layers are (1) the thin *platysma muscle* in the subcutaneous tissue of the neck, (2) the bulging *sternocleidomastoid muscle,* (3) the *sternohyoid* and *omohyoid* muscles, which are in the same lateral plane, and (4) the *sternothyroid* muscle.

Surrounded by the thyroid gland are first the *trachea* and then the *esophagus*. Behind the esophagus is the buccopharyngeal fascia, a connective tissue structure enclosing the upper part of the alimentary canal. Behind the thyroid gland, to the left and right, are the *carotid sheaths*. Within each carotid sheath are three important structures: the *common carotid artery,* the *internal jugular vein,* and the *vagus nerve*.

Ascending between the platysma and the sternocleidomastoid muscles is the external jugular vein.

Consult Figure 16–1 as you find necessary in order to answer the questions which follow.

Viewed from anterior to posterior, the esophagus is *anterior to/posterior to* (circle one) the trachea.

---

posterior to

The contents of the carotid sheath include the _____ _____ artery, the _____ _____ vein, and the _____ nerve.

Posterior

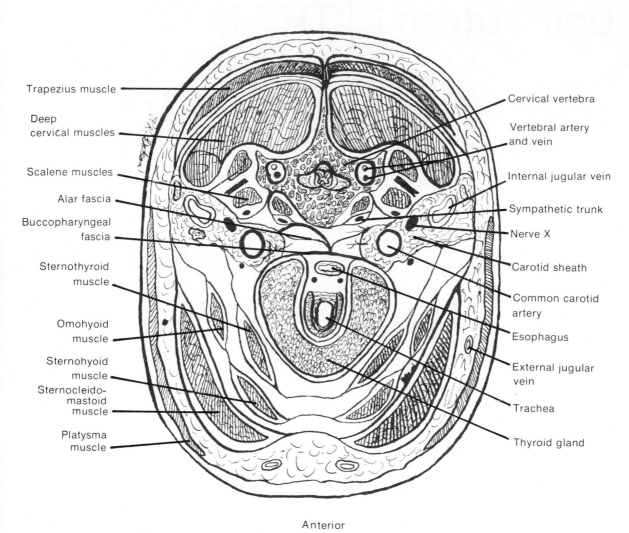

Trapezius muscle

Deep cervical muscles

Scalene muscles

Alar fascia

Buccopharyngeal fascia

Sternothyroid muscle

Omohyoid muscle

Sternohyoid muscle

Sternocleido-mastoid muscle

Platysma muscle

Cervical vertebra

Vertebral artery and vein

Internal jugular vein

Sympathetic trunk

Nerve X

Carotid sheath

Common carotid artery

Esophagus

External jugular vein

Trachea

Thyroid gland

Anterior

Figure 16–1.   Schematic cross section of the neck at the isthmus of the thyroid gland. (Redrawn from Woodburne: Essentials of Human Anatomy. 4th Ed. New York, Oxford University Press.)

ANSWER   common carotid . . . internal jugular . . . vagus

QUESTION
3
The external jugular vein rises between the _____ muscle and the _____ muscle.

ANSWER   platysma . . . sternocleidomastoid

QUESTION
4
Proceeding from superficial to deep, the order of succession of the muscles in the anterior part of the neck is as follows:

1. _____ muscle
2. _____ muscle
3. _____ and _____ muscles
4. _____ muscle

1. platysma
2. sternocleidomastoid
3. sternohyoid . . . omohyoid
5. sternothyroid

ANSWER

Posterior

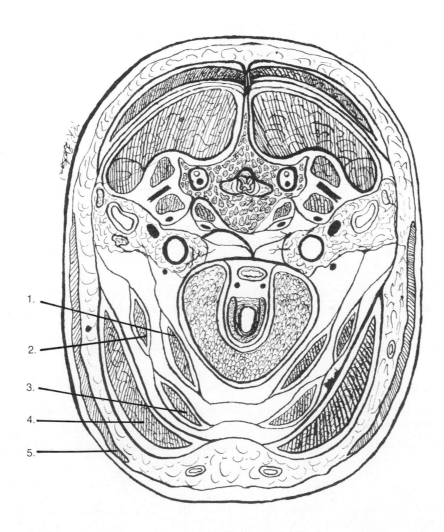

Anterior

(Redrawn from Woodburne: Essentials of Human Anatomy. 4th Ed. New York, Oxford University Press.)

QUESTION
5

In the numbered blank labels below, write the names of the corresponding numbered muscles in the diagram, page 621.

Labels

1. _____ muscle
2. _____ muscle
3. _____ muscle
4. _____ muscle
5. _____ muscle

ANSWER

Check your labels with Figure 16–1.

ITEM 2   OVERVIEW OF THE NECK: THE POSTERIOR HALF

Examine Figure 16–1 again. This time, begin your observation of the structural succession posteriorly, and move from superficial structures to deep.

The outermost structure, the *trapezius muscle,* is followed by two masses of *deep cervical muscles* dorsolateral to the *cervical vertebra.* Lateral to the cervical vertebra, the *scalene muscles* appear. The *vertebral artery* and *vein* can be seen rising in the transverse process of the cervical vertebra. Anterior to the cervical vertebra, you can see the cervical *sympathetic nerve trunk.* Finally, notice the *alar fascia* attaching along the midline of the buccopharyngeal fascia and extending in a lateral direction to terminate in the carotid sheath.

Consult Figure 16–1 as you find necessary in order to answer the questions which follow.

QUESTION
6

Proceeding from the posterior aspect inward, the order of succession of the neck muscles is: (1) the _____ muscle, (2) the deep _____ muscles, and (3) the _____ muscles.

ANSWER

trapezius . . . cervical . . . scalene

QUESTION
7

The cervical sympathetic trunk is located *ventral to/dorsal to* (circle one) the vertebral column.

ANSWER

ventral to

QUESTION
8

The vertebral vein and artery run inside the _____ _____ of cervical vertebrae.

ANSWER

transverse processes

In the numbered spaces below write the names of the corresponding numbered structures in the accompanying diagram.

Labels

1. _____ muscle
2. _____ _____ muscles
3. _____ artery and vein
4. _____ muscles
5. _____ trunk

Check your labels with Figure 16–1.

ANSWER

Posterior

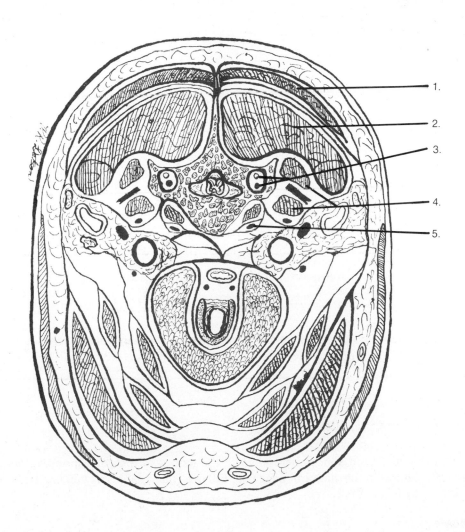

Anterior

(Redrawn from Woodburne: Essentials of Human Anatomy. 4th Ed. New York, Oxford University Press.)

ITEM
3

TRIANGLES OF THE NECK

Location of deeper structures of the neck is facilitated by reference to triangles defined by muscular, bony, and cartilaginous landmarks. Figure 16–2 illustrates these triangles and the landmarks which define them.

The most conspicuous muscular landmark of the neck is the *sternocleidomastoid muscle*. This muscle derives its name from three of the four bones to which it attaches, the sternum and clavicle below and the mastoid process and occipital bone above. The sternocleidomastoid muscle, bisecting the neck diagonally, divides the neck into the *anterior triangle* and the *posterior triangle*. The anterior margin of the anterior triangle is the median line of the neck; the superior border, the lower margin of the body of the mandible; the posterior border, the sternocleidomastoid muscle. The anterior border of the posterior triangle is the sternocleidomastoid muscle; the posterior border, the trapezius muscle; the inferior border, the middle third of the clavicle. The omohyoid and digastric muscles and the hyoid bone subdivide the main triangles into smaller triangles.

QUESTION
10

The kinds of structures which serve as landmarks for localization of deep structures of the neck are _____, _____, and _____.

ANSWER

muscles . . . bones . . . cartilage (in any order)

QUESTION
11

The inferior points of attachment of the sternocleidomastoid muscle are the _____ and the _____.

ANSWER

sternum . . . clavicle (in either order)

QUESTION
12

The superior points at which the sternocleidomastoid muscle attaches are the _____ bone and the _____ process.

ANSWER

occipital . . . mastoid

QUESTION
13

In the numbered spaces below, write the names of the corresponding numbered structures in the diagram, page 626. Fill in as many labels as you can without referring to Figure 16-2.

Labels

1. _____ muscle
2. _____ bone

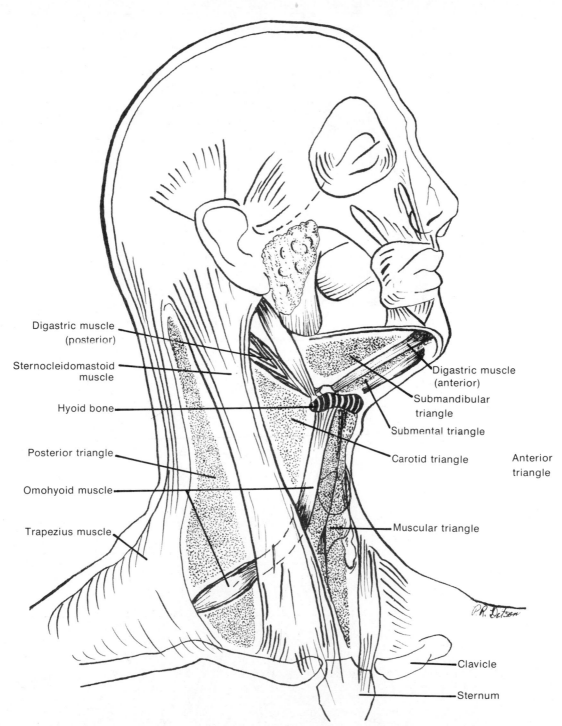

Figure 16–2. The anterior and posterior cervical triangles. (Redrawn from Woodburne: Essentials of Human Anatomy. 4th Ed. New York, Oxford University Press.)

3. _____ muscle
4. _____ muscle
5. _____ muscle

Check your labels with Figure 16–2.

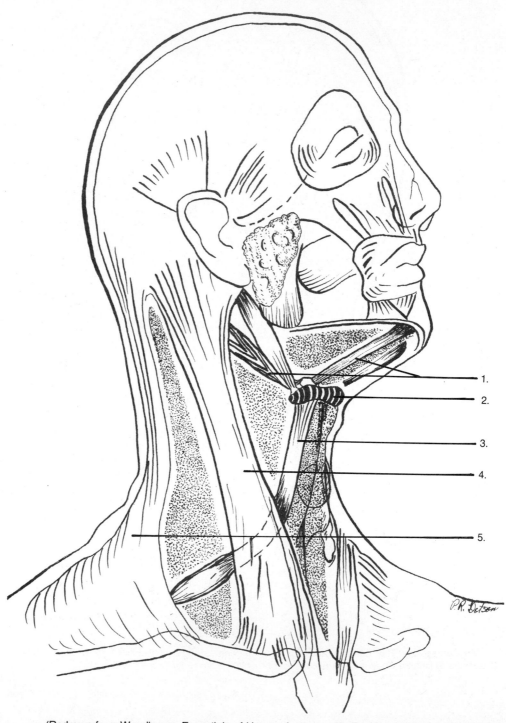

1.

2.

3.

4.

5.

(Redrawn from Woodburne: Essentials of Human Anatomy. 4th Ed. New York, Oxford University Press.)

THE ANTERIOR TRIANGLE: THE SUPRAHYOID SUBDIVISIONS

ITEM 4

Look back to Figure 16–2 and notice how the portion of the anterior triangle above the hyoid bone, the suprahyoid part, is subdivided by the digastric muscle into a *submandibular triangle* above and a *submental triangle* below.

Refer to Figure 16–2 as necessary to answer questions 14 and 15.

The submental triangle is bounded by the midline of the neck, the _____ _____muscle, and the _____ bone.

QUESTION
14

---

digastric . . . hyoid

ANSWER

The submandibular triangle is bounded by the lower border of the _____ _____, the _____ bone, and the _____ muscle.

QUESTION
15

---

mandible . . . hyoid . . . digastric

ANSWER

THE ANTERIOR TRIANGLE: THE INFRAHYOID SUBDIVISIONS

ITEM 5

Look back to Figure 16–2 again and examine the infrahyoid subdivisions of the anterior triangle, which are below the hyoid bone. The omohyoid muscle, crossing deep to the sternocleidomastoid muscle, divides the infrahyoid portion into the *carotid triangle* above the omohyoid and the *muscular triangle* below.

Refer to Figure 16–2 as necessary to answer the following questions.

The carotid triangle is bounded above by the posterior belly of the _____ muscle, anteriorly by the _____ muscle, and posteriorly by the _____ muscle.

QUESTION
16

---

digastric . . . omohyoid . . . sternocleidomastoid

ANSWER

The muscular triangle is bounded superiorly by the _____ bone, anteriorly by the midline of the neck, posterosuperiorly by the _____ muscle, and posteroinferiorly by the _____ muscle.

QUESTION
17

---

hyoid . . . omohyoid . . . sternocleidomastoid

ANSWER

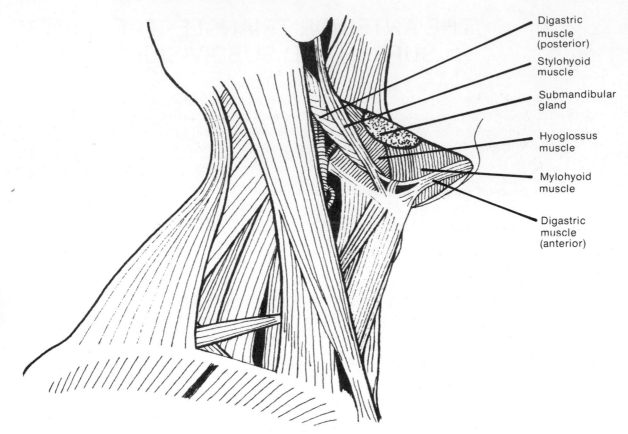

Figure 16-3. Muscles of the submandibular triangle. (Modified from Wolf-Heidegger: Atlas of Systematic Human Anatomy. Vol. I. Basel, S. Karger AG.)

ITEM 6   THE SUBMANDIBULAR TRIANGLE: THE MUSCLES

Figure 16–3 shows the following muscles of the submandibular triangle: the *mylohyoid, hyoglossus, stylohyoid,* and *digastric* muscles. The mylohyoid and hyoglossus muscles enter into formation of the floor of the triangle. The stylohyoid and digastric muscles, together with the mylohyoid, work in concert to raise the hyoid bone in swallowing, for example. With the hyoid bone held in place by the infrahyoid muscles, the stylohyoid, mylohyoid, and digastric are involved in depressing the mandible.

QUESTION 18

The infrahyoid muscles must hold the _____ bone in place in order for the suprahyoid muscles to depress the mandible; the infrahyoid muscles must relax in order for the suprahyoid muscles to raise the _____ bone.

ANSWER   hyoid . . . hyoid

Suprahyoid muscles forming the floor of the submandibular triangle are the _____ muscle and the _____ muscle.

mylohyoid . . . hyoglossus (in either order)

The suprahyoid muscles which work together with the mylohyoid muscles to raise the hyoid bone are the _____ and the _____ muscles.

stylohyoid . . . digastric (in either order)

THE SUBMANDIBULAR TRIANGLE: THE CONTENTS

The submandibular gland lies in the submandibular triangle between the angle of the mandible and the mylohyoid muscle. Deep to the submandibular gland are the hypoglossal nerve and the facial artery. Within the triangle, the facial artery gives off the submental artery. The lingual artery runs across the submandibular triangle before going deep to the hyoglossus muscle on its way to the tongue.

Arteries found in the submandibular triangle include the _____ artery, the _____ artery, and the _____ artery.

facial . . . submental . . . lingual (in any order)

Deep to the submandibular gland in the submandibular triangle are found the _____ nerve and the _____ artery.

hypoglossal . . . facial

THE SUBMENTAL TRIANGLE

The submental triangle is the central region above the hyoid bone between the two anterior bellies of the digastric muscles. Figure 16–4 shows the submental triangle from the ventral aspect of the neck. The floor of the submental triangle is the anteromedial part of the mylohyoid muscle. The triangle contains submental lymph nodes and the beginning of the anterior jugular vein.

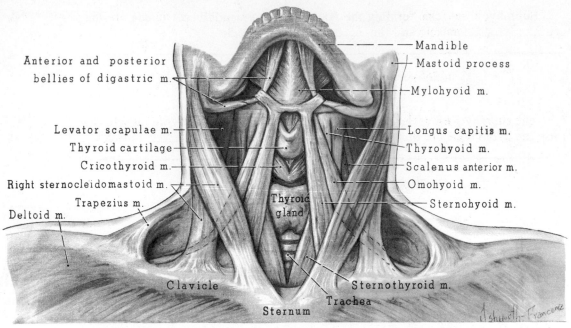

Figure 16–4. The infrahyoid region of the neck, ventral aspect. (From Jacob and Francone: Structure and Function in Man. 3rd Ed. Philadelphia, W. B. Saunders Co.)

QUESTION 23

The lateral boundaries of the submental triangle are the _____ _____ of the right and left digastric muscles.

ANSWER

anterior bellies

QUESTION 24

The submental triangle is bounded anteriorly by the border of the _____ and posteroinferiorly by the _____ bone.

ANSWER

mandible . . . hyoid

QUESTION 25

The anteromedial part of the _____ muscle forms the floor of the submental triangle.

ANSWER

mylohyoid

QUESTION 26

The submental triangle contains submental _____ _____ and the beginning of the _____ _____ vein.

ANSWER

lymph nodes . . . anterior jugular

THE MUSCULAR TRIANGLE   ITEM 9

Figure 16–4 shows the front of the neck with cartilages and muscles of the infrahyoid region in the muscular triangle. The infrahyoid region comprises the area from the hyoid bone above to the manubrium below. The floor of the infrahyoid region is formed from the trachea and the thyroid and cricoid cartilages. The right and left omohyoid muscles form the lateral boundaries of the region.

The lower border of the infrahyoid region is the _____; the upper margin is the _____ bone.

QUESTION
27

---

manubrium . . . hyoid

ANSWER

The trachea and the thyroid and cricoid cartilages form the _____ of the muscular triangle; the _____ muscles constitute the lateral boundaries.

QUESTION
28

---

floor . . . omohyoid

ANSWER

THE INFRAHYOID MUSCLES   ITEM 10

The infrahyoid muscles are four in number and serve the function of stabilizing the hyoid bone and the larynx. The four muscles of this group appear in Figure 16–4: the *sternohyoid* and *omohyoid* superficially, and the *sternothyroid* and *thyrohyoid* in a deeper plane.

The sternohyoid extends from the manubrium and medial clavicle to the anterior body of the hyoid bone. A tendinous sling at the clavicle divides the omohyoid muscle into superior and inferior bellies; the superior belly extends from the clavicle up to the hyoid bone and the inferior belly from the clavicle posterolaterally to the scapula.

The sternothyroid muscle extends from the manubrium to the oblique line of the thyroid cartilage; the thyrohyoid muscle, from the oblique line of the thyroid cartilage upward to the greater horn of the hyoid bone.

The two structures which are stabilized by the infrahyoid muscles are the _____ bone and the _____.

QUESTION
29

ANSWER

hyoid . . . larynx

QUESTION
30

The superior belly of the omohyoid muscle extends from the tendinous sling at the clavicle to the anterior body of the _____ bone; the inferior belly, from the tendinous sling to the _____.

ANSWER

hyoid . . . scapula

QUESTION
31

The muscle extending from the oblique line of the thyroid cartilage to the hyoid bone is the _____ muscle; that from the sternum to the thyroid cartilage is the _____ muscle.

ANSWER

thyrohyoid . . . sternothyroid

ITEM 11   THE CAROTID TRIANGLE: MUSCULAR BOUNDARIES AND FLOOR

The superior part of the anterior triangle is the *carotid triangle,* the area bounded by the sternocleidomastoid muscle, the omohyoid muscle, and the posterior belly of the digastric muscle. The floor of the carotid triangle is formed from the hyoglossus and thyrohyoid muscles together with the middle and inferior pharyngeal constrictor muscles. Except the pharyngeal constrictor muscles, these muscles can be seen in Figure 16–5.

QUESTION
32

The carotid triangle is bounded anteriorly by the _____ muscle; posteriorly, by the _____ muscle, and superiorly by the _____ muscle.

ANSWER

omohyoid . . . sternocleidomastoid . . . digastric

QUESTION
33

Two infrahyoid muscles make up the floor of the carotid triangle, the _____ muscle and the _____ muscle.

ANSWER

hyoglossus . . . thyrohyoid

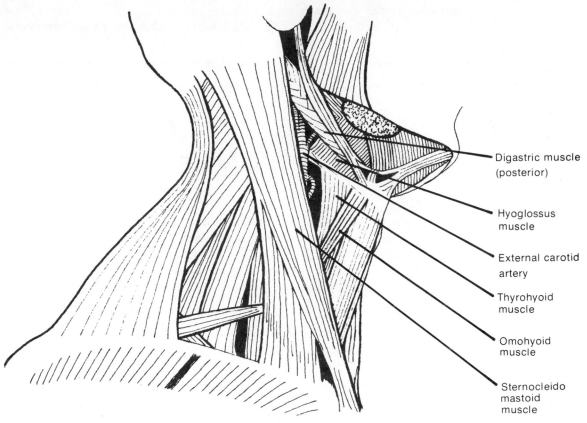

Figure 16-5. Muscles of the carotid triangle. (Modified from Wolf-Heidegger: Atlas of Systematic Human Anatomy. Vol. I. Basel, S. Karger AG.)

Digastric muscle (posterior)

Hyoglossus muscle

External carotid artery

Thyrohyoid muscle

Omohyoid muscle

Sternocleido mastoid muscle

THE CAROTID TRIANGLE: THE CONTENTS   ITEM 12

The *carotid triangle* derives its name from its position in approaching the carotid arterial system. If you will refer to Figure 16–5, you will notice a segment of the external carotid artery running deep to the sternocleidomastoid muscle in the carotid triangle. The internal jugular vein also extends through the carotid triangle. Nerves extending through the carotid triangle include the vagus, accessory, and hypoglossal nerves, and the cervical part of the sympathetic trunk.

Blood vessels in the carotid triangle include the _____ arteries and the _____ _____ veins.

QUESTION 34

carotid . . . internal jugular

ANSWER

QUESTION 35

Nerves in the carotid triangle include the _____ nerve, the _____ nerve, the _____ nerve, and the cervical sympathetic trunk.

ANSWER

vagus . . . accessory . . . hypoglossal (in any order)

ITEM 13 THE POSTERIOR TRIANGLE

The posterior triangle, enclosed between the trapezius and sterno-cleidomastoid muscles, contains lymph nodes and the transverse cervical and suprascapular blood vessels. Deep to the prevertebral fascia, which constitutes the floor of the posterior triangle, are the deep back muscles, the subclavian artery, and the cervical and brachial nerve plexuses.

QUESTION 36

Contents of the posterior triangle include _____ nodes of the neck as well as the transverse _____ artery and the _____ artery.

ANSWER

lymph . . . cervical . . . suprascapular

QUESTION 37

The anterior border of the posterior triangle is formed by the _____ muscle; the posterior border, by the _____ muscle.

ANSWER

sternocleidomastoid . . . trapezius

QUESTION 38

Structures deep to the floor of the posterior triangle include the _____ and _____ nerve plexuses and the _____ artery.

ANSWER

cervical . . . brachial . . . subclavian

ITEM 14 MUSCLES OF THE BACK OF THE NECK

Figure 16–6 shows the superficial muscles of the back of the neck. The *semispinalis capitis, splenius capitis,* and *trapezius muscles* extend the head when acting bilaterally; these muscles rotate the head when acting singly. Another action of the trapezius muscle is abduction of the scapula and elevation of the shoulder girdle. The sternocleidomastoid muscle inserts at its posteriormost limit at the

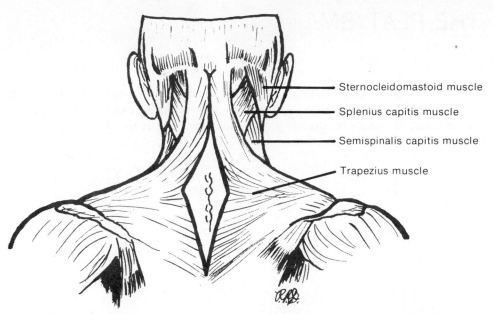

Figure 16–6. Superficial muscles of the back of the neck. (Modified from Wolf-Heidegger: Atlas of Systematic Human Anatomy. Vol. I. Basel, S. Karger AG.)

lateral part of the superior nuchal line of the occipital bone, and therefore is partially visible from the back of the head even though it is a lateral muscle. The sternocleidomastoid muscle also extends or rotates the head.

Superficial muscles of the back of the neck which extend or rotate the head are the _____ muscle and the _____ capitis and _____ capitis muscles.

QUESTION 39

trapezius . . . semispinalis . . . splenius

ANSWER

Besides extending or rotating the head, the trapezius muscle also effects elevation of the _____ and abduction of the _____.

QUESTION 40

shoulder . . . scapula

ANSWER

Although the sternocleidomastoid is a muscle of the side of the neck, it is partially visible from the back of the head because its posterior insertion is in the superior nuchal line of the _____ bone.

QUESTION 41

occipital

ANSWER

ITEM 15   THE PLATYSMA

The *platysma,* a broad, thin sheet of muscle in the subcutaneous tissue of the neck, is pictured in Figure 16–7. This muscle extends across the neck from the fascia below the clavicle, inserting near the corner of the mouth.

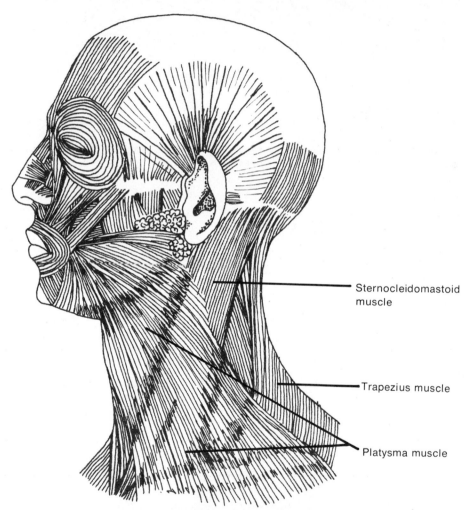

Sternocleidomastoid muscle

Trapezius muscle

Platysma muscle

Figure 16–7. Platysma muscle, lateral aspect. (Redrawn from Anson, Ed: Morris' Human Anatomy. 12th Ed. New York, McGraw-Hill Book Co., Inc.)

QUESTION
42

Being an extremely superficial neck muscle, the platysma lies in the _____ _____ of the neck.

ANSWER   subcutaneous tissue

THE PHARYNX   ITEM 16

The pharynx, pictured in Figure 16–8, is a muscular, fibrous tube which serves both the respiratory and the digestive systems. The region above the level of the soft palate is known as the *nasopharynx;* that between the soft palate and the opening of the larynx, as the *oropharynx;* that between the laryngeal orifice and the esophagus, as the *laryngopharynx*.

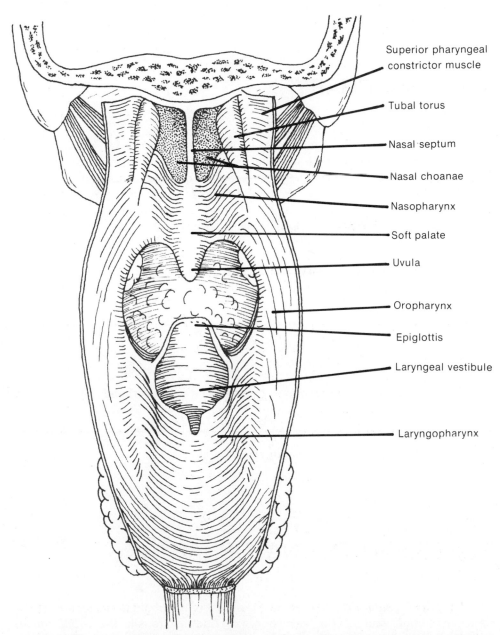

Superior pharyngeal constrictor muscle

Tubal torus

Nasal septum

Nasal choanae

Nasopharynx

Soft palate

Uvula

Oropharynx

Epiglottis

Laryngeal vestibule

Laryngopharynx

Figure 16–8. The pharynx, posterior aspect, shown with the posterior wall removed (Redrawn from Woodburne: Essentials of Human Anatomy. 4th Ed. New York, Oxford University Press.)

QUESTION
43
Match the area of the pharynx in Column A with the appropriate description from Column B.

Column A	Column B
( ) 1. nasopharynx	A. region between laryngeal orifice and esophagus
( ) 2. oropharynx	B. region above the soft palate
( ) 3. laryngopharynx	C. region between laryngeal orifice and soft palate

ANSWER
1.—(B); 2.—(C); 3.—(A)

ITEM 17   THE NASOPHARYNX

The nasopharynx is continuous with the nasal choanae, the *superior pharyngeal constrictor* muscle forming its lateral and posterior walls and the soft palate, its anterior floor. The passage between the pharynx and the middle ear, the *auditory tube,* opens in the lateral wall of the nasopharynx. A hoodlike cartilaginous overhang of the auditory tube called the *tubal torus* rises posterosuperior to the opening. Locate these structures on Figure 16–8.

QUESTION
44
The floor of the nasopharynx is formed by the _____ _____; its posterior and lateral walls, by the superior pharyngeal _____ muscle.

ANSWER
soft palate . . . constrictor

QUESTION
45
The tubal torus is an elevation of cartilage which overhangs the orifice of the _____ _____.

ANSWER
auditory tube

ITEM 18   TONSILS IN THE NASOPHARYNX

The *pharyngeal tonsil,* or adenoids, is a mass of lymphoid tissue located in the upper posterior wall of the nasopharynx. Another tonsil, the *tubal tonsil,* is located behind the opening of the auditory tube. Both these tonsillar groups are more prominent in children than in adults. Inflammation and enlargement, obviously, can partly occlude the upper respiratory passageways and block the opening of the auditory tube, which equalizes air pressure in the middle ear.

Adenoids is another term applied to the *pharyngeal/tubal* (circle one) tonsil.

pharyngeal

The function of the auditory tube is to equalize _____ pressure in the _____ ear.

air . . . middle

Enlargement of pharyngeal and tubal tonsils following inflammation can block the orifice of the _____ tube and partially occlude the _____ passages.

auditory . . . respiratory

THE OROPHARYNX ITEM 19

The oropharynx is the region extending from the soft palate above to the upper border of the epiglottis below. Notice in Figure 16–9 how the oropharynx is continuous with the mouth through the oropharyngeal orifice, or *fauces*. The fauces is bounded laterally by the palatoglossal and palatopharyngeal folds. Between these folds lie the *palatine tonsils*.

The tonsillar folds are the two arches formed by the _____ and _____ muscles.

palatoglossal . . . palatopharyngeal (in either order)

Between the palatoglossal and palatopharyngeal folds are found the _____ _____ tonsils.

palatine

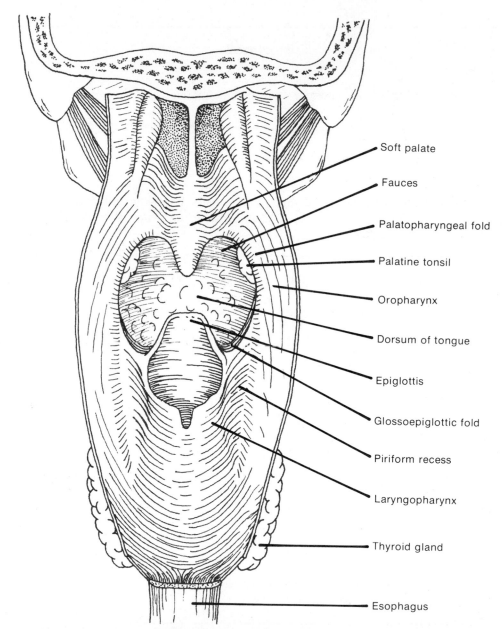

Figure 16–9. The oropharynx and laryngopharynx, posterior aspect, shown with the posterior wall removed. (Redrawn from Woodburne: Essentials of Human Anatomy. 4th Ed. New York, Oxford University Press.)

THE EPIGLOTTIS ITEM 20

Re-examine Figure 16–9 and observe the position of the *epiglottis* at the extreme lower border of the tongue. The free surface of this cartilaginous structure extends upward during breathing, leaving the opening of the larynx patent. During swallowing, the free surface of the epiglottis is pulled downward to cover the larynx so that food is deflected posteriorly to the esophagus. A single median and two lateral *glossoepiglottic folds* connect the anterior border of the epiglottis with the tongue.

The epiglottis is located at the root of the _____.

tongue

ANSWER

The glossoepiglottic folds connect the _____ with the lower posterior border of the _____.

epiglottis . . . tongue

ANSWER

The epiglottis extends upward during _____ to open the larynx; it swings downward during _____ to close the larynx.

breathing . . . swallowing

ANSWER

THE LARYNGOPHARYNX ITEM 21

The position of the *laryngopharynx* can be seen in Figure 16–9. This region of the pharynx is continuous with the oropharynx, extending from the epiglottis above to the esophagus below. The anterior part of the laryngopharynx is formed by the epiglottis, the opening into the larynx, and the posterior part of the cricoid cartilage of the larynx. The laryngopharynx extends laterally and anteriorly around the larynx, leaving the *piriform recess* in the space between the pharynx and the lateral surface of the thyroid cartilage.

QUESTION
54

The uppermost portion of the laryngopharynx is composed of the epiglottis and the back part of the _____ cartilage of the larynx; the lower continuation of the laryngopharynx is the _____.

ANSWER

cricoid . . . esophagus

QUESTION
55

The piriform recess is the space enclosed between the _____ and the lateral surface of the _____ cartilage.

ANSWER

pharynx . . . thyroid

ITEM 22   THE PHARYNX: THE MUSCLES

The muscles of the pharynx are shown in Figure 16–10. These muscles include one longitudinal muscle, the *stylopharyngeus,* and three lateral *constrictors:* the *inferior, middle,* and *superior.* Notice how the constrictor muscles overlap one another as they terminate posteriorly in the pharyngeal raphe.

The stylopharyngeus muscle elevates the pharynx to receive food driven backward by the tongue. Serial contractions of the constrictor muscles, in turn, drive the food down into the esophagus.

QUESTION
56

The muscles which insert at the pharyngeal raphe are the _____, _____, and _____ constrictor muscles.

ANSWER

inferior . . . middle . . . superior (in any order)

QUESTION
57

The stylopharyngeus muscle runs in a *lateral/vertical* (circle one) direction.

ANSWER

vertical

QUESTION
58

The function of the stylopharyngeus muscle is to _____ the pharynx to receive food from the tongue; that of the constrictor muscles, to move food down to the _____.

ANSWER

elevate . . . esophagus

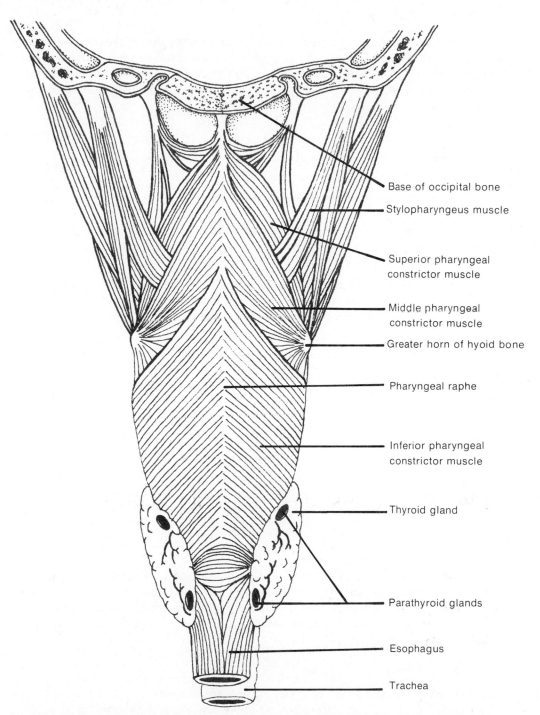

Base of occipital bone

Stylopharyngeus muscle

Superior pharyngeal
constrictor muscle

Middle pharyngeal
constrictor muscle

Greater horn of hyoid bone

Pharyngeal raphe

Inferior pharyngeal
constrictor muscle

Thyroid gland

Parathyroid glands

Esophagus

Trachea

Figure 16–10.   Muscles of the pharynx, posterior aspect. (Redrawn from Wolf-Heidegger: Atlas of Systematic Human Anatomy. Vol. II. Basel, S. Karger AG.)

ITEM 23 THE PHARYNX: THE NERVE SUPPLY

The nerve supply to the pharynx is derived from the *pharyngeal plexus*, except for a branch of the glossopharyngeal nerve which supplies the stylopharyngeus muscle. The pharyngeal plexus contains motor fibers from the vagus nerve, sensory fibers predominantly from the glossopharyngeal nerve, and vasomotor fibers from the superior cervical sympathetic ganglion.

QUESTION 59

Innervation of the stylopharyngeus muscle is from fibers of the _____ _____ nerve.

ANSWER

glossopharyngeal

QUESTION 60

The vagus nerve in the pharyngeal plexus supplies *afferent/efferent* (circle one) fibers to the pharynx; the glossopharyngeal nerve in the plexus supplies *afferent/efferent* (circle one) fibers; the superior cervical ganglion supplies *sympathetic/parasympathetic* (circle one) fibers.

ANSWER

efferent . . . afferent . . . sympathetic

ITEM 24 THE PHARYNX: THE BLOOD SUPPLY

The principal blood supply to the pharynx is through the *ascending pharyngeal* and *superior thyroid* branches of the external carotid artery. The *ascending palatine* branch of the facial artery provides additional blood supply to the pharynx, as do the *descending palatine* and *pharyngeal* branches of the maxillary artery.

QUESTION 61

Blood is supplied to the pharynx through the ascending _____ _____ and superior _____ arteries, and the ascending and descending _____ arteries.

ANSWER

pharyngeal . . . thyroid . . . palatine

THE LARYNX   ITEM 25

The larynx is located between the pharynx above and the trachea below. It is composed of cartilage, ligaments, and intrinsic muscles, covered by mucous membrane. The thyroid gland covers part of the lateral surface of the larynx. Skeletal support is by the hyoid bone and the thyroid and cricoid cartilages.

The larynx serves two purposes, that of an open airway to the trachea and that of an instrument of phonation by means of the vocal folds. Variation of the tension and shape of the vocal folds determines pitch and other qualities of phonation.

The kinds of tissue that comprise the larynx include _____, _____, _____, and _____ membrane.

QUESTION 62

cartilage . . . ligament . . . muscle . . . mucous

ANSWER

The twofold function of the larynx is to admit _____ to the trachea and to produce various sounds by alteration of the shape and tension of the _____ _____.

QUESTION 63

air . . . vocal folds

ANSWER

THE LARYNX: THE VOCAL FOLDS   ITEM 26

Figure 16–11 shows a frontal section through the larynx and upper trachea with posterior parts of the constrictor muscles cut away. Note the epiglottis superiorly and the cut edges of the thyroid and cricoid cartilages laterally. Ventricular folds and vocal folds are shown extending anteroposteriorly across the laryngeal orifice. The more inferior of the folds, the *true vocal folds*, extend from the arytenoid cartilages posteriorly to the thyroid cartilage anteriorly. These folds overlie muscles which are active in phonation. The laterally directed space between the folds is the *ventricle*. Also observe in Figure 16–11 the cut surface of the thyroid gland extending from the thyroid cartilage above to the upper trachea below.

The vocal folds extend from the _____ cartilages to the _____ cartilage.

QUESTION 64

arytenoid . . . thyroid

ANSWER

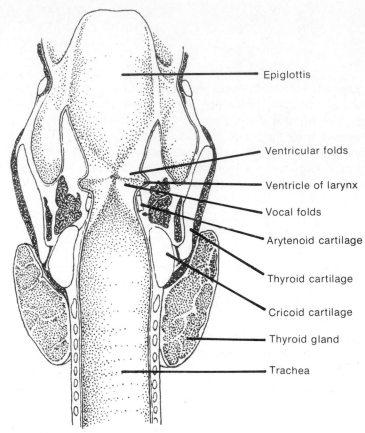

Epiglottis

Ventricular folds

Ventricle of larynx

Vocal folds

Arytenoid cartilage

Thyroid cartilage

Cricoid cartilage

Thyroid gland

Trachea

Figure 16–11.   Frontal section through the larynx and upper part of the trachea. (Redrawn from Wolf-Heidegger: Atlas of Systematic Human Anatomy. Vol. II. Basel, S. Karger AG.)

QUESTION
65

The thyroid gland extends from the _____ cartilage to the upper _____ .

ANSWER

thyroid . . . trachea

ITEM 27   THE LARYNX: THE NERVE AND BLOOD SUPPLY

All muscles of the larynx are innervated by the *inferior laryngeal branch* (the recurrent branch) of the vagus nerve, with the sole exception of the cricothyroid muscle, which is supplied by the *external branch of the superior laryngeal nerve* of the vagus nerve. Sensory innervation of the larynx is provided by both the internal branch of the superior laryngeal nerve and the inferior (recurrent) branch of the vagus nerve.

The blood supply of the larynx is derived from the *superior* laryngeal branch of the *superior* thyroid artery and the *inferior* laryngeal branch of the *inferior* thyroid artery.

All innervation of the larynx, both sensory and motor, is supplied by branches of the _____ nerve.

QUESTION
66

vagus

ANSWER

The external branch of the superior laryngeal nerve provides *sensory/motor* (circle one) innervation of the larynx; the internal branch of the superior laryngeal nerve provides *sensory/motor* (circle one) innervation.

QUESTION
67

motor . . . sensory

ANSWER

Sensory innervation of the larynx is derived from the _____ laryngeal and the _____ laryngeal branches of the vagus nerve.

QUESTION
68

superior . . . inferior (recurrent)

ANSWER

The blood supply to the larynx comes by way of laryngeal branches of the superior and inferior _____ arteries.

QUESTION
69

thyroid

ANSWER

SUMMARY OF UNIT SIXTEEN

THE TRIANGLES OF THE NECK

Triangles of the neck, demarcated by various bones and superficial muscles, constitute reference areas for locating deeper structures. The sternocleidomastoid muscle bisects the neck diagonally into anterior and posterior triangles. The superior part of the anterior triangle is subdivided by the anterior belly of the digastric muscle into a submandibular triangle and a submental triangle. The inferior part of the anterior triangle is subdivided by the omohyoid muscle into a carotid triangle above and a muscular triangle below.

The muscles of the submandibular triangle are the mylohyoid, hyoglossus, stylohyoid, and digastric. The first three of these muscles either raise the hyoid bone, as in swallowing, or help to depress the mandible. The submandibular triangle contains the submandibular gland, the hypoglossal nerve, and the facial artery.

The submental triangle, between the anterior bellies of the two digastric muscles, contains lymph nodes and the beginning of the anterior jugular vein.

The muscular triangle contains the four infrahyoid muscles: the sternohyoid, omohyoid, sternothyroid, and thyrohyoid. These muscles stabilize the hyoid bone and the larynx. The carotid triangle contains the carotid artery and the internal jugular vein. Nerves running through the carotid triangle include the vagus, accessory, and hypoglossal nerves, and the cervical sympathetic trunk.

The posterior triangle, between the trapezius and sternocleidomastoid muscles, contains lymph nodes as well as transverse cervical and suprascapular blood vessels. Deep to the floor of the posterior triangle are the subclavian artery, cervical and brachial plexuses, and the deep back muscles.

Superficial muscles of the back of the neck, involved in extending and rotating the head, include the trapezius, splenius capitis, and semispinalis capitis. The most superficial anterior neck muscle is the broad, thin platysma, lying in the subcutaneous tissue and extending from the clavicle to the lower part of the face and corners of the mouth.

THE PHARYNX

The pharynx, a muscular, fibrous tube extending from the soft palate down to the esophagus, serves both respiratory and digestive systems. Its uppermost part is the nasopharynx; the area posterior to the fauces is the oropharynx; the part between the laryngeal orifice and the esophagus is the laryngopharynx.

The nasopharynx contains the opening of the auditory tube and the pharyngeal and tubal tonsils. Swelling of these tonsils can occlude the opening of the auditory tube and partially block respiratory passageways. The fauces, where the oropharynx begins, is bounded by the tonsillar pillars and palatoglossal and palatopharyngeal folds. The epiglottis swings down to cover the opening of the larynx when food is swallowed and extends upward to open the larynx during breathing. The laryngopharynx extends around the larynx, leaving the piriform recess as a space between the pharynx and the thyroid cartilage.

The muscles of the pharynx include the longitudinal stylopharyngeus, which elevates the pharynx to receive food, and the three constrictors, which drive food down into the esophagus. The glossopharyngeal nerve provides motor supply to the stylopharyngeus muscle as well as sensory supply to most of the rest of the pharynx. The vagus nerve innervates the constrictor muscles. Blood supply to the pharynx is through the ascending pharyngeal and superior thyroid arteries, the ascending palatine branch of the facial artery, and the descending palatine and pharyngeal branches of the maxillary artery.

THE LARYNX

The larynx serves as an air passage to the trachea and as an instrument of phonation. Its main skeletal support is by the hyoid bone and the thyroid and cricoid cartilages. Inside the larynx, vocal folds extend from arytenoid cartilages posteriorly to the thyroid cartilage anteriorly. Innervation of the larynx is by both external and internal branches of the superior laryngeal part of the vagus nerve, as well as by the recurrent (inferior) laryngeal branch of the vagus. Blood supply to the larynx comes through laryngeal branches of the superior and inferior thyroid arteries.

The contents of the submandibular triangle include the _____ gland, the _____ nerve, and the _____ artery.

QUESTION **70**

---

submandibular . . . hypoglossal . . . facial

ANSWER

The submandibular triangle contains, in addition to the bordering digastric muscle, the _____ muscle, the _____ muscle, and the _____ muscle.

QUESTION **71**

---

mylohyoid . . . hyoglossus . . . stylohyoid (any order)

ANSWER

The suprahyoid muscles are involved in _____ the hyoid bone or in _____ the mandible.

QUESTION **72**

---

raising . . . depressing

ANSWER

The submental triangle contains _____ nodes and the beginning of the anterior _____ _____.

QUESTION **73**

---

lymph . . . jugular vein

ANSWER

The four infrahyoid muscles are the _____, the _____, the _____, and the _____.

QUESTION **74**

---

sternohyoid . . . omohyoid . . . sternothyroid . . . thyrohyoid (in any order)

ANSWER

QUESTION
75

Acting in unison, the infrahyoid muscles stabilize either the _____ _____ or the _____.

ANSWER

hyoid bone . . . larynx

QUESTION
76

Nerves which travel through the carotid triangle include the _____, the _____, the _____, and fibers of the cervical _____ trunk.

ANSWER

vagus . . . accessory . . . hypoglossal . . . sympathetic

QUESTION
77

Vessels in the carotid triangle are the _____ _____ vein and the _____ arteries.

ANSWER

internal jugular . . . carotid

QUESTION
78

The trapezius, splenius capitis, and semispinalis capitis are superficial muscles at the _____ of the neck; the platysma is a superficial muscle of the _____ and _____ of the neck.

ANSWER

back . . . front . . . sides

QUESTION
79

The nasopharynx is that part of the pharynx above the level of the _____ _____; the oropharynx, the area continuous with the _____ of the mouth; the laryngopharynx, the part which extends to the _____.

ANSWER

soft palate . . . fauces . . . esophagus

QUESTION
80

The tubal torus is a cartilaginous overhang above the site where the _____ _____ opens into the _____.

ANSWER

auditory tube . . . nasopharynx

QUESTION
81

The tonsillar pillars which bound the fauces are the _____ and the _____ folds.

ANSWER

palatoglossal . . . palatopharyngeal

QUESTION
82

The piriform recess is a space in the laryngopharynx between the pharynx itself and the _____ cartilage.

ANSWER

thyroid

QUESTION
83

The stylopharyngeus muscle elevates the _____ to receive food; food is driven into the esophagus by the _____ _____ muscles.

ANSWER

pharynx . . . pharyngeal constrictor

QUESTION
84

Innervation of the pharyngeal constrictor muscles is from the _____ nerve; innervation of the stylopharyngeus muscle, from the _____ nerve.

ANSWER

vagus . . . glossopharyngeal

QUESTION
85

The main blood supply to the pharynx comes through the ascending _____ artery and the superior _____ artery.

ANSWER

pharyngeal . . . thyroid

QUESTION
86

The skeletal support of the larynx is provided by the _____ bone and the _____ and _____ cartilages.

ANSWER

hyoid . . . thyroid . . . cricoid

QUESTION
87

The vocal folds attach posteriorly to the _____ cartilages and anteriorly to the _____ cartilage.

ANSWER

arytenoid . . . thyroid

QUESTION
88

Blood supply is brought to the larynx by laryngeal branches of the superior and inferior _____ arteries.

ANSWER

thyroid

QUESTION
89

Innervation of the larynx is by the superior and inferior laryngeal branches of the _____ nerve.

ANSWER

vagus

PART FOUR
□
CLINICAL APPLICATIONS

Unit Seventeen □ ROUTES OF SPREAD OF DENTAL INFECTION

MEANS OF PROPAGATION OF DENTAL INFECTIONS

An infection which originates in a tooth, in supporting structures, or in bone can spread to adjacent structures, and even to parts of the body far removed from the original site.

One route by which infections may spread from the primary site is through continuity of tissue. Once the infection has spread outside the tooth and alveolar processes, its route of propagation is determined largely by the location of loose connective tissue planes, with infection spreading into those facial spaces which offer the line of least resistance.

Secondly, bacteria may propagate through vascular channels, producing a systemic infection.

Thirdly, infection can spread from the dental area through the lymphatic system, as was mentioned in Unit Twelve.

The three principal means by which dental infections may spread are (1) through continuity of _____, (2) through _____ channels, and (3) through the _____ system.

QUESTION
1

tissues . . . vascular . . . lymphatic

ANSWER

QUESTION
2

Loose connective tissue planes of the face invite spread of infection because of their lack of _____ to invasion.

ANSWER

resistance

QUESTION
3

Systemic bacterial infections spread via *continuity of tissue/vascular channels/lymphatic system* (circle one).

ANSWER

vascular channels

QUESTION
4

Sites of dental infection may be the _____ itself, the _____ region, or _____ bonc.

ANSWER

tooth . . . periodontal . . . alveolar

ITEM 2   ROUTE FROM UPPER INCISORS TO THE NASAL REGION

In the maxillary area, the density and height of alveolar bone vary with the region. The alveolar process is made up of thin outer plates of compact bone and an inner core of cancellous bone. Obviously, the thinner the alveolar process, the more readily an infection can penetrate to deeper structures. The upper central incisor tooth is usually longer, and extends nearer to the nasal plate of compact bone, than the lateral incisor. A periapical abscess of the central incisor may therefore penetrate into the nasal region.

QUESTION
5

The direction in which dental infection may spread is determined in part by the thickness of the _____ _____ in a particular area.

ANSWER

alveolar process

QUESTION
6

Because the central incisor extends near the _____ plate of the alveolar process, an abscess of this tooth is apt to spread into the _____ region.

ANSWER

nasal . . . nasal

ROUTE FROM MAXILLARY LATERAL INCISORS TO THE LABIAL REGION

In the region of the maxillary lateral incisors, the labial plate of bone is usually thin in comparison to the lingual plate because the roots of these teeth slant toward the labial surface. Consequently, infections which originate at the roots of the upper lateral incisors are likely to penetrate anteriorly, following the line of least resistance to reach the labial vestibule.

The roots of upper lateral incisors usually slant toward the _____ surface of the alveolar process, making spread of infection from these teeth apt to move toward the _____ vestibule.

labial . . . labial

PROXIMITY OF UPPER MOLARS TO THE MAXILLARY SINUS

The premolar and molar teeth, and sometimes even the canine teeth, are located below the bony floor of the maxillary sinus, as is shown in Figure 17–1. Whether or not the roots of these teeth are in close proximity to the floor of the sinus depends on the depth of the alveolar process in given individuals.

In general, the first and second premolars are farthest from the sinus because their roots are shorter than molar roots, and because the floor of the sinus slopes upward in this region. The floor of the maxillary sinus normally slopes closest to the apices of the molar teeth, leaving the thinnest plate of bone between the molars and the floor of the sinus. Occasionally the floor of the sinus has conical projections conforming to the contour of the roots of the teeth. In cases where the invasion of the sinus into the alveolar bone is extreme, the bony floor of the sinus may be altogether absent above the roots of the teeth, so that periodontal tissue is in direct contact with the mucosa of the sinus.

Of the teeth below the bony floor of the maxillary sinus, the ones most removed from the floor of the sinus are the
  A. molars
  B. first premolars
  C. second premolars

The correct answer is B. Look at Figure 17–1 again, and notice the shortness of the roots of the first premolar tooth and the upward slant of the floor of the sinus.

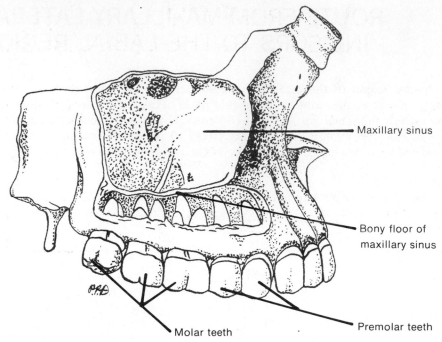

Figure 17–1.   Lateral view of a large maxillary sinus in relation to the roots of maxillary molar and premolar teeth. (Redrawn from Sicher, Harry, and DuBrul, E. Lloyd: Oral Anatomy, ed 6, St. Louis, 1975, The C. V. Mosby Co.)

QUESTION
9

When the bone of the floor of the maxillary sinus is absent, there is immediate contact between the _____ tissue surrounding roots of the maxillary teeth and the _____ of the sinus.

ANSWER

periodontal . . . mucosa

QUESTION
10

The bony floor of the maxillary sinus is thinnest above the roots of the _____ teeth.

ANSWER

molar

ITEM 5   THE MAXILLARY SINUS: INFECTION

Infection of the maxillary sinus may be caused by infected maxillary teeth extending into its lower regions. Infection may also result from a generalized sinus infection spreading from one sinus to another because of the proximity of the ostia in the lateral nasal wall. The closeness of the superior alveolar nerves to the lower border of the maxillary sinus may cause misinterpretations as to whether pain is originating in the sinus or in the teeth.

Infection of the maxillary sinus may be traceable to (circle one)
A. infection of the maxillary teeth
B. infection spreading from other sinuses
C. both of the above.

The correct answer is C. Either the maxillary teeth or other infected sinuses may infect the maxillary sinus.

Confusion as to whether pain is originating in the maxillary sinus or in the maxillary teeth is caused by the close proximity of the superior _____ _____ to the lower margin of the maxillary sinus.

alveolar nerves

Generalized sinus infection can easily occur because of the closeness of the _____ of the paranasal sinuses in the lateral nasal wall.

openings (ostia)

THE MANDIBULAR ALVEOLAR PROCESS: CHARACTERISTICS

ITEM 6

The alveolar process of the mandible is generally stronger than its maxillary counterpart. The labial surface in the region of the lower incisors, however, may be extremely thin and is usually penetrated by variably sized openings near the apices of the teeth.

The roots of the premolar and first molar mandibular teeth are usually inclined toward the buccal surface, making the outer alveolar plate relatively thin. In contrast, the roots of the second and third molars in the mandibular alveolar process are inclined lingually, resulting in a thinner inside layer of alveolar bone. As is the case in the maxillary region, the thickness of the alveolar process of the mandible usually determines the direction a periapical abscess will take as it follows the line of least resistance.

The thinnest part of the alveolar process of the mandible is near the lower _____ teeth.

incisor

QUESTION
15

Roots of the lower premolar and first molar teeth incline to the *lingual/buccal* (circle one) side of the alveolar process; roots of the second and third lower molars incline to the *lingual/buccal* (circle one) side.

ANSWER

buccal . . . lingual

QUESTION
16

Periapical abscess of a second or third lower molar is likely to spread toward the _____ side because of the thinness of alveolar bone on that side.

ANSWER

lingual

QUESTION
17

Periapical abscess of a lower premolar or first molar tooth is apt to go to the _____ side because the alveolar bone is _____ on that side.

ANSWER

buccal . . . thinner

ITEM 7   PROXIMITY OF LOWER TEETH TO THE MANDIBULAR CANAL

The mandibular canal, shown in Figure 17–2, is the channel in which the inferior alveolar nerve and blood vessels run through the mandible. Near the premolars, the mandibular canal splits into the narrow incisive canal, which continues anteriorly, and the wider mental canal, which turns anteriorly and opens at the mental foramen.

The relationship of the lower teeth to the mandibular canal is important. The incisors and canines are near the incisive canal; the first premolar is near the mental canal; the last premolar and the molar teeth are in close proximity to the mandibular canal. Because of the close proximity of the third molar, in particular, to the mandibular canal, involvement of the roots of this tooth can be extremely distressing. With the entire inferior alveolar nerve implicated, the patient is frequently unable to pinpoint the source of pain.

QUESTION
18

Proximity to the mandibular canal is most apt to cause particular problems of involvement of the roots of the (circle one)
A. first premolar tooth
B. third molar tooth
C. incisor and canine teeth

ANSWER

The correct answer is B.

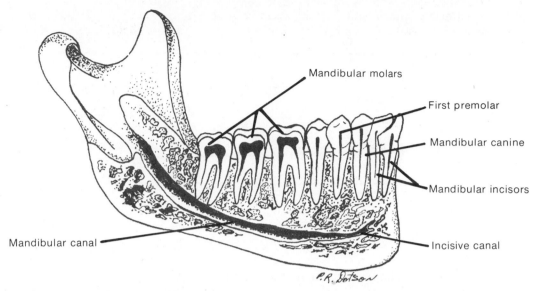

Figure 17–2. Sagittal section through the mandible, showing relationship of mandibular teeth to the mandibular canal. Note the close proximity of the apices of the third molar to the mandibular canal. (Redrawn from Sicher, Harry and DuBrul, E. Lloyd: Oral Anatomy, ed 6, St. Louis, 1975, The C. V. Mosby Co.)

The contents of the mandibular canal which may be affected by the roots of molar teeth are the _____ _____ nerve and blood vessels.

QUESTION
19

---

inferior alveolar

ANSWER

Difficulty in pinpointing the source of distress involving roots of the lower molars results from the fact that the entire inferior _____ _____ may be affected.

QUESTION
20

---

alveolar nerve

ANSWER

RELATIONSHIP OF FACIAL MUSCLES   ITEM
TO SPREAD OF INFECTION   8

The position of attachment of the muscles of the face influences the route of propagation of infection. Muscles present a relatively effective barrier against bacterial invasion, whereas the loose connective tissue fascia between muscles provides the route of least resistance. Infections which have penetrated the outer layer of the alveolar process may surface either in the vestibule or in subcutaneous tissues, depending on the location of the fascial planes separating muscles.

QUESTION
21

Muscle attachments of the face present a *barrier to/route of* spread of dental infection (circle one).

ANSWER

barrier to

QUESTION
22

Loose connective tissue *resists/invites* (circle one) propagation of infection.

ANSWER

invites

QUESTION
23

Depending on the location of muscle attachments, abscesses of the teeth may appear either in the _____ of the oral cavity or in _____ tissue.

ANSWER

vestibule . . . subcutaneous

ITEM 9

ROUTE FROM LOWER CANINES AND LOWER INCISORS

Dental abscesses are more likely to become cutaneous in regions where the roots of the teeth extend beyond the origin of muscles. Examine the anterior region of the lower jaw in Figure 17–3, and notice where the *lower incisive* and *mentalis muscles* arise from the base of the alveolar process. If the roots of the lower canines and lower incisors are long, an abscess is likely to penetrate the loose connective tissue below these muscles and appear as a cutaneous abscess instead of extending through the muscles to the submucosal space of the vestibule.

QUESTION
24

Situations in which a dental abscess tends to become cutaneous are those in which the roots of teeth extend beyond the attachment of the _____ _____.

ANSWER

facial muscles

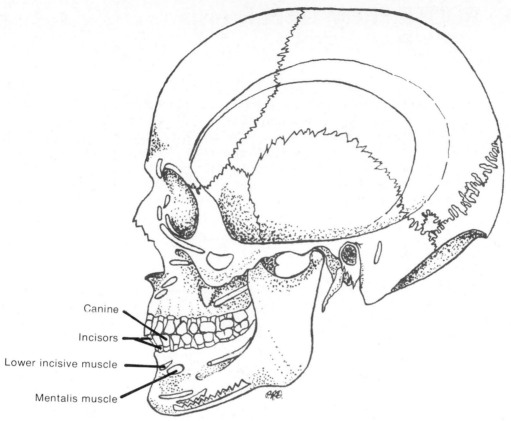

Figure 17–3. Mentalis and lower incisive muscles in relationship to mandibular incisor and canine teeth. (Redrawn from Sicher, Harry, and DuBrul, E. Lloyd: Oral Anatomy, ed 6, St. Louis, 1975, The C. V. Mosby Co.)

When roots of teeth do not extend beyond the origin of muscles, the muscles block the spread of infection to the _____, so that the infection moves instead toward the _____ of the mouth.

QUESTION
25

---

skin . . . vestibule

ANSWER

The facial muscles which attach below the lower canine and lower incisor teeth are the lower _____ muscle and the _____ muscle.

QUESTION
26

---

incisive . . . mentalis

ANSWER

Abscesses of the lower canine and lower incisor teeth surface cutaneously when the roots of these teeth extend *above/below* (circle one) the lower incisive and mental muscles.

QUESTION
27

---

below

ANSWER

ITEM 10
ROUTE FROM UPPER AND LOWER MOLARS

When the roots of the upper and lower molar teeth are long, as they are in some individuals, abscesses of these teeth are apt to be cutaneous. Note that the maxillary and mandibular attachments of the *buccinator muscles,* shown in Figure 17–4, are located near the base of the alveolar processes. In young persons whose molars have not yet erupted, and in adults who have long molar roots, these apices extend below the mandibular origin and above the maxillary origin of the buccinator muscle. In such cases a periapical abscess would tend to be barred from the vestibular mucosa, but would be free to move into subcutaneous tissue.

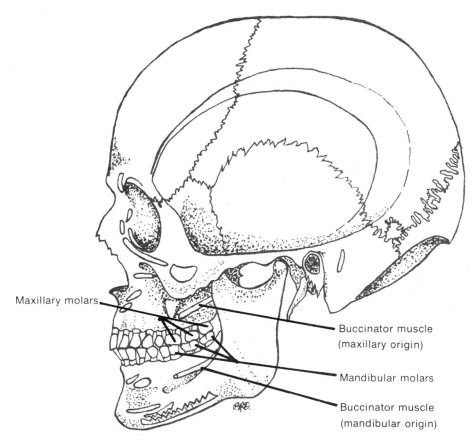

Maxillary molars

Buccinator muscle
(maxillary origin)

Mandibular molars

Buccinator muscle
(mandibular origin)

Figure 17–4. Upper and lower molar teeth in relationship to maxillary and mandibular origins of the buccinator muscle. (Redrawn from Sicher, Harry, and DuBrul, E. Lloyd: Oral Anatomy, ed 6, St. Louis, 1975, The C. V. Mosby Co.)

QUESTION
28

Spread of abscesses of the upper and lower molar teeth to subcutaneous tissue occurs when roots of these teeth are long enough to extend above the maxillary attachment or below the mandibular attachment of the _____ muscle.

ANSWER

buccinator

When roots of the upper or lower molars extend beyond the attachments of the buccinator muscle, a periapical abscess *does/does not* (circle one) tend to invade the submucosa of the vestibule of the mouth.

Does not. (If you missed this question, reread Question 28. When roots of teeth extend beyond the attachments of the buccinator, an abscess extends anteriorly to subcutaneous tissue, rather than to the vestibule.)

ROUTE FROM UPPER CANINES TO THE VESTIBULE

ITEM 11

Figure 17–5 indicates the position of muscles in relationship to the maxillary canine teeth. Levator muscles arise high on the maxilla, separated by a fascial plane. Usually a periapical abscess of an upper canine tooth will perforate the lateral alveolar plate below the origin of the levator muscles and spread to submucosa of the vestibule. In some individuals, roots of maxillary canine teeth

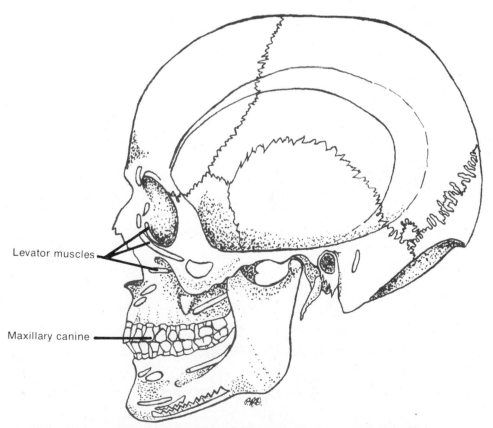

Levator muscles

Maxillary canine

Figure 17–5. Maxillary canine tooth in relationship to levator muscles. (Redrawn from Sicher, Harry, and DuBrul, E. Lloyd: Oral Anatomy, ed 6, St. Louis, 1975, The C. V. Mosby Co.

extend above the origin of some of the levator muscles. In these patients, an infection may spread to subcutaneous tissue rather than to the vestibule.

QUESTION
30

Usually the levator muscles *prevent/invite* (circle one) spread of abscesses of the maxillary canine teeth to subcutaneous tissue.

ANSWER

prevent

QUESTION
31

When abscesses of the maxillary canines are blocked by muscle attachments from surfacing cutaneously, they follow the line of least resistance through loose connective tissue to surface in the _____.

ANSWER

vestibule

ITEM 12   ROUTE FROM MANDIBULAR PREMOLARS

In Figure 17–6, examine the positions of the *depressor muscles* on the lower jaw. These muscles arise near the base of the mandible at a point below the apices of the lower premolar teeth. The depressor muscles, then, restrict an abscess from reaching subcutaneous tissue, but permit it to spread to the submucosa of the vestibule.

QUESTION
32

The depressor muscles arise near the base of the mandible *above/below* (circle one) the roots of the lower premolar teeth.

ANSWER

below

QUESTION
33

Abscesses of the mandibular premolar teeth usually spread to the *vestibule/subcutaneous tissue* (circle one).

ANSWER

vestibule

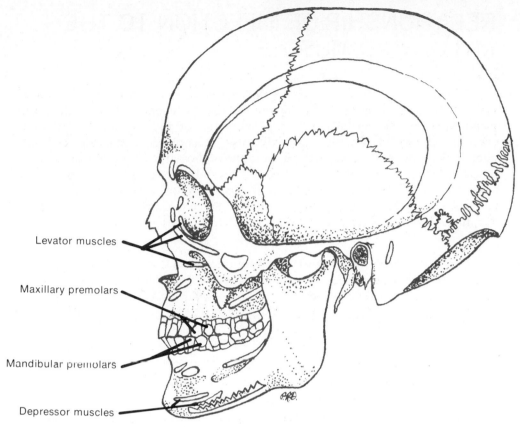

Figure 17–6. Relationships of maxillary and mandibular premolar teeth to muscle attachments. (Redrawn from Sicher, Harry and DuBrul, E. Lloyd: Oral Anatomy, ed 6, St. Louis, 1975, The C. V. Mosby Co.)

ROUTE FROM THE MAXILLARY PREMOLARS

ITEM 13

Look back to Figure 17–6 and notice how the *levator muscles* are situated above the maxillary premolar teeth and are attached superior to the apices of the roots. An abscess of the upper premolars is therefore barred from spreading cutaneously and almost always appears in the superior vestibule.

Facial muscles in the region of the upper premolars arise *above/below* (circle one) the roots of these teeth, so that abscesses spread to the *vestibule/subcutaneous tissue* (circle one).

QUESTION **34**

above . . . vestibule

ANSWER

ITEM 14   RELATIONSHIP OF INFECTION TO THE MYLOHYOID MUSCLE

The mylohyoid muscle constitutes the floor of the oral cavity, and the roots of most of the mandibular teeth are superior to the attachment of this muscle to the mandible. This arrangement confines infections of the mandibular incisors, canines, and premolars to the oral cavity. Also, this arrangement usually confines infections of the first and second molars to the oral cavity. If a periapical abscess of any of these teeth extends through the lingual alveolar plate, it remains in connective tissue between the mylohyoid muscle and the sublingual mucosa and appears as a swelling in the floor of the mouth. Since there is no definitive midline partition, this type of abscess usually spreads to the opposite side.

QUESTION 35   Infections of most of the lower teeth are restrained from spreading below the oral cavity by the _____ muscle because the roots of these teeth are _____ to this muscle.

ANSWER   mylohyoid . . . superior

QUESTION 36   Abscesses reach the connective tissue between the mylohyoid muscle and the sublingual mucosa by spreading through _____ _____ bone.

ANSWER   lingual alveolar

QUESTION 37   Abscesses of lower teeth spread through connective tissue to the opposite side because of the absence of a _____ _____.

ANSWER   midline partition

ITEM 15   RELATIONSHIP OF THE THIRD MOLAR TO THE MYLOHYOID MUSCLE

Because the mylohyoid muscle is somewhat shorter than the oral cavity, the roots of the third molar always extend behind and below the mylohyoid muscle. The same is true of the roots of the second molar in many individuals, but rarely is this the case with the first molar. Abscesses originating at the lingual side of the third molar almost invariably extend to the fascial plane lateral to the hyoglossus muscle, and frequently further down into the lower regions of the neck. Abscesses anterior to the third molar may spread to both submandibular and sublingual space.

Abscesses of the third molar may spread into lower regions of the neck because its roots extend _____ and _____ the mylohyoid floor of the oral cavity.

---

behind (posterior to) . . . below (inferior to)

Spaces into which abscesses anterior to the third molar may extend are the _____ space and the _____ space.

---

submandibular . . . sublingual (in either order)

Roots of the third molar extend to the fascia lateral to the hyoglossus muscle *rarely/often/invariably* (circle one); roots of the second molar, *rarely/often/invariably* (circle one); roots of the first molar, *rarely/often/invariably* (circle one).

---

invariably . . . often . . . rarely

PROPAGATION OF THROMBOPHLEBITIS OF THE FACE AND JAW

ITEM 16

Thrombophlebitis is the infection of a blood clot brought on by an inflammatory process in a vein. Infected clots, or *thrombi,* can break from their original sites and travel through the vascular channels to other vulnerable areas. A displaced clot, or *embolus,* in the face or jaws may move from its point of origin to extremely sensitive areas within the cranium. If the infection extends to the dural sinuses, a fatal meningitis could ensue. If it extends to the cavernous sinus, it is not only very inaccessible but it also endangers cranial nerves located in that sinus.

A thrombus is a blood _____ in a vein; an embolus is a displaced _____.

---

clot . . . thrombus (clot)

Potentially fatal meningitis may result if an infected embolus makes its way to the _____ sinuses, and cranial nerves may be endangered if it reaches the _____ sinus.

---

dural . . . cavernous

QUESTION
43

An additional complication of thrombophlebitis of the sinuses within the cranial cavity is posed by the _____ of the infection to treatment.

ANSWER

inaccessibility

ITEM 17   COMMUNICATION OF EXTRACRANIAL WITH INTRACRANIAL VENOUS NETWORKS

The channels through which an infected embolus from the face or jaws actually enters the dural sinuses are veins which connect extracranial with intracranial venous networks. There are three such routes: the emissary veins, the superior ophthalmic vein, and the inferior ophthalmic vein.

QUESTION
44

To reach the dural sinuses an embolus travels through veins which connect _____ venous networks with _____ venous networks.

ANSWER

extracranial . . . intracranial (in either order)

QUESTION
45

The veins through which extracranial veins communicate with intracranial veins are the _____ veins and the superior and inferior _____ veins.

ANSWER

emissary . . . ophthalmic

ITEM 18   PROPAGATION OF THROMBOPHLEBITIS THROUGH EMISSARY VEINS

Direct connections between extracranial and intracranial veins are established by the short *emissary veins* which pass through the cranium at certain regions. The most constant of the emissary veins are the *parietal vein* at the superior midline of the skull and the *mastoid vein* in the mastoid region. The parietal vein connects extracranial veins with the superior sagittal sinus; the mastoid vein connects extra-

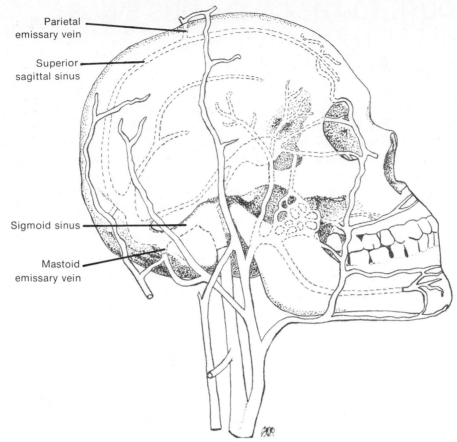

Parietal
emissary vein

Superior
sagittal sinus

Sigmoid sinus

Mastoid
emissary vein

Figure 17–7. Emissary veins and their connections with dural sinuses. (Redrawn from Sicher, Harry, and DuBrul, E. Lloyd: Oral Anatomy, ed 6, St. Louis, 1975, The C. V. Mosby Co.)

cranial veins with the sigmoid sinus. Look at Figure 17–7 and locate the parietal and mastoid emissary veins and the sinuses with which they communicate.

Typical regions where emissary veins pass through the cranium are the _____ region and the _____ region.

QUESTION
46

parietal . . . mastoid

ANSWER

The parietal emissary vein leads into the _____ sinus; the mastoid emissary vein, into the _____ sinus.

QUESTION
47

sagittal . . . sigmoid

ANSWER

ITEM 19   ROUTE TO THE CAVERNOUS SINUS THROUGH THE SUPERIOR OPHTHALMIC VEIN

Of utmost concern in cases of thrombophlebitis of the face and jaws is the possibility of propagation of an infected embolus to the cavernous sinus. This may occur either by way of the superior ophthalmic vein, or by way of the pterygoid plexus of veins. As you read this and the next item, trace these pathways on Figure 17–8.

In traveling the first route, an embolus will move through the facial vein and into the angular vein, from which it will pass into the superior ophthalmic vein. This vein empties directly into the cavernous sinus. In such a case, obvious orbital infection would precede complications in the cavernous sinus, providing an advance warning of sinus involvement. Fortunately, the availability of antibiotics for control of infections makes involvement of the cavernous sinus a rarity in modern dentistry.

The pterygoid plexus route of thrombophlebitis is discussed in Item 20.

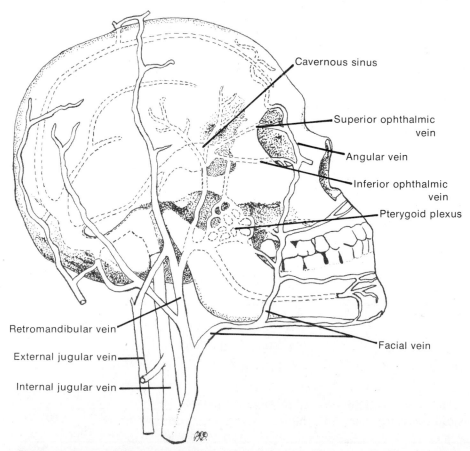

Figure 17–8. The veins of the face, showing the superior and inferior ophthalmic vein routes to the cavernous sinus. (Redrawn from Sicher, Harry, and DuBrul, E. Lloyd: Oral Anatomy, ed 6, St. Louis, 1975, The C. V. Mosby Co.)

One route by which an infected embolus travels from the face or jaws to the cavernous sinus is through the facial vein to the _____ vein, and then through the superior _____ vein into the cavernous sinus.

---

angular . . . ophthalmic

When an infected embolus travels through the superior ophthalmic vein route, an advance danger signal of impending cavernous sinus involvement is _____ infection.

---

orbital

ROUTE THROUGH THE PTERYGOID PLEXUS

ITEM 20

Again refer to Figure 17–8 to trace the second route by which an infected embolus may reach the cavernous sinus: through the *pterygoid plexus of veins*. The pterygoid plexus communicates with the cavernous sinus either by way of an emissary vein at the foramen ovale or through the inferior orbital fissure to the inferior ophthalmic vein.

Unlike cases of thrombophlebitis communicated through the superior ophthalmic vein, cases in which an infected embolus invades the cavernous sinus and the meninges by way of the pterygoid plexus display no advance signal of danger.

A second route of spread of infection to the cavernous sinus is through the _____ plexus of veins by way of the inferior _____ vein.

---

pterygoid . . . ophthalmic

VENOUS DRAINAGE OF THE UPPER JAW

ITEM 21

In Figure 17–8, notice the many cross channels connecting veins of the face with those of the jaws. Because of this extensive network of veins, there is no way to predetermine which direction an infected embolus will take. The drainage of upper and lower jaws through deep anastomoses provides potential routes for the passage of an infected thrombus.

Veins of the anterior upper jaw drain into the infraorbital veins. The infraorbital veins join the facial veins at the infraorbital foramen and join the pterygoid plexus in the infratemporal fossa. Veins of the posterior upper jaw drain into the superior alveolar veins, which, in turn, enter the pterygoid plexus of veins.

QUESTION
51

The extensive maze of interconnecting veins of the face and jaws makes it impossible to predict the _____ in which a displaced venous clot in the face will travel.

ANSWER

direction

QUESTION
52

At the infraorbital foramen, the infraorbital veins communicate with the _____ veins; in the infratemporal fossa, they communicate with the _____ _____.

ANSWER

facial . . . pterygoid plexus

QUESTION
53

The superior alveolar veins drain into the *pterygoid plexus/facial veins* (circle one).

ANSWER

pterygoid plexus

QUESTION
54

The superior alveolar veins receive drainage from the *anterior/posterior* (circle one) upper jaw; the infraorbital veins, from the *anterior/posterior* (circle one) upper jaw.

ANSWER

posterior . . . anterior

ITEM 22   VENOUS DRAINAGE OF THE LOWER JAW

Veins of the lower jaw drain primarily into the *inferior alveolar veins,* which extend to the pterygoid plexus. Additionally, they drain anteriorly through the mental foramen into the *inferior labial vein* and thus into the facial vein.

QUESTION
55

For the most part, drainage of the lower jaw is received into the inferior _____ veins which, in turn, connect with the pterygoid plexus; however, the lower jaw also drains anteriorly into the inferior _____ vein, which is continuous with the facial vein.

---

alveolar . . . labial   *ANSWER*

DAMAGING EFFECTS OF THROMBOPHLEBITIS IN THE CAVERNOUS SINUS

ITEM 23

    Besides the threat of meningitis posed by thrombophlebitis in any of the dural sinuses, the deleterious effect of this infection in the cavernous sinus is compounded by the danger of damage to several of the cranial nerves. Figure 17–9 shows the cranial nerves in the cavernous sinus. The abducens nerve runs through the cavernous sinus, while the oculomotor nerve, the trochlear nerve, and the ophthalmic and maxillary branches of the trigeminal nerve are located in the connective tissue of the sinus wall. Consequently the abducens nerve is the most immediately and severely affected by thrombophlebitis of the cavernous sinus.

    The abducens nerve supplies motor innervation to a single muscle, the *lateral rectus muscle* of the eye. Consequently, the first symptom of an infected cavernous sinus is paresis or paralysis of the lateral rectus muscle.

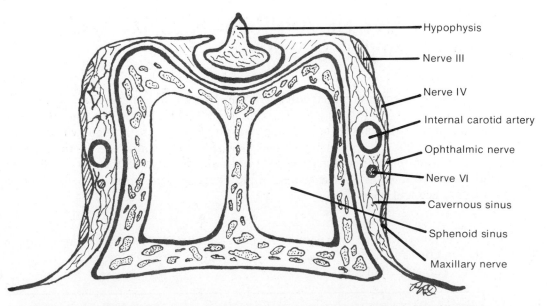

Figure 17–9. Coronal section through the cavernous sinus, showing locations of cranial nerves. (Redrawn from Woodburne: Essentials of Human Anatomy. 4th Ed. New York, Oxford University Press.)

QUESTION
56

Two possible harmful effects of thrombophlebitis of the cavernous sinus are _____ and damage to some of the _____ _____.

ANSWER

meningitis . . . cranial nerves

QUESTION
57

Malfunction of the lateral rectus muscle of the eye results from damage to the _____ nerve.

ANSWER

abducens

QUESTION
58

Place a check mark in the parentheses before each of the cranial nerves which is found in the cavernous sinus.

( ) olfactory   ( ) abducens
( ) optic   ( ) facial
( ) oculomotor   ( ) vestibulocochlear
( ) trochlear   ( ) glossopharyngeal
( ) ophthalmic branch, trigeminal   ( ) vagus
( ) maxillary branch, trigeminal   ( ) accessory
( ) mandibular branch, trigeminal   ( ) hypoglossal

ANSWER

You should have placed check marks before the following five nerves: oculomotor, trochlear, ophthalmic, maxillary, and abducens.

ITEM 24   SUMMARY OF APPROACHES TO THE CAVERNOUS SINUS

The dangerous potential outcome of an infected cavernous sinus is damage to the cranial nerves or meningitis. The vulnerability of the cavernous sinus to thrombophlebitis is apparent, considering the many avenues through which an infected embolus can approach this sinus. The cavernous sinus receives the superior and inferior ophthalmic veins from the front and connects with the pterygoid plexus of veins from below. These routes, in turn, receive veins from virtually all areas of the face and jaws.

QUESTION
59

Venous drainage from dental structures can enter the cavernous sinus through the superior and inferior _____ veins and through the _____ _____ of veins.

ANSWER

ophthalmic . . . pterygoid plexus

SUMMARY OF UNIT SEVENTEEN

Dental infections can spread from their origins to other parts of the body through continuity of tissues, through vascular channels, and through the lymphatic system.

SPREAD OF INFECTION THROUGH BONE

Some infections arise in the alveolar process, which is composed of an inner core of cancellous bone covered by a thin outer plate of compact bone on both lingual and buccal surfaces. When an abscess penetrates to the outside of the alveolar process, it tends to spread in the direction where the compact bone is thinnest. Contributing to the thinness of a given surface are the roots of the teeth which incline toward that surface.

An abscess of a central incisor may penetrate the nasal region. At the site of the upper lateral incisor, the plate is thinner on the labial side, so infections of these teeth will migrate to the labial vestibule. In the area of the mandibular incisor teeth, the labial plate of alveolar bone is also thin. In the area of the premolars and first molar, the thinner plate is on the buccal side; near the second and third molars, the lingual surface is the thinner. Running horizontally below the lower molars is the mandibular canal through which runs the inferior alveolar nerve. Involvement of the roots of the third mandibular molar with the canal can affect the entire inferior alveolar nerve, so that the source of pain cannot be pinpointed by the patient.

The maxillary sinus, located above the upper premolar and molar teeth, may become enlarged and invade the alveolar process, leaving the bony floor of this sinus separated from the roots of the molars only by a very thin osseous partition. In extreme cases, there may be no bony separation at all, leaving the mucosa of the sinus in direct contact with periodontal structures. In cases of enlarged maxillary sinuses, infections of an upper molar can penetrate the sinus.

RELATIONSHIP OF MUSCLE ATTACHMENT TO SPREAD OF INFECTION

Muscles of the face present a barrier to the spread of infection, but loose connective tissue offers the line of least resistance. Once an abscess has penetrated the outer layer of the alveolar process, it tends to spread to the skin if the roots of the teeth extend beyond the muscle attachment. The abscess moves toward the vestibule of the mouth if the roots of the teeth do not reach the origins of muscles which block its spread to subcutaneous tissue. Because of the particular positions of muscle attachments relative to roots of the teeth, almost all cutaneous abscesses originate in upper or lower molars or the lower incisors. Less frequently, they originate in lower or upper canines. On the other hand, abscesses of upper or lower premolars and upper incisors almost invariably move to the vestibule.

The mylohyoid muscle constitutes a floor for all but the posterior portion of the oral cavity. This muscular floor confines infections of most of the teeth to the area above the oral cavity. The roots of the third lower molar, however, always extend behind and below the mylohyoid floor, so that infections of this tooth are unimpeded from spreading to the submandibular and sublingual spaces and even into lower regions of the neck. In many individuals, the relationship of the roots of the second molar to the mylohyoid muscle is like that of the third molar.

PROPAGATION OF THROMBOPHLEBITIS

An inflammatory process in a vein may form clots, or thrombi, which may break away from their place of origin and migrate through blood vessels to other parts of the body. An infected embolus, or displaced thrombus, may originate in the face or jaws and travel through the veins of the face by way of a variety of routes to find its way to the dural sinuses, propagating its infection in these sensitive structures. Meningitis can ensue, and in cases of the cavernous sinus involvement, cranial nerves can be damaged.

The network of veins in the face is so extensive that it is impossible to predict which channels an embolus might pass through. The immediate approaches to the dural sinuses are through the short emissary veins, which connect extra-cranial with intracranial venous networks; through the ophthalmic veins; and through the pterygoid plexus of veins. Although the number of emissary veins is variable, two are fairly constant: the parietal emissary vein, which leads into the superior sagittal sinus, and the mastoid emissary vein, which leads into the sigmoid sinus. The most clinically significant routes of approach to intravenous networks are the ophthalmic veins, which empty directly into the cavernous sinus. One route by which an infected embolus moves is through the facial vein into the angular vein at the orbit, and on through the superior ophthalmic vein to the cavernous sinus. A second route is through the pterygoid plexus of veins to the inferior ophthalmic vein or to an emissary vein at the foramen ovale, and then into the cavernous sinus.

The drainage channels of the upper and lower jaws form potential routes of infection. The anterior upper jaw drains through the infraorbital veins into the facial vein, and also drains into the plexus. The posterior upper jaw drains into the superior alveolar veins, then into the pterygoid plexus. Principal drainage of the lower jaw is into the inferior alveolar veins, and on to the pterygoid plexus. Additional drainage of the lower jaw goes through the inferior labial vein and into the facial vein.

Thrombophlebitis of the cavernous sinus not only poses the threat of meningitis, but also endangers the cranial nerves located in this sinus: the oculomotor and trochlear nerves, the ophthalmic and maxillary divisions of the trigeminal nerve, and the abducens nerve. The abducens nerve, which supplies the lateral rectus muscle of the eye, is the most exposed cranial nerve in the cavernous sinus. Damage to this nerve will impair function of the lateral rectus muscle, an impairment signified by the drooping of the axis of the iris and pupil. The cavernous sinus is vulnerable to thrombophlebitic invasion from several approaches: from the superior and inferior ophthalmic veins anteriorly and from a connection to the pterygoid plexus of veins inferiorly.

QUESTION
60

Abscesses which penetrate outside the alveolar process tend to do so through the thinnest part of the outer *compact/cancellous* (circle one) bone.

ANSWER

compact

QUESTION
61

An abscess of a maxillary central incisor tooth tends to penetrate the _____ region; an abscess of a maxillary lateral incisor tends to penetrate the _____ vestibule.

nasal . . . labial

ANSWER

Abscesses of mandibular premolar and first molar teeth tend to penetrate the *buccal/lingual* (circle one) alveolar plate; abscesses of mandibular third molar teeth, the *buccal/lingual* (circle one) alveolar plate.

QUESTION
62

---

buccal . . . lingual

ANSWER

The maxillary sinus is situated above the upper _____ and _____ teeth, and descends closest to the apices of the _____ teeth.

QUESTION
63

---

premolar . . . molar . . . molar

ANSWER

The space within bone most vulnerable to infection from the second and third lower molars is the _____ canal; the space above the second and third molars is the _____ sinus.

QUESTION
64

---

mandibular . . . maxillary

ANSWER

When the roots of teeth do not extend beyond the confines of facial muscle attachments, periapical abscesses tend to spread to the _____; when the roots do extend beyond these muscle attachments, abscesses tend to spread to the _____.

QUESTION
65

---

vestibule . . . skin

ANSWER

Periapical abscesses which most frequently spread to the skin are those of the maxillary _____ teeth, the mandibular _____ teeth, and the mandibular _____ teeth.

QUESTION
66

---

molar . . . molar . . . incisor

ANSWER

Periapical abscesses which almost always spread to the vestibule of the mouth are those of maxillary and mandibular _____ teeth.

QUESTION
67

---

premolar

ANSWER

Periapical abscesses of the upper incisors frequently spread to the _____; those of the lower incisors, to the _____.

QUESTION
68

ANSWER

vestibule . . . skin

QUESTION
69

The muscle which prevents abscesses of most of the teeth from spreading below the floor of the mouth is the _____ muscle.

ANSWER

mylohyoid

QUESTION
70

Abscesses of the third, and often the second, molars are able to descend to the submandibular space and even lower because these roots extend beyond the confining barrier of the _____ muscle.

ANSWER

mylohyoid

QUESTION
71

Thrombophlebitis is a condition of infection of a _____ in the veins.

ANSWER

clot (thrombus)

QUESTION
72

A displaced thrombus from the face or jaws can reach various dural sinuses through the short _____ veins and can reach the cavernous sinus directly through the _____ veins or through the _____ _____ of veins.

ANSWER

emissary . . . ophthalmic . . . pterygoid plexus

QUESTION
73

Extracranial venous networks communicate with the superior sagittal sinus through the _____ emissary vein, and with the sigmoid sinus through the _____ emissary vein.

ANSWER

parietal . . . mastoid

QUESTION
74

When an embolus makes its way to the cavernous sinus via the superior ophthalmic route, it passes sequentially through the following veins: (1) the _____ vein, (2) the _____ vein, and (3) the superior ophthalmic vein.

ANSWER

facial . . . angular

QUESTION
75

When an embolus makes its way to the cavernous sinus via the facial route, it passes through the _____ _____ of veins en route to the inferior ophthalmic vein.

Damage to the abducens nerve by thrombophlebitis impairs function of   *QUESTION*
the _____ _____ muscle of the eye, causing the axis of the   **76**
_____ and _____ to droop.

Cranial nerves in the cavernous sinus which may be damaged by thrombo-   *QUESTION*
phlebitis include the following   **77**
  1. _____ nerve
  2. _____ nerve
  3. _____ division of the trigeminal nerve
  4. _____ division of the trigeminal nerve
  5. _____ nerve

---

  1. oculomotor
  2. trochlear
  3. ophthalmic
  4. maxillary
  5. abducens

Unit Eighteen □ ANATOMICAL TOPOGRAPHY FOR DENTAL INJECTIONS

ITEM 1   ANATOMICAL LANDMARKS AND INDIVIDUAL VARIATIONS

Successful injection of local anesthetics requires a knowledge of certain relatively invariable landmarks, usually bone, and the topography of the nerves which are the objects of oral anesthesia. Because there may be considerable size variation from one person to another, the relationship of the landmarks to each other is more significant than absolute measurements. Correlation of superficial landmarks in a given individual may be done visually or by means of palpation.

QUESTION 1

The exact site and direction of injection is determined by (circle one)
A. calculating average distances and angles of bony landmarks in the mouth.
B. correlating landmarks in the mouth to one another in each individual.

ANSWER

The correct answer is B.

QUESTION 2

Because of size variations among normal individuals, absolute measurements are less important than the _____ of structures to each other.

ANSWER

relationship

QUESTION 3

The palpating finger and the eye suffice for recognition of _____ landmarks.

ANSWER

superficial

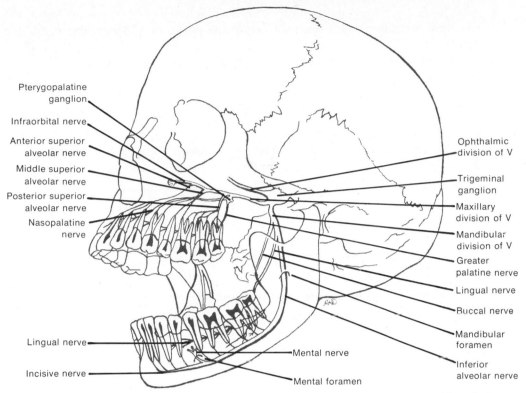

Figure 18–1. Nerves supplying the teeth and adjacent structures. (Redrawn from Manual of Local Anesthesia in General Dentistry. New York, Cook-Waite Laboratories, Inc.)

TARGET NERVES FOR ANESTHETIZING MAXILLARY TEETH

ITEM 2

Figure 18–1 shows the nerves which are the targets for anesthesia of various teeth and adjacent structures. Nerves supplying the maxillary teeth are branches of the maxillary division of the trigeminal nerve. These branches include (1) the posterior superior alveolar nerve, supplying the third and second molar teeth and the distal and palatal roots of the first molar; (2) the middle superior alveolar nerve, supplying the first and second premolar teeth and the mesial root of the first molar, and (3) the anterior superior alveolar nerve, which innervates the canine teeth and the lateral and central incisors.

Note that two nerves are targets for anesthetizing the first maxillary molar, because the distal and palatal roots of this tooth are innervated by the posterior superior alveolar nerve, and the mesial root is supplied by the middle superior alveolar nerve.

The second and third maxillary molars and part of the first maxillary molar are innervated by the _____ _____ _____ nerve.

QUESTION
4

───────────────────────────────

posterior superior alveolar

ANSWER

QUESTION
5

The first maxillary molar tooth is innervated by two different branches of the maxillary division of the trigeminal nerve: the posterior superior alveolar nerve supplies the _____ and _____ roots of the first maxillary molar; the middle superior alveolar nerve, the _____ root.

ANSWER

distal . . . palatal . . . mesial

QUESTION
6

Maxillary premolar teeth are innervated by the _____ _____ _____ nerve.

ANSWER

middle superior alveolar

QUESTION
7

The anterior superior alveolar nerve supplies the _____ teeth and the _____ teeth.

ANSWER

incisor . . . canine

ITEM 3   TARGET NERVES FOR ANESTHETIZING MANDIBULAR TEETH

Examine Figure 18–1 again, and notice the innervation of the mandibular teeth. Among other branches, the mandibular division of the trigeminal nerve gives off the inferior alveolar nerve, which extends through the mandibular canal giving off small dental branches which supply the lower molar and premolar teeth. At the mental foramen, the inferior alveolar nerve bifurcates to form the incisive nerve, which continues forward to supply the lower canine and incisor teeth, and the mental nerve, which passes outward through the mental foramen to supply the chin and lower lip.

QUESTION
8

Nerve supply to the lower molar and premolar teeth is derived from small nerves which branch off the _____ _____ nerve.

ANSWER

inferior alveolar

QUESTION
9

The continuation of the inferior alveolar nerve mesial to the mental foramen is the _____ nerve, which supplies the mandibular _____ and _____ teeth.

ANSWER

incisive . . . canine . . . incisor

The mental nerve branches off the inferior alveolar nerve and passes outward through the mental foramen to supply the _____ and lower _____.

chin . . . lip

TARGET NERVES FOR ANESTHETIZING TISSUES ADJACENT TO MAXILLARY TEETH

ITEM
4

Soft tissue of the palate is supplied by two nerves which leave the maxillary nerve at the pterygopalatine ganglion: the nasopalatine nerve, which innervates the anterior third of the palatal mucoperiosteum, and the greater palatine nerve, which innervates the posterior two thirds. Terminal branches of the two nerves overlap in the region of the canine teeth. Extractions or surgical procedures involving the maxillary teeth require anesthetizing of either the nasopalatine or the greater palatine nerve, depending on the region. Examine Figure 18–1 again and notice the origin and course of the nasopalatine and greater palatine nerves.

For dental surgery, in addition to anesthetizing nerves supplying the teeth, it is also necessary to anesthetize the _____ adjacent to the teeth.

mucoperiosteum (soft tissue)

Nerves supplying the mucoperiosteum of the palate are the _____ nerve and the greater _____ nerve, both of which are given off the maxillary division of the trigeminal nerve at the _____ ganglion.

nasopalatine . . . palatine . . . pterygopalatine

Sensory innervation of the posterior two thirds of the palate is supplied by the _____ _____ nerve; innervation of the anterior third of the palate, by the _____ nerve, with some overlapping of nerve supply in the region of the _____ teeth.

greater palatine . . . nasopalatine . . . canine

ITEM 5

TARGET NERVES FOR ANESTHETIZING TISSUES ADJACENT TO MANDIBULAR TEETH

Look back to Figure 18–1 and find the locations of two branches of the mandibular division of the trigeminal nerve which supply tissue adjacent to mandibular teeth: the buccal nerve and the lingual nerve. A separate buccal injection will anesthetize the buccal tissues in the mandibular molar region. A lingual injection will anesthetize the soft tissues on the lingual surface of the mandible.

QUESTION
14

Besides supplying the anterior two thirds of the tongue, the _____ nerve also supplies lingual gingiva.

ANSWER

lingual

QUESTION
15

The buccal nerve supplies soft tissues on the buccal surface of mandibular _____ teeth.

ANSWER

molar

ITEM 6

TYPES OF INJECTION: PLEXUS ANESTHESIA

The target of injections may be nerve endings in the region of particular teeth or the main trunk of an alveolar nerve. The network of nerves at the apices of the teeth is called the *alveolar* (or *dental*) *plexus*. Blocking of conduction at any nerve plexus site is variously termed *plexus anesthesia, supraperiosteal injection,* or *infiltration*. This type of oral anesthesia is confined to a small area of the jaw and to a few teeth or even a single tooth. The anesthetic solution deposited on the periosteum spreads through the periosteum and bony plate by diffusion, penetrating nerve fibers which supply the periodontal membrane and those which enter the apices.

While alveolar bone of the maxilla is thin enough for plexus anesthesia, the density of the bone of the mandible makes this method impractical for all mandibular teeth except the lower incisors.

QUESTION
16

Plexus anesthesia is more effective in the _____ region, because of the _____ of bone in that area.

maxillary . . . thinness   *ANSWER*

With plexus anesthesia, the solution reaches nerve fibers to teeth and peri-   *QUESTION*
odontal membranes by means of _____.   **17**

---

diffusion   *ANSWER*

BLOCK INJECTIONS   ITEM 7

With a *block injection,* the anesthetic solution is introduced at a point where it blocks conduction through a nerve trunk. Block anesthesia has the advantage of effecting a rapid analgesia to an extensive area. The commonest block injections are: (1) mandibular injection for a complete block of the inferior alveolar nerve and anesthesia of all mandibular teeth on one side; (2) mental injection for anesthesia of the incisor, canine, and premolar mandibular teeth; (3) trunk injection for blocking the posterior superior alveolar nerve supply to the second and third maxillary molars and two roots of the first molar; and (4) infraorbital injection to block the area supplied by the anterior and middle superior alveolar nerves, namely, the maxillary incisors, canines, premolars, and the mesial root of the first molar.

Two advantages of block injections are the _____ area anesthetized   *QUESTION*
and the _____ with which anesthesia develops.   **18**

---

extensive . . . speed   *ANSWER*

An infraorbital injection blocks conduction from the maxillary area supplied   *QUESTION*
by the _____ and the _____ superior alveolar nerves.   **19**

---

anterior . . . middle   *ANSWER*

The teeth blocked by a trunk injection of the posterior superior alveolar nerve   *QUESTION*
include the _____ and _____ maxillary molars and two roots   **20**
of the _____ maxillary molar.

---

second . . . third . . . first   *ANSWER*

A mandibular injection blocks the entire _____ _____ nerve, anesthetizing all the mandibular teeth on one side.

inferior alveolar

A mental injection blocks the _____, _____, and _____ mandibular teeth.

incisor . . . canine . . . premolar

ITEM 8   PLEXUS ANESTHESIA OF THE MAXILLARY TEETH

Plexus anesthesia of the maxillary teeth can be effected by injecting into the vestibule near the mucogingival junction. Alveolar bone in this region is relatively thin and porous, except for the thicker column at the zygomatic process of the maxilla in the area of the first molar tooth. The injection should be at the apical third of the root length rather than at or above the apices. One reason for this site of injection is that the higher the injection, the greater the thickness of bone encountered. The second reason favoring injection somewhat below the apices is that the connective tissue here is more dense and less vascular and therefore more apt to keep the anesthetic solution localized. Above the mucogingival junction, the loose and vascular connective tissue tends to permit the spread of the solution, with consequent dilution and rapid removal.

For plexus anesthesia of the maxillary teeth, the injection should be somewhat below the apices because at a higher level the bone is _____ and the connective tissue is _____.

thicker . . . looser

The disadvantage of injecting into very loose and vascular connective tissue is that the solution is _____ and rapidly _____.

diluted . . . removed

PLEXUS ANESTHESIA OF THE POSTERIOR SUPERIOR ALVEOLAR NERVE

ITEM 9

Figure 18–2 shows the site of injection for plexus anesthesia of the posterior superior alveolar nerve, with the needle introduced in the region of the second maxillary molar. This injection will block conduction from the third and second maxillary molars as well as from the distal and palatal roots of the first molar. An injection near the apex of the second premolar will anesthetize the mesial root of the first molar, completing anesthesia of that tooth. A posterior palatine injection, described in Items 17 and 18, is needed for extraction or periodontal surgery, in order to anesthetize the mucoperiosteum of the palate.

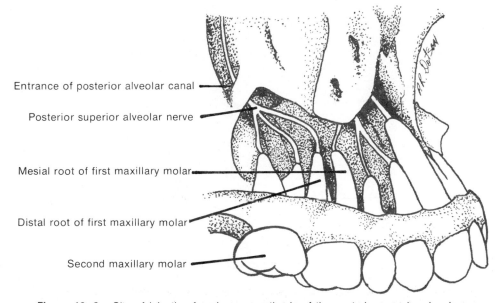

Entrance of posterior alveolar canal

Posterior superior alveolar nerve

Mesial root of first maxillary molar

Distal root of first maxillary molar

Second maxillary molar

Figure 18–2. Site of injection for plexus anesthesia of the posterior superior alveolar nerve. (Redrawn from Manual of Local Anesthesia in General Dentistry. New York, Cook-Waite Laboratories, Inc.)

Anesthesia of the posterior superior alveolar nerve blocks conduction from the _____ and _____ maxillary molars and two roots of the _____ maxillary molar.

QUESTION 25

---

third . . . second . . . first

ANSWER

For extraction of a maxillary molar tooth it is necessary to anesthetize the palatal mucoperiosteum by blocking conduction of the _____ _____ nerve.

QUESTION 26

---

greater palatine

ANSWER

ITEM 10   PLEXUS ANESTHESIA OF THE MIDDLE SUPERIOR ALVEOLAR NERVE

Figure 18–3 shows the site of injection for plexus anesthesia of the middle superior alveolar nerve. Anesthesia of this nerve blocks conduction from both maxillary premolars and the mesial root of the first molar. A partial posterior palatine injection is also necessary to anesthetize palatine mucoperiosteum for extraction or periodontal surgery.

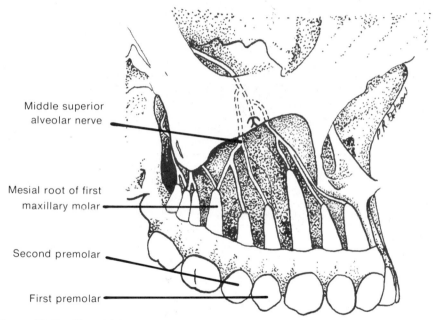

Figure 18–3. Site of injection for plexus anesthesia of the middle superior alveolar nerve. (Redrawn from Manual of Local Anesthesia in General Dentistry. New York, Cook-Waite Laboratories, Inc.)

QUESTION 27

Partial blocking of conduction of the greater palatine nerve is needed in order to anesthetize the _____ _____ for extraction involving maxillary premolar teeth.

ANSWER   palatine mucoperiosteum

QUESTION 28

Plexus anesthesia of the maxillary premolars requires blocking conduction of the _____ superior alveolar nerve.

ANSWER   middle

QUESTION
29

Plexus anesthesia of the middle superior alveolar nerve blocks conduction from the mesial root of the maxillary _____ _____ tooth.

first molar

ANSWER

PLEXUS ANESTHESIA OF THE ANTERIOR SUPERIOR ALVEOLAR NERVE

**ITEM
11**

Figure 18–4 shows the site of injection for plexus anesthesia of the anterior superior alveolar nerve, with the needle introduced at the mucolabial fold, mesial to the maxillary canine tooth. Injections over the roots of the canine teeth on both sides will anesthetize overlapping fibers from the anterior superior alveolar nerve of the opposite side, as well as blocking conduction from the maxillary canine and incisor teeth on both sides. Extraction or periodontal surgery requires additional anesthesia of the nasopalatine nerve at the incisive canal.

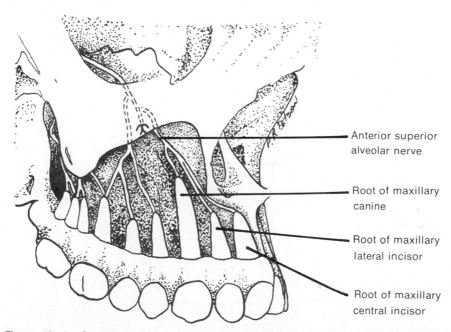

Anterior superior
alveolar nerve

Root of maxillary
canine

Root of maxillary
lateral incisor

Root of maxillary
central incisor

Figure 18–4. Site of injection for plexus anesthesia of the anterior superior alveolar nerve. (Redrawn from Manual of Local Anesthesia in General Dentistry. New York, Cook-Waite Laboratories, Inc.)

QUESTION
30

Plexus anesthesia of the anterior superior alveolar nerve requires injections on both sides because nerve fibers from each side _____ with fibers from the other side.

ANSWER   overlap (intermingle)

QUESTION   Plexus anesthesia of the anterior superior alveolar nerve blocks conduction
31   from the maxillary _____ and _____ teeth.

ANSWER   canine . . . incisor (in either order)

ITEM 12   PLEXUS ANESTHESIA OF MANDIBULAR INCISORS

Although bone density of the mandible precludes plexus anesthesia of most of the mandibular teeth, the bone in the area of the lower central and lateral incisors is porous enough to permit infiltration of the nerve endings of these teeth. Figure 18–5 shows the site of injection.

The incisive nerve, the anterior continuation of the inferior alveolar nerve, is found at approximately the level of the mental fossa. Injection into the vestibular mucosa anterior to the mandible and below the apices of the teeth is effective in blocking the plexus. For extraction, it is necessary to inject the lingual nerve to anesthetize the soft tissue on the lingual surface of the mandible. This procedure is described in Items 25 and 26.

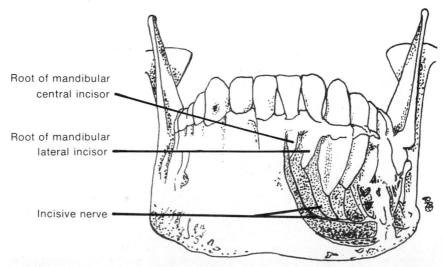

Root of mandibular central incisor

Root of mandibular lateral incisor

Incisive nerve

Figure 18–5. Site of injection for plexus anesthesia of mandibular incisor teeth. (Redrawn from Manual of Local Anesthesia in General Dentistry. New York, Cook-Waite Laboratories, Inc.)

QUESTION   For most mandibular teeth, plexus anesthesia is (circle one)
32   A. practical because of the porosity of the bone of the mandible.
                 B. impractical because of the density of the bone of the mandible.

The correct answer is B. Only in the area of the mandibular incisor teeth is the bone porous and thin enough to allow effective plexus anesthesia.

ANSWER

The mandibular incisor teeth are supplied by the _____ nerve, which is the forward continuation of the _____ _____ nerve.

QUESTION
33

incisive . . . inferior alveolar

ANSWER

The point of injection for plexus anesthesia of the mandibular incisors is the _____ _____ anterior to the _____.

QUESTION
34

vestibular mucosa . . . mandible

ANSWER

In addition to plexus anesthesia, extraction also requires a _____ injection to anesthetize the soft tissue on the lingual surface of the mandible.

QUESTION
35

lingual

ANSWER

TRUNK INJECTION OF THE POSTERIOR SUPERIOR ALVEOLAR NERVE   ITEM 13

Besides using the plexus anesthesia described in the preceding items, it is sometimes necessary to anesthetize larger areas by block injections of the main trunk of an alveolar nerve or the entire maxillary or mandibular nerve.

The posterior superior alveolar nerve may be blocked before it enters the posterior alveolar canal on the posterior aspect of the maxilla. The needle is introduced opposite the second maxillary molar, and then follows an oblique route, since the injection site cannot be reached from below. Look back to Figure 18–2 and notice where the posterior superior alveolar nerve enters the posterior alveolar canal.

A trunk injection of the posterior superior alveolar nerve is approached from the _____ opposite the _____ maxillary molar tooth.

QUESTION
36

vestibule . . . second

ANSWER

QUESTION
37
The posterior superior alveolar nerve is blocked with a trunk injection before the nerve enters the _____ _____ canal.

ANSWER
posterior alveolar

ITEM 14   CONTROL OF BLEEDING WITH A POSTERIOR SUPERIOR ALVEOLAR BLOCK

With a posterior superior alveolar block, the needle is routed along the lateral surface of the maxilla, in contact with bone, to avoid rupture of a vessel in the pterygoid plexus of veins. Although routing close to bone usually avoids the pterygoid venous plexus, the posterior superior alveolar artery occasionally ruptures near the periosteum. If this happens, a hematoma forms and spreads to the loose connective tissue of the cheek. Bleeding is controlled by pressing the cheek against bone at the anterior border of the masseter muscle at a level just below the zygomatic arch.

QUESTION
38
The pterygoid plexus of veins is avoided in a posterior superior alveolar nerve block by routing the needle against _____.

ANSWER
bone

QUESTION
39
If it occurs with a posterior superior alveolar nerve block, bleeding is controlled by pressure against the bone just below the _____ arch at the anterior border of the _____ muscle.

ANSWER
zygomatic . . . masseter

ITEM 15   INFRAORBITAL TRUNK INJECTION

The anterior and middle superior alveolar nerves branch from the *infraorbital nerve* within the infraorbital canal, as shown by the dotted lines in Figure 18–6. Effective infraorbital anesthesia blocks conduction from all the maxillary teeth supplied by the middle and anterior superior alveolar nerves: the mesial root of the first molar, the second and first premolars, the canines, and the lateral and

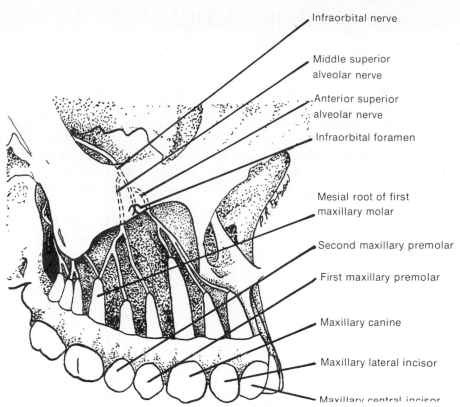

Infraorbital nerve

Middle superior
alveolar nerve

Anterior superior
alveolar nerve

Infraorbital foramen

Mesial root of first
maxillary molar

Second maxillary premolar

First maxillary premolar

Maxillary canine

Maxillary lateral incisor

Maxillary central incisor

Figure 18–6. Site of injection for infraorbital block injection. Intraosseous portions of nerves indicated by broken lines. (Modified from Manual of Local Anesthesia in General Dentistry. New York, Cook-Waite Laboratories, Inc.)

central incisors. An unavoidable but harmless extension of anesthesia occurs in the upper lip, anterior cheek, nose, and lower eyelid.

Accessibility to the root of the infraorbital nerve is through the infraorbital foramen, seen in Figure 18–6. This foramen can be palpated as a rough spot in most individuals. The infraorbital foramen is usually on a vertical plane with the pupil, when the eye is fixed straight ahead. The height of the injection is measured to avoid penetrating the orbit.

The anterior superior alveolar nerve supplies the maxillary _____ and _____ teeth; the middle superior alveolar nerve supplies the first and second _____ teeth and the mesial root of the first _____ tooth.

QUESTION
40

incisor . . . canine . . . premolar . . . molar

ANSWER

The trunk of the infraorbital nerve can be reached through the _____ foramen, but care must be taken to prevent the needle from entering the _____.

QUESTION
41

infraorbital . . . orbit

ANSWER

ITEM 16   NASOPALATINE INJECTION

Besides blocking conduction from the anterior maxillary teeth, an infraorbital injection anesthetizes the labial mucosa and gingiva adjacent to the maxillary incisor and canine teeth. If any sensitivity remains on the lingual side, the mucosa and gingiva of this area can be anesthetized by a *nasopalatine block*. The nasopalatine block is also preferred in some cases where infections of the anterior maxillary teeth are involved. The rationale for the nasopalatine block in this instance is avoidance of the infraorbital area because of its susceptibility to spreading infection to the cavernous sinus.

The *nasopalatine nerve* emerges onto the hard palate through the incisive canal just posterior to the maxillary central incisors, as shown in Figure 18–7. With infiltration of the nasopalatine nerve, the anesthetic is deposited at the incisive canal.

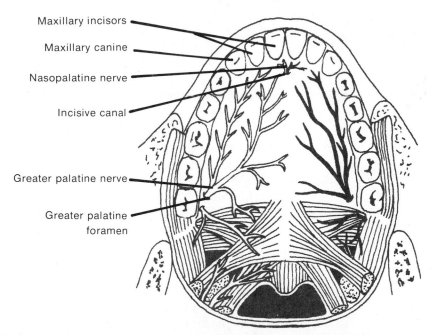

Maxillary incisors

Maxillary canine

Nasopalatine nerve

Incisive canal

Greater palatine nerve

Greater palatine foramen

Figure 18–7. Sites of nasopalatine and greater palatine injections. (Modified from Leeson and Leeson: Human Structure. Philadelphia, W. B. Saunders Co.)

QUESTION 42

In the area of the maxillary incisor and canine teeth, the anterior superior alveolar nerve supplies mucosa and gingiva on the _____ side; the nasopalatine nerve supplies mucosa and gingiva on the _____ side.

ANSWER   labial . . . lingual

GREATER PALATINE NERVE BLOCK   ITEM 17

The *greater palatine nerve* innervates the soft tissues of the posterior two thirds of the palate. A palatine nerve block is required for extraction of maxillary teeth. Look at Figure 18–7 and observe the greater palatine nerve emerging through the greater palatine foramen, then extending forward in a groove medial to the alveolar process. Notice also in Figure 18–7 that the terminal branches of the greater palatine nerve overlap those of the nasopalatine nerve in the region of the maxillary canine teeth. The lingual gingiva of the hard palate is supplied by the greater palatine nerve up to the region of the maxillary canines.

The middle and posterior regions of the lingual gingiva and mucosa of the hard palate are supplied by the _____ _____ nerve; the anterior region is supplied by the _____ nerve.

QUESTION 43

---

greater palatine . . . nasopalatine

ANSWER

The greater palatine nerve lies in a groove between the hard palate and the _____ process.

QUESTION 44

---

alveolar

ANSWER

SITE OF INJECTION FOR PALATINE NERVE BLOCK   ITEM 18

The greater palatine nerve is blocked close to the greater palatine foramen. This foramen lies at the suture between the palatine part of the maxilla and the horizontal plate of the palatine bone, just medial to the alveolar process adjacent to the last maxillary molar. In the region of the foramen, the greater palatine nerve is embedded in a limited amount of loose connective tissue. Anterior or medial to this area, however, the connective tissue is so dense and so closely adherent to bone that effective diffusion cannot take place. Therefore, a rapid, forced injection into this dense connective tissue causes undue postoperative pain and even necrosis of tissue.

The location of the greater palatine foramen is just medial to the alveolar process between the _____ part of the maxilla and the horizontal plate of the _____ bone.

QUESTION 45

ANSWER

palatine . . . palatine

QUESTION
46

The greater palatine foramen lies at the level of the maxillary _____ _____ tooth.

ANSWER

third molar

QUESTION
47

Injection of fluid into dense connective tissue is to be avoided because such injection results in ineffective _____, postoperative _____, and _____ of tissue.

ANSWER

diffusion . . . pain . . . necrosis

ITEM 19   MAXILLARY NERVE BLOCK

A major operation on the upper jaw requires blocking of all branches of the maxillary nerve. For this block, fluid can be deposited in the pterygopalatine fossa where the main trunk of the maxillary nerve divides into its terminal branches. The preferred approach to the pterygopalatine fossa is from the cheek through the ptery-gopalatine fissure. With this buccal approach, the needle is routed anterior to the coronoid process along the maxillary tuberosity to the lateral pterygoid plate, and then redirected into the fossa. The advantage of first contacting the lateral ptery-goid plate is that it insures entry at a level low enough to avoid puncturing the max-illary artery. Care is necessary also to avoid puncturing the superior alveolar artery at the maxillary tuberosity and the descending palatine artery in the lower ptery-gopalatine fossa.

QUESTION
48

The best route of entry to reach the main trunk of the maxillary nerve in the pterygopalatine fossa is a buccal approach through the _____ fissure.

ANSWER

pterygopalatine

QUESTION
49

The reason for a low level of entry into the pterygopalatine fossa is to avoid puncturing the _____ _____.

ANSWER

maxillary artery

INFERIOR ALVEOLAR NERVE BLOCK

When it is desirable to anesthetize all the mandibular teeth, the inferior alveolar nerve may be blocked before it enters the bony canal of the mandible. Entry is made into the pterygomandibular space superior to the entrance of the nerve into the mandibular foramen. As shown in Figure 18–8, the pterygomandibular space lies between the ramus of the mandible laterally and the medial pterygoid muscle medially.

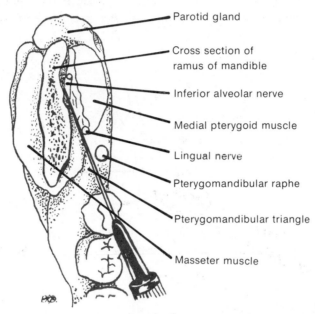

Figure 18–8. Horizontal section of the ramus of the mandible, showing the pterygomandibular space. (Redrawn from Manual of Local Anesthesia in General Dentistry. New York, Cook-Waite Laboratories, Inc.)

For an inferior alveolar nerve block, the needle enters the _____ space to reach the _____ foramen.

---

pterygomandibular . . . mandibular

The lateral boundary of the pterygomandibular space is the _____ of the mandible; the medial boundary is the _____ _____ muscle.

---

ramus . . . medial pterygoid

ITEM 21
SITE OF INJECTION FOR INFERIOR ALVEOLAR NERVE BLOCK

With an inferior alveolar nerve block, injection is made as close to the mandibular foramen as possible. The needle is inserted medial and posterior to the deep tendon of the temporalis muscle and lateral to the lateral pterygoid muscle. The deep tendon of the temporalis can be palpated as it inserts on the anterior border of the mandibular ramus. Once bone is contacted behind the tendon, the syringe is rotated anteriorly so that the needle glides against bone until the mandibular foramen is reached. The mandibular foramen is bounded by bone laterally and by the sphenomandibular ligament medially. Notice in Figure 18–9 that the top of the mandibular foramen is on a plane level with the occlusal surface of the lower molars.

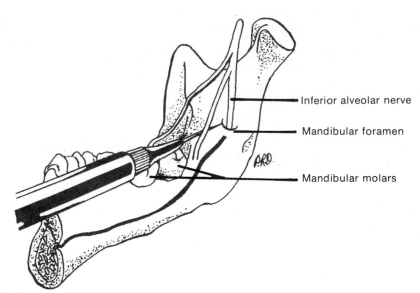

Figure 18–9.   Inner surface of the ramus, right mandible, showing the inferior alveolar nerve. (Redrawn from Manual of Local Anesthesia in General Dentistry. New York, Cook-Waite Laboratories, Inc.)

QUESTION
52

With an inferior alveolar nerve block, solution is deposited as close as possible to the _____ foramen.

ANSWER

mandibular

QUESTION
53

The point of insertion of the needle for an inferior alveolar nerve block is medial and posterior to the deep tendon of the _____ muscle.

ANSWER

temporalis

QUESTION
54

The height of the mandibular foramen reaches the level of the occlusal surface of the lower _____ teeth.

ANSWER

molar

QUESTION
55

The lateral boundary of the mandibular foramen is the bone of the _____ of the mandible; the medial boundary is the _____ ligament.

ANSWER

ramus . . . sphenomandibular

CAUTIONS CONCERNING INFERIOR ALVEOLAR NERVE BLOCKS

**ITEM
22**

A constant danger with an inferior alveolar nerve block is the possibility of entering a blood vessel. Injection of anesthetic drugs into the venous circulation has a depressant effect on cardiac muscle and is therefore to be avoided absolutely. The course of the inferior alveolar artery and veins is closer to bone than the course of the inferior alveolar nerve. Therefore, when the bone is used as a landmark, there is an ever present possibility of puncturing a vessel. For this reason, it is imperative that the operator aspirate to determine whether blood will enter the syringe in a particular location. If so, the needle must be withdrawn and relocated before the injection is made.

An occasional occurrence with an inferior alveolar nerve block is simultaneous blockage of the sensory auriculotemporal nerve and the motor branches of the facial nerve. When this happens, the patient loses voluntary control of the muscles of facial expression until the anesthetic solution is absorbed.

QUESTION
56

The possibility of injecting anesthetic into a blood vessel at the region of the mandibular foramen is present because of the proximity of blood vessels to _____.

ANSWER

bone

QUESTION
57

Once the needle is in position for an injection it is imperative to _____ in order to determine whether the needle is in a blood vessel.

ANSWER

aspirate

QUESTION
58

Occasionally, the _____ and _____ nerves are blocked along with the inferior alveolar nerve.

ANSWER

auriculotemporal . . . facial (in either order)

QUESTION
59

Blockage of the facial nerves causes temporary paralysis of the muscles of _____ _____ lasting until the anesthetic wears off.

ANSWER

facial expression

ITEM 23   MENTAL NERVE BLOCK

Rarely, it is desirable to anesthetize the anterior mandibular teeth, but an inferior alveolar block is not possible due to injury. The region from premolar to premolar can be blocked effectively by injecting into the mental canal, as illustrated in Figure 18–10.

The needle should be directed posteriorly three fourths of an inch below the crest of the gingiva between the two premolar teeth. If teeth are missing and alveolar bone has been resorbed, the mental foramen is located at a higher plane than usual, and can sometimes be palpated.

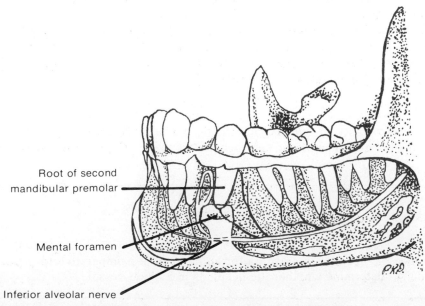

Root of second
mandibular premolar

Mental foramen

Inferior alveolar nerve

Figure 18–10. Location of the mental foramen. (Redrawn from Manual of Local Anesthesia in General Dentistry. New York, Cook-Waite Laboratories, Inc.)

Injection into the mental canal can effectively anesthetize anterior teeth from _____ tooth to _____ tooth.

premolar . . . premolar

The location of the mental foramen is below and between the two mandibular _____ teeth.

premolar

When alveolar bone has been resorbed, the mental foramen will be found at a somewhat _____ plane than usual in reference to the crest of the gingiva.

higher

SITE OF INJECTION FOR MENTAL NERVE BLOCK

ITEM 24

Once the buccal mucosa is entered and the location of the mental foramen is determined, the needle for a mental nerve block is directed toward the contour of the mental canal. Slow injection of a few drops of fluid as the needle is pushed forward helps prevent injury to the nerve, since the projected solution helps to push the nerve out of the way of the needle.

To block the mental nerve, the needle is inserted into the _____ canal and advanced to follow the contour of the _____.

mental . . . canal

With a mental injection, slowly depositing a small amount of fluid as the needle is advanced prevents _____ to the nerve.

injury

ITEM 25   LINGUAL NERVE INJECTION

The lingual nerve diverges from the inferior alveolar nerve in the infratemporal fossa, descends through the pterygomandibular space anterior and slightly medial to the inferior alveolar nerve, then turns anteriorly and medially in the floor of the mouth. The lingual nerve extends forward medial to the alveolar process to supply all the lingual gingiva and mucous membranes of the floor of the mouth. This nerve must be blocked in all operative procedures on the lower jaw not strictly confined to the teeth.

QUESTION
65

The position of the lingual nerve relative to the inferior alveolar nerve is _____ and _____.

ANSWER

anterior . . . medial

QUESTION
66

The lingual nerve supplies lingual _____ and the _____ membranes of the floor of the mouth.

ANSWER

gingiva . . . mucous

ITEM 26   SITE OF LINGUAL NERVE INJECTION

At the level of the mandibular foramen, the lingual nerve lies medial and anterior to the inferior alveolar nerve, as can be seen in Figure 18–11. In the usual approach to the lingual nerve, the needle is directed across the opposite second premolar into the retromolar area. Injection of a small amount of solution as the needle touches bone suffices to anesthetize the lingual nerve.

QUESTION
67

The position of the lingual nerve with reference to the inferior alveolar nerve is _____ and _____ to the inferior alveolar nerve.

ANSWER

anterior . . . medial (in either order)

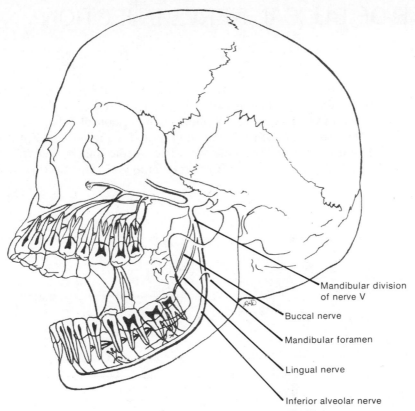

Mandibular division
of nerve V

Buccal nerve

Mandibular foramen

Lingual nerve

Inferior alveolar nerve

Figure 18–11. Site of injection for lingual nerve block. (Redrawn from Manual of Local Anesthesia in General Dentistry. New York, Cook-Waite Laboratories, Inc.)

BUCCAL NERVE INJECTION   ITEM 27

Part of the innervation of the soft tissues on the buccal aspect of the mandibular molar teeth is received from the *buccal branch* of the mandibular nerve. This buccal branch, a part of the trigeminal nerve, is not to be confused with the buccal branch of the facial nerve, which is motor to muscles of this area. Anesthetizing adjacent soft tissues is required for extraction of mandibular molars. The structures anesthetized with a buccal injection include the mucous membrane of the cheek, the mandibular gingiva, and the skin of the cheek.

The buccal nerve which is sensory to tissues adjacent to the mandibular molars is a branch of the _____ division of the _____ nerve.

QUESTION
68

---

mandibular . . . trigeminal

ANSWER

The buccal nerve innervates _____ _____ of the cheek, _____ of the cheek, and mandibular _____.

QUESTION
69

---

mucous membrane . . . skin . . . gingiva

ANSWER

ITEM 28   SITE OF BUCCAL NERVE INJECTION

The location of the buccal branch of the mandibular nerve in relation to the lingual and inferior alveolar nerves can be seen in Figure 18–12. Notice the area to which the buccal nerve distributes. The region of soft tissues on the buccal aspect anesthetized with this injection includes the area adjacent to the first, second, and third mandibular molars. The needle can be inserted at the base of the ascending ramus; however, various techniques of injection may be used.

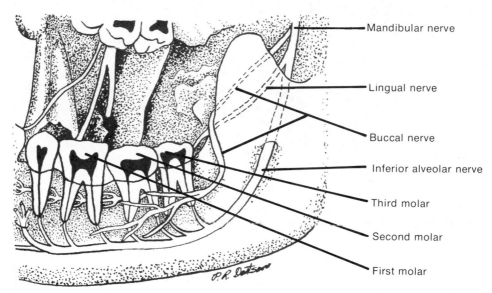

Figure 18–12.   Location of the buccal branch of the mandibular nerve. (Redrawn from Manual of Local Anesthesia in General Dentistry. New York, Cook-Waite Laboratories, Inc.)

QUESTION
70

A common point for insertion of anesthesia of the buccal nerve is the base of the _____ _____.

ANSWER

ascending ramus

QUESTION
71

A buccal injection anesthetizes mucous membrane and skin of the cheek and mandibular gingiva from the _____ _____ tooth to the _____ _____ tooth.

ANSWER

first molar . . . third molar

SUMMARY OF UNIT EIGHTEEN

Prior to learning injection techniques, the student must be familiar with the locations of nerves and bony landmarks along the routes of injection.

INNERVATION OF THE MAXILLARY AND MANDIBULAR REGIONS

Branches of the maxillary division of the trigeminal nerve innervate the entire maxillary region. The posterior superior alveolar nerve supplies the second and third molars and the distal and palatal roots of the first molar. The middle superior alveolar nerve supplies the mesial root of the first molar and the premolar teeth. The anterior superior alveolar nerve innervates canines and incisors. Palatine mucoperiosteum and gingiva adjacent to the maxillary molars and premolars are innervated by the greater palatine nerve; mucoperiosteum and gingiva adjacent to maxillary canines and incisors, by the nasopalatine nerve.

The inferior alveolar branch of the mandibular division of the trigeminal nerve, and its anterior continuation, the incisive nerve, supply mandibular teeth. The lingual nerve innervates soft tissue on the lingual surface; the buccal nerve, soft tissue on the posterior buccal surface.

TYPES OF INJECTIONS

Anesthesia intended to stop conduction from a local region is variously termed plexus anesthesia, supraperiosteal anesthesia, or infiltration. With this method, the anesthetic solution diffuses through soft tissue and porous bone to reach the nerve network. Infiltration is effective for operative procedures on maxillary teeth and mandibular incisors, but is ineffective for the remainder of the mandibular teeth because of the density of adjacent bone.

Block anesthesia is introduced at a site which is proximal to an entire nerve trunk; therefore, a large area is effectively anesthetized. Common sites for block injections are the zygomatic area for blocking the distribution of the posterior superior alveolar nerve; the infraorbital area for blocking the distribution of the middle and anterior superior alveolar nerves; the posterolateral palate for blocking the greater palatine nerve; the anteromedial palate for blocking the nasopalatine nerve; the mandibular foramen for an inferior alveolar nerve block; and the mental foramen for an incisive nerve block.

Block Injections.   A posterior superior alveolar nerve block involves introducing the needle into the vestibule near the second maxillary molar, and continuing obliquely to a site near the posterior superior alveolar foramen on the maxillary tuberosity. For an infraorbital nerve block, the infraorbital foramen is reached through the labial vestibule with the needle introduced superior to the maxillary canine and directed to a point on a vertical plane with the pupil of the eye. The infraorbital foramen is palpated and the height from the vestibule gauged so that penetration of the orbit is avoided. The greater palatine block, required for surgery, is approached through the mucoperioxteum in the posterolateral palate adjacent to the last maxillary molar tooth. The naso-palatine block is appraoched in the anterior midline of the palate. To block all branches of the maxillary nerve for a major operation, fluid is deposited in the pterygopalatine fossa where the main trunk of the maxillary nerve divides into its terminal branches. The approach to the fossa is from the cheek through the pterygopalatine fissure.

The inferior alveolar nerve is anesthetized all along its length by a block injection at the mandibular foramen. This foramen is bounded by the medial surface of the ramus of the mandible laterally and the sphenomandibular ligament medially. The mental nerve is blocked by directing the needle through the mental foramen and depositing the solution in the mental canal. The lingual nerve is anesthetized by directing the needle across the opposite premolar into the retromolar area. For a buccal injection, the needle can be inserted at the base of the ascending ramus.

With injections of any sort, care must be exercised to avoid entering a blood vessel. This is particularly likely in the case of the posterior superior alveolar nerve block, the infraorbital block, the nasopalatine block, and the inferior alveolar block, where blood vessels are in close proximity to nerves. The chance of injecting into a blood vessel is minimized considerably by aspiration before injection.

QUESTION
72

The second and third maxillary molars and the distal and palatal roots of the first molar are innervated by the _____ _____ _____ nerve.

ANSWER

posterior superior alveolar

QUESTION
73

Maxillary premolars and the mesial root of the first molar are innervated by the _____ _____ _____ nerve.

ANSWER

middle superior alveolar

QUESTION
74

The anterior superior alveolar nerve innervates the maxillary _____ and _____ teeth.

ANSWER

canine . . . incisor (in either order)

QUESTION
75

Posterior palatine mucoperiosteum is supplied by the _____ _____ nerve; anterior palatine mucoperiosteum, by the _____ nerve.

ANSWER

greater palatine . . . nasopalatine

QUESTION
76

Mandibular teeth are innervated by the _____ _____ nerve and the _____ nerve.

ANSWER

inferior alveolar . . . incisive

Soft tissue in the floor of the mouth is innervated by the _____ nerve; that at the posterior buccal region, by the _____ nerve.

lingual . . . buccal

Anesthesia restricted to a local region is termed _____ anesthesia, _____ anesthesia, or _____.

plexus . . . supraperiosteal . . . infiltration (in any order)

Anesthesia intended to prevent pain conduction over an extensive area by blocking a major nerve trunk is termed _____ anesthesia.

block

To avoid injecting anesthetic solution into a blood vessel, it is imperative that the operator _____.

aspirate

INDEX

Note: Items are listed under nouns rather than under descriptive adjectives. For example, *facial nerve* is listed under *Nerve* rather than *Facial*. Page numbers in italics refer to illustrations.